Business Mastery³

Third Edition

A Guide for Creating a Fulfilling, Thriving Business and Keeping It Successful

Cherie Sohnen-Moe

Business Mastery³

A Guide for Creating a Fulfilling, Thriving Business
and Keeping It Successful

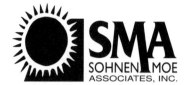

Published by Sohnen-Moe Associates, Inc.
3906 W. Ina Road #200-367
Tucson, Arizona 85741-2295
520-743-3936 • 800-786-4774
sma@sohnen-moe.com • www.sohnen-moe.com

The publisher does not assume and hereby disclaims any liability to any party for any loss or damage caused by errors or omissions in *Business Mastery³*. This book is designed to be a planning guide. It is sold with the understanding that the publisher is not engaged in rendering legal, accounting or other professional advice.

Publisher's Cataloging in Publication
(Prepared by Quality Books, Inc.)

Sohnen-Moe, Cherie.
　　Business mastery: a guide for creating a fulfilling, thriving business and keeping it successful/ Cherie Sohnen-Moe. -- 3rd ed.
　　p. cm.
　　Includes index.
　　Preassigned LCCN: 97-62132.
　　ISBN: 0-9621265-4-3

　　1. Business-Management--Handbooks, manuals, etc. 2. Management--Handbooks, etc.
I. Title.

HD31.S64 1997　　　　658
　　　　　　　　　　QBI97-41368

Cover illustration and design by Nancy Parker, Jim Moe and Rich Foster.
Clip art provided by: ClickArt © 1996, 1995, 1994, 1993, T/Maker Company; Clip Art © 1990-1997, RT Computer Grapics, Inc., NM.; Corel Draw! 5 © 1994, Corel Corporation.

Printed in the United States of America

Preface

• Overview •

You can have an enjoyable, profitable fulfilling career without sacrificing your values. For the past decade, *Business Mastery* has supported business owners in all realms to reach new levels of success.

This book is written specifically for wellness professionals. If you are a massage therapist, chiropractor, counselor, esthetician, social worker, acupuncturist, homeopath, Rolfing® practitioner, nutritionist, naturopath, polarity therapist, Reiki practitioner, psychiatrist, aromatherapist, personal trainer, physician, reflexologist, physical therapist, or a practitioner of any of the numerous allied health care professions, this book is for you!

Business Mastery is also endorsed by other business owners. Many people embrace the principles and holistic approach to life and business that is the foundation of this book.

Tremendous shifts are occurring in the wellness industry and are reflected in this book—which is broader in scope than previous editions. The marketing chapter is greatly expanded, the practice management chapter has been split into several chapters; plus there are two new chapters titled Therapeutic Communications and Conscious Business. I've added more than 200 new pages of material, including samples of ads, promotional materials and contracts. In addition the forms have been updated and the layout revamped. I hope you find this edition even more useful and fun to use. I was unable to include specific examples for each type of practice—otherwise this book would have contained thousands of pages. It's my hope that everyone can easily relate to the examples provided.

Business Mastery covers the major aspects of building and maintaining a successful practice. You may find that you only need to concentrate on certain sections of this book depending on your business experience and the degree of clarity you possess. Some of the topics may not be relevant to you now, and may become so in the future. These business skills are fundamental to your success—whether you work for someone else or are self-employed. It's beyond the scope of this book to thoroughly educate you in all of these areas. Some skills are extremely difficult to illustrate in a book (such as the delivery components in public speaking). Other topics such as insurance reimbursement may require several books to cover procedures and codes. My intent is to convey the fundamentals for business success and to familiarize you with the other principles and skills so that you can appropriately decide which areas you want or need to pursue.

I welcome any comments you may have about the content, style or layout of this book. I will do my best to incorporate your suggestions in subsequent editions of *Business Mastery*.

I wish you great happiness, health, prosperity, success and balance!

• Acknowledgments •

So many people have supported me in making this book a reality. Much of the material for this book has been developed and refined over the past 20 years in my coaching practice, in courses and seminars I've facilitated, and through my own process of personal and professional development.

I am grateful for the content suggestions, editing assistance, quotes, artistic creation, inspiration and general support I received from Dominick Angiulo, Margaret Avery Moon, Simi Aziz, Barb Baun, Terry Belville, Phyllis Bloom, Jacque Dailey, Robert Decker, Rich Foster, Kalyn Gibbens, Julie Goodwin, Janice Hollender, Rochelle Jewell, Jamie Lee, Kenneth Lund, Mark Moseley, Nancy Parker, Bob Sexton and Helen Sohnen. Thank you all!

I give special appreciation to Barbara Buchanan, Lorie Eufemiese, Cathy Harless, M.A. LaBrash, David Lauterstein, Melissa Mower, Heather Nicoll, Dianne Polseno, Christine Rosche, Karen Wilhelmsen, Tracy Williams, Tracy Wise and Jan Zobel. Lorie brainstormed ideas with me and assisted in writing the sections on employees, legal issues and technology. Dianne allowed me to adapt her Informed Consent form. The procrastination section is based on an article that Barbara and I co-authored. Melissa provided direction and excellent editing suggestions. M.A., Jan and Christine graciously allowed me to include sections from their books. Karen shared great quotes and created the layout design. Tracy Williams provided important information on working with people with disabilities. Heather allowed me to use her brochure as an example. David and Cathy read the draft and gave me invaluable feedback. Tracy Wise also gave me excellent feedback, allowed me to adapt his independent contractor agreement and supplied me with many inspirational quotes.

I acknowledge all of my friends who encourage me to pursue my dreams and keep me laughing. Most of all I am so thankful for my wonderful husband Jim. He has assisted in every phase of this book—from copy editing to layout to cover design. His unconditional love and total support for whatever I choose to do has given me the courage to follow my heart.

• About the Author •

I am an author, business coach, international workshop facilitator and successful business owner since 1978. I hold a bachelor's degree in psychology from UCLA and have extensive experience in business management, training, communication and creative problem solving—which combines well with my ability to assist others in achieving what they want in life.

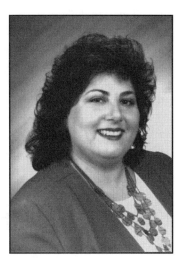

I was a massage practitioner for six years and still keep a part-time rebirthing practice. I have served as a faculty member of several schools. Currently my major focus is on writing, coaching and facilitating workshops. I am an internationally published author, writing articles for several journals and magazines. I am an active member of numerous professional and community organizations. Among my honors I have received the Distinguished Service Award and the Professional Achievement Award from the American Society for Training and Development, Outstanding Instructor at the Desert Institute of the Healing Arts and am listed in several editions of Who's Who.

I am dedicated to supporting people reach the levels of success they desire...personally, financially and professionally.

• How to Use This Book •

No matter where you are in your career, if you are willing to take a new look at your life and challenge some of your old thought patterns, you will find that reading this book from beginning to end is an incredibly valuable process.

Business Mastery has been designed to follow a pattern—the chapters build upon each other. You may need to read a specific chapter and then go back to the beginning of the book. For instance, if you are considering going into partnership, proceed directly to chapters six and seven. Maybe you have been in practice for a while now; you have a business plan, you know what you want out of life, and you still aren't accomplishing your goals. In that case you may want to start with chapter three, Success Strategies.

The major culmination of this book is the business plan. Even if you decide to skip the previous chapters and go right to the business plan, please skim through the entire book to get a sense of the flow. Some sections include aspects of business that may not pertain to you—such as product sales, group practice, employees or working for someone else. Just review them (someday, you may decide to incorporate those areas) and complete the sections that are appropriate to *your* business/career.

This is not a book to sit and read in one evening. It's filled with numerous exercises and soul-searching questions. It may take a while to complete this manual. One way to make this more manageable (and less overwhelming) is to allot a specific amount of time each day to work through the book.

One of the first activities is to create a business journal. Ideally use a three-ring binder so you can easily add information. Items to keep in this journal are your responses to the exercises, your business plan and samples of your marketing materials (you can put cards and brochures in plastic sleeves). Even if you do the written work on computer, you may want to keep printed copies in the notebook.

Appendix A contains business forms. Please feel free to make copies of these templates (for your personal use only). Appendix B contains valuable information on working with people with disabilities as well as a business organization directory, professional association registry and listings of IRS and SBA resources.

This is not a book to read and put on a shelf. *Business Mastery* is a handbook—a resource tool for you to use regularly. It will help you create the success that you truly deserve!

Pictograph Glossary

The following icons signal tips, resources and exercises.

 Exercise: Most of the exercises involve writing. This is your cue to get out your business journal or go to your computer.

 Idea: Quick tips or suggestions for other ways to utilize the information.

 Publication Resources: Books, magazines and other publications with more information on specific topics.

 Miscellaneous Resources: Contact these companies for information on their products and services.

 Internet Resources.

 Inspirational Quotes.

 Step Forward: Lets you know where you can find related information in a subsequent section.

 Step Back: Refers you to an earlier section.

Table of Contents

Appendix B

Index

Other Offerings

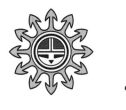

1

Initial Considerations

Exploration
Self-Employment
Clearing
Scope

• Exploration •

Achieving success in the business world while staying true to the principles of healing and service to others may at times seem like a contradiction in terms. The business world is often portrayed as being heartless, as indeed it can be if you don't know the rules. The exciting thing is that once you do learn the rules, you can choose which ones you want to incorporate in your life and determine how to circumvent many of the ones you don't like. Many people who choose a career in the health care field don't like the business facets at all and thus don't take the time to learn the rules for success or rebel against them. Unfortunately, that attitude rarely leads to success.

Most people stumble through their lives, not really knowing how or why things happen around them. We experiment with jobs, friends and hobbies until we find something (or someone) we can master; and then we are inclined to stick with that same thing. It's as though, deep down, we are terrified that we'll never be able to be good at much of anything, thinking that once we've somehow found something we do well, we better not let it go. It can be very scary to take risks and make changes; particularly if your life is finally on an even keel. So, we end up living the old (and extremely limiting) cliché : A bird in the hand is worth two in the bush.

One of the most important traits that successful people have in common is the dedication to knowledge. Knowledge is power. Self-awareness is the foundation of that knowledge. So, before you even begin to create or update a plan for your career or business, it's vital that you assess your current state. It is extremely difficult to know how to get to your destination if you don't know your starting point. Including the personal aspects of your life as well as the professional ones is important. You are a whole being and your career is only one—albeit very significant—part of your life. This chapter contains several activities designed to assist you in assessing yourself, clearing obstacles and visualizing your future.

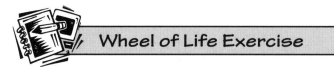

Wheel of Life Exercise

Figure 1.1 is a completed example of an exercise called the "Wheel of Life." Its purpose is to support you in evaluating your life. The chart for you to fill out is on the page following the example. Imagine that the center point (A) is the least desirable state and the outside of the circle (B) is the most desirable state. Look at each category. Take a moment to think about where you are right now. Where is that in relation to where you want to be? Then mark along the line (for each of the 10 categories) where you feel you are right now. Next, connect the dots. Do you have a balanced wheel or does it look like a starburst? Keep in mind that it can be very difficult to smoothly roll through life when your wheel (life) isn't balanced.

Consider this wheel from two points of view. First, notice any categories that are proportionately nearer the center than others. Those are the areas to concentrate on improving. The object is to bring more balance to your wheel. The second aspect is to enhance all the categories so that they are toward the outside (most desirable) of the circle.

Figure 1.1

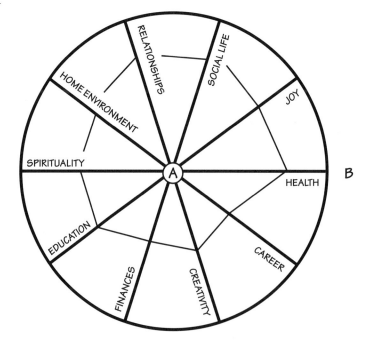

Wheel of Life

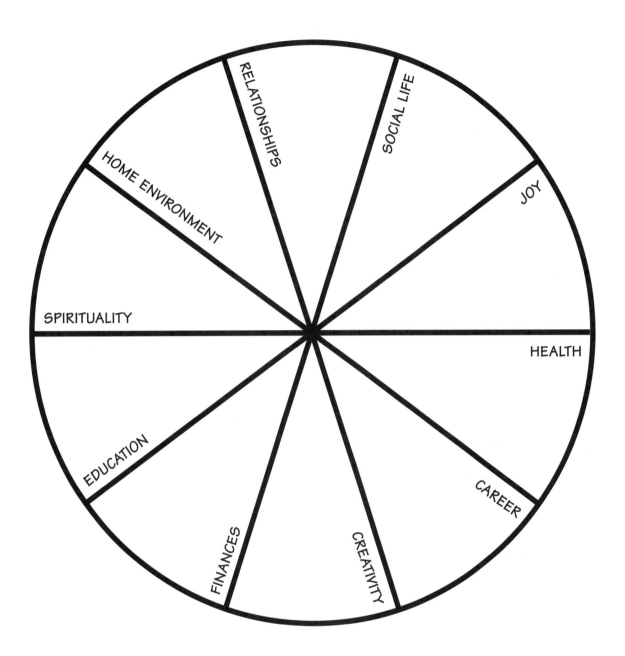

Suggestion: *Date this wheel and do this exercise every few months. It's a great way to chart your progress! An additional copy of the Wheel of Life is in Appendix A.*

Take out your business journal or go to your computer to do these exercises.

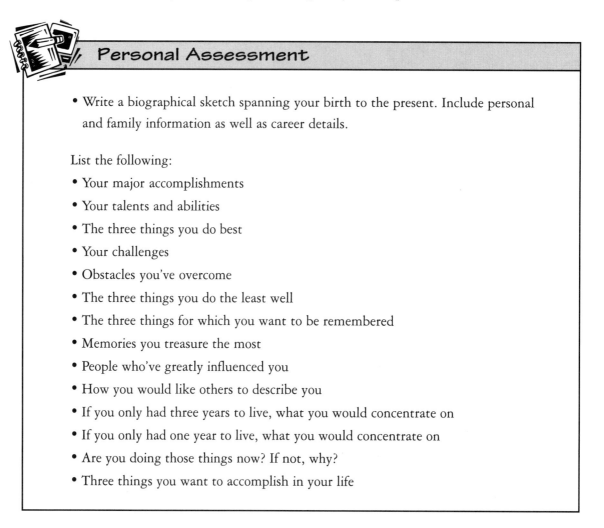

Personal Assessment

• Write a biographical sketch spanning your birth to the present. Include personal and family information as well as career details.

List the following:
• Your major accomplishments
• Your talents and abilities
• The three things you do best
• Your challenges
• Obstacles you've overcome
• The three things you do the least well
• The three things for which you want to be remembered
• Memories you treasure the most
• People who've greatly influenced you
• How you would like others to describe you
• If you only had three years to live, what you would concentrate on
• If you only had one year to live, what you would concentrate on
• Are you doing those things now? If not, why?
• Three things you want to accomplish in your life

Career Assessment

• Describe the current state of your career/business. Include length of time in your field, average yearly income and number of clients.

List the following:
• What is working well
• Three attributes of your business of which you're the most proud
• What isn't working well
• Three attributes of your business of which you're the least proud
• The changes you would like to see occur
• What you would like people to say about your business

• Self-Employment •

The job market is beginning to broaden for health care providers. Some practitioners work in clinics, hospitals, spas, gyms, hotels and salons. Others work for cruise lines, corporations, other health care providers or even travel with athletes or celebrities. Still, private practice is the most prevalent option, although not everyone is suited for private practice. Many advantages and disadvantages exist in being self-employed. It takes a certain personality type to be truly successful in one's own business. Successful business owners are inventive and follow through with their plans. They respect money. They possess considerable expertise in their particular career field and have broad experience in several others. They have very good oral and written communication skills, and are usually considered very personable. The major factors in their success are their attitudes (they are positive thinkers), determination, self-discipline, service orientation and their persistence—they don't quit! Think about yourself. Do you possess these qualities? In most instances (unless, for example, you have a partner with a lot of business acumen) it's not enough just to have talent, you need to manage the "business." Many of the small businesses that don't succeed are examples of this problem—talent without proper business skills.

Some of the advantages of being self-employed are having a potentially flexible schedule, being independent, being your own boss and the possibility of receiving tax advantages. Frequently you are more creative and experience increased personal satisfaction with a greater sense of achievement. Self-employment may also offer you a better opportunity to contribute to others.

Some of the disadvantages of being self-employed are the long hours—usually 10 to 14 hours per day, six to seven days a week. As a business owner, not only will you be working with clients, you will also be actively marketing and managing your practice. In the beginning, you may need to devote two to three hours in business promotion and development for every hour of client interaction. Sometimes the start-up costs are greater than you've anticipated. Just printing business cards and mailing notices adds up. You may also experience a deep sense of "aloneness." The income is usually not steady and there are financial risks. Finally, the statistics for success for small businesses aren't exactly inspiring.

According to a study by Bruce D. Phillips of the U.S. Small Business Administration and Bruce A. Kirchhoff of Babson College, survival rates for service businesses are only average and the percentage of service businesses that grow is below average in comparison to small businesses in general. In doing this study, they have found that two out of five new small businesses actually survive at least six years—instead of the more often cited (but inaccurate) statistics that claim that four out of five businesses fail within five years.

Many of life's failures are people who did not realize how close they were to success when they gave up.
— Thomas Edison

Though the odds are improving, these statistics can still seem quite depressing. At the very least, they are cause for concern. The two major reasons for failure are mismanagement and undercapitalization. Mismanagement is generally a result of poor planning, not realistically evaluating strengths and weaknesses, failing to anticipate obstacles, improper budgeting and lacking the necessary business skills. Undercapitalization is not having enough start-up capital and/or needing to take draw (salary) before the business is firmly established.

The U.S. Small Business Administration is a wonderful source of information. The people are friendly and do their best to assist you. The following (revised) questions and worksheets are used with permission from their Management Aids MP12.

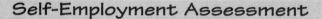

Self-Employment Assessment

- Are you willing to take the risks in being self-employed?
- Do you know how much credit you can get from your suppliers?
- Do you know where you are going to get your start-up funding?
- Have you talked to a banker about your plans?
- If you need/want a partner with money or skills that you don't have, do you know someone who is qualified and appropriate?
- Have you talked to a lawyer about your business?
- Does your family support your plan to be in business?
- Have you figured out whether you could net more money working for someone else?

Self-Employment Checklist Scoring Key

After completing the checklist on page seven, count the checks you made beside the answers to each question in the Self-Employment Checklist. How many checks are beside the first answer? How many checks are beside the second answer? How many checks are beside the third answer?

If most of your checks are beside the first answer, you probably have what it takes to run a business. If not, you're likely to have more trouble than you can handle by yourself. Better find a partner who is strong on the points in which you experience challenges. If many checks are beside the third answer, not even a good partner could shore you up.

Under each question, check the answer that says what you feel or comes closest to it. Be honest with yourself.

Are you a self starter?
- ❑ I do things on my own, nobody has to tell me to get going.
- ❑ If someone gets me started, I keep going all right.
- ❑ Easy does it. I don't put myself out until I have to.

How do you feel about other people?
- ❑ I like people. I can get along with just about everybody.
- ❑ I have plenty of friends—I don't need anyone else.
- ❑ Most people irritate me.

Can you lead others?
- ❑ I can get most people to go along when I start something.
- ❑ I can give the orders if someone tells me what we should do.
- ❑ I let someone else get things moving. Then I go along if I feel like it.

Can you take responsibility?
- ❑ I like to take charge of things and see them through.
- ❑ I'll take over if I have to, but I'd rather let someone else be responsible.
- ❑ There's always some eager beaver around wanting to show how smart s/he is. I say let him/her.

How good an organizer are you?
- ❑ I like to have a plan before I start. I'm usually the one to get things lined up when the group wants to do something.
- ❑ I do all right unless things get too confused. Then I quit.
- ❑ I get all set and then something comes along and presents too many problems. So I just take things as they come.

How good a worker are you?
- ❑ I can keep going as long as I need to. I don't mind working hard for something I want.
- ❑ I'll work hard for a while, but when I've had enough, that's it.
- ❑ I can't see that hard work gets you anywhere.

Can you make decisions?
- ❑ I can make up my mind in a hurry if I have to. It usually turns out okay, too.
- ❑ I can if I have plenty of time. If I have to make up my mind fast, I think later I should have decided the other way.
- ❑ I don't like to be the one who has to decide things.

Can people trust what you say?
- ❑ You bet they can. I don't say things I don't mean.
- ❑ I try to be on the level most of the time, but sometimes I just say what's easiest.
- ❑ Why bother if the other person doesn't know the difference?

Can you stick with it?
- ❑ If I make up my mind to do something, I don't let anything stop me.
- ❑ I usually finish what I start—if it goes well.
- ❑ If it doesn't go right away, I quit. Why beat your brains out?

How good is your health?
- ❑ I never run down!
- ❑ I have enough energy for most things I want to do.
- ❑ I run out of energy sooner than most of my friends seem to.

Suggestion: *Before you fill out this checklist, photocopy it for use in your journal.*

At this point you still may be uncertain about being self-employed or working for someone else. The next sections on Clearing and Scope are designed to assist you in discerning what you really want in your life and career. Hopefully that will support you in resolving any residual self-employment dilemma.

• Clearing •

Before you can effectively create your career/business plan, it's necessary to clear the impediments to choosing what you want. People are greatly influenced by events that have happened to them throughout their lifetime. All too often we allow (subconsciously or consciously) our past mistakes, incompletions and even our successes to obstruct the creation and accomplishment of new goals. We are not always aware of the degree of the impact our past has on our present and future.

A lot of the events and conditions were unpleasant and many decisions and attitudes were developed in response, popularly referred to as "negative conditioning" or "survival skills." Conclusions that were made in the past may have been based upon false information or a situation that was only valid at that time. Just because particular actions were effective in past situations doesn't mean they will continue to be in the future. In general, those types of decisions and beliefs are very limiting and do not enhance well-being. Also, it's extremely difficult to be creative and spontaneous when shouldering the burden of the past.

It's not always easy to release negative thought patterns, but the results of doing so are worth the effort. When you are detached from those past beliefs and attitudes, you can replace them with new supportive thoughts that contribute to having your life be the way YOU want. Frequently, this clearing stage is overlooked (or worse, considered irrelevant or too time consuming) and people attempt to move directly into repatterning. This is one reason why setting goals, writing affirmations, doing visualizations and listening to tapes doesn't always work. Sometimes the conflicts, contradictions and conditioning need to be unearthed, acknowledged and accepted before they can be replaced. For clearing to be truly effective, it must take place on all levels: mental, emotional, physical and spiritual. The clearing process requires recognizing that a block exists and being willing to go through whatever it takes to fully release it, even if that means re-experiencing the buried negativity and pain.

Many techniques are available for clearing. You may choose different ones or a combination depending upon the issue. Also, you may respond better to one type of clearing technique than another. Experiment! Some of the techniques for clearing include psychotherapy, bodywork/massage, yoga, rebirthing, some forms of martial arts, energy balancing, flotation, counseling, hypnotherapy, meditation, cognitive therapy, psychic work and written/verbal clearing exercises. If you do clearing work and follow-through on your own and aren't getting the results you want, it may be appropriate to get the support of a therapist.

It is the commonest of mistakes to consider that the limit of our power of perception is also the limit of all there is to perceive.
— C. W. Leadbeater

If you bring forth what is inside you, what you bring forth will save you.
— The Gospel according to Thomas

Sentence Completions ⌁

An example of one technique for releasing old thought patterns is called "sentence completions." This clearing process is designed to elicit conscious and unconscious thoughts, attitudes, beliefs and feelings so that they can be recognized and released, thus enabling you to be more free to achieve what you really desire.

You can do these exercises alone by writing or verbally with a partner. If you want to do it verbally, have your partner ask you the question(s) and you let your answers come out uncensored. Your partner's role is to keep you moving through the process.

The directions for written sentence completions are: Designate one page for each question. At the top of the first page, write down the first question. Answer the question with the first thoughts that come to your mind. Don't try to figure out the "right" answers. It's important to let your thoughts and feelings come out uncensored.

Continue to list your thoughts. Fill the whole page. It isn't necessary to write complete sentences. Occasionally reread the question and list any new or different thoughts. Some of your answers may not make sense and that's okay. When you think that the list is finished, go over it again. Add any additional thoughts.

See Chapter Three, page 45
included is an exercise to dissolve specific issues.

Example

The things that are important to me are...

Being able to do what I want	*Success*
Feeling good about myself	*Having fun*
Making a difference in the world	*Being healthy*
Friends	*Tacos*
Money	*Movies*
Traveling	*Happiness*

Remember, it might not make sense—but if that's what's there, you must respect it.

Notice any unconscious defense mechanisms that may occur to distract you (e.g., thoughts about the other things you really ought to be doing, how hungry you are, how silly this exercise is, or daydreaming, falling asleep and going blank). If you are experiencing these defenses, acknowledge to yourself what is happening and then continue with the exercise.

Do this same procedure for each question. It's common to find that some of your answers are the same or quite similar for different questions. It's important to not restrict any of the answers that come up.

The following sentence completions exercise is designed to assist you in removing obstacles to fulfilling your dreams.

The clearing exercises in this manual are geared toward career, but this process can be utilized for any area in your life. Feel free to adapt the lists or create your own.

Great men are they who see that spiritual is stronger than any material force, that thoughts rule the world.
— Emerson

Go to your business journal. Set aside 21 pages and follow the preceding instructions.

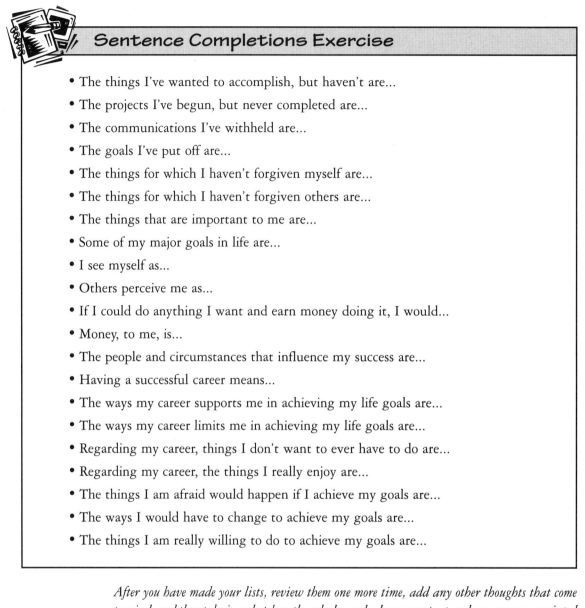

Sentence Completions Exercise

- The things I've wanted to accomplish, but haven't are...
- The projects I've begun, but never completed are...
- The communications I've withheld are...
- The goals I've put off are...
- The things for which I haven't forgiven myself are...
- The things for which I haven't forgiven others are...
- The things that are important to me are...
- Some of my major goals in life are...
- I see myself as...
- Others perceive me as...
- If I could do anything I want and earn money doing it, I would...
- Money, to me, is...
- The people and circumstances that influence my success are...
- Having a successful career means...
- The ways my career supports me in achieving my life goals are...
- The ways my career limits me in achieving my life goals are...
- Regarding my career, things I don't want to ever have to do are...
- Regarding my career, the things I really enjoy are...
- The things I am afraid would happen if I achieve my goals are...
- The ways I would have to change to achieve my goals are...
- The things I am really willing to do to achieve my goals are...

After you have made your lists, review them one more time, add any other thoughts that come to mind, and then take in a deep breath, exhale, and release your past and any energy associated with it by shredding or (preferably) burning the lists.

• Scope •

This section is designed to encourage you to visualize your potential future. Allow yourself the freedom to state your desires, dreams and goals. Remember, this is about your **IDEALS**, not necessarily what you think is realistic. We will forge some of these dreams into goals in the next chapter. Make any notes in your business journal.

Visualization Exercise

Visualization assists you in gauging where you are in relation to where you want to be. If you prefer to visualize with your eyes closed, you may want to have a friend read you these questions, or you could make an audio tape of the exercise—leaving ample time for thought between questions.

Envisioning your life is one of the most enjoyable aspects of long-range planning. This is where you let your imagination range free. Put aside any concerns about whether your vision is realistic or attainable. If you have any negative thoughts about your ability or worthiness to have this life, acknowledge those thoughts and continue with the exercise. Encompass all areas of your life, including your career, environment, relationships, finances, education, spirituality, health and social life.

Your Ideal Life Description

- *Imagine that you are living the life of your dreams right now. Describe where you live: Where do you reside—what city, state or country? What type of home do you live in? How is it furnished? What is the ambiance? Think about yourself: What do you look like? What are your attitudes toward life? How do you nurture yourself? How do you feel about yourself? Contemplate your relationships: Who are your friends? How do you interact with your family? How do you impact others? What are the important characteristics of your romantic relationship? What is your social life like?*

- *Now think about your career: What profession are you in? What are your responsibilities and activities? What type of business atmosphere do you have? Who do you work with? What are your business relationships like? What is your financial status?*

- *Reflect upon your personal growth: What types of activities do you engage in to take care of your well-being? How are you furthering your education? What do you do to foster your spirituality? How do you spend your leisure time?*

- *Lastly, consider any other areas that are important to you: What do you do to make certain these things happen? What are your attitudes about them?*

In summary, the question to ask yourself is: "If I could be anywhere doing anything, where would I be and what would I be doing?" Be sure to note any realizations in your journal. Sometimes what's important are the qualities of life and not necesarily the specific activities. For instance, your future vision might not have "looked" dramatically different from your current status, but perhaps it "felt" different. Maybe you were more relaxed, energetic and happier. The following exercise continues to add depth to your visualization.

1. Where do you want to practice? What city, state or country?
2. Do you want to have multiple locations? ❑ Yes ❑ No ❑ Maybe If yes, where?
3. Do you want to travel as part of your career? ❑ Yes ❑ No ❑ Maybe If yes, where?
4. What type of work location do you want? Do you want to have a private office or work at a medical facility? Do you want an office in your home? Would you rather just do outcalls only? Perhaps you would like to have a combination of the above?
5. How many hours per week do you want to work? Hours doing what specifically? In addition to client interaction, include the other business-related activities such as marketing, bookkeeping, networking and planning.
6. Do you want any associates? ❑ Yes ❑ No ❑ Maybe
   How many? What would they do?
7. What type of business atmosphere do you want?
8. How much do you want the net business profit to be annually? $_____
9. How much money do you want for your salary/draw after taxes? $_____
10. What benefits do you want your business to have (e.g., health insurance, paid vacations, retirement fund)?
11. What type(s) of people do you want to have as clients?
12. Which professions could provide referrals to your business?*
13. For which professions can you be a good source of referrals? *
    * Please note that although these questions sound the same, they aren't. Of course there will be some duplication, but not always. For example, let's say you are a chiropractor or a massage therapist. A competition weight-lifting instructor might be an excellent source of client referrals. Probably every one of his/her clients could use your services. But, it is highly unlikely that the majority of your clients would benefit from competition weight-lifting training.
14. Describe your ideal office/location in detail including external features, the style of decorations, equipment and ambiance.

If you plan to work for someone else, answer the following questions:
15. What is the lowest fee or percentage you will accept? $_____ or _____%
16. List at least five places or people for whom you'd like to work.
17. Describe the ideal business agreement. What would you like your employer to offer? What are you willing to provide?

Courage is very important. Like a muscle, it is strengthened by use.
— Ruth Gordon

Now comes the difficult part—determining whether you are on the path to making your dreams become reality and ascertaining the extent to which you are willing to do whatever is necessary to have your life be that of your dreams. It's perfectly okay to not work on everything at once—actually you will probably drive yourself (and those around you) crazy if you attempt to change too many things too quickly.

You may also find that you are not willing to take some of the required steps to achieve an aspect of your dream. Give yourself permission to set your own boundaries and priorities. This is where dreams become differentiated from goals. And thus, Chapter Two.

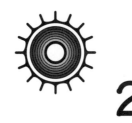

2

Life Planning

Goal Setting
Strategic Planning
Follow-Through

• Goal Setting •

Now that you have assessed your current status, done some earnest clearing work, envisioned your ideal life and considered the scope of your business, it's time to set clear purposes, priorities and goals for your life and your business. Goal setting is the means of turning your dreams into reality. Dreams are similar to wishes: they are things we fantasize about, yet do little to make certain they occur (but we're certainly ecstatic when they do). Goals are those things to which you commit and take action to ensure their attainment.

Goal setting is tied into the reticular activating system. Our senses (particularly sight) are constantly flooded with a vast amount of stimuli, yet we are consciously aware of only a fraction of that data. Most of that information is not necessary for our well-being, so it gets screened. In essence, we have programmed directional signalers (or in some cases, blinders) in our brains. Although this may seem like an over-simplification, it's indeed how it functions. For example, recall the last time you decided to get a new car. You finally chose the model and color, and lo and behold, it seemed like everywhere you went, you saw "your car." Now, all of those people didn't just go out and purchase those cars when you did. They were already on the road. You just hardly noticed them before because it wasn't significant to you. This is the magnificence of goal setting. By establishing clear goals, you are programming your brain to be aware and notify your conscious mind of the information and opportunities that YOU DESIRE.

The inability to actualize goals is usually related to unclear goals, lack of commitment, conflict or negative conditioning. Very few people write goals, and those who do, don't always write their goals in a way that easily produces results. Sometimes they write what they think they should want or what their spouse, parent, boss or peers think they should want. Other times they claim to want something, but what they really want is what that "thing" represents. Occasionally conflicts exist in relation to the achievement of their goals. The attainment of one goal may preclude the fulfillment of another, or the consequences may not be viewed favorably by their immediate family and colleagues. Quite often people have a lot of negative conditioning that they need to overcome.

There are people who write goals that aren't real for them—they "know" that they could never achieve them. They set unrealistic deadlines or have goals that are dependent on other people. Some have page after page of goals and yet hardly ever accomplish anything. And then other people are so detail oriented that they lose sight of the big picture.

We have a tendency to get so caught up in the list-making and the things we "ought to do" and "should do" that we don't always take into account the overall picture and consider what would be the most appropriate action to take. Life isn't about just getting by, making it from day to day. It's about reaching for and attaining our full potential at all levels. Often we do things out of habit or because it's easy, or because we do it well. Doing well at what you currently do might not be the most beneficial thing if your main focus is personal and professional growth.

You need a context for your goals, something to connect them. Otherwise they become chores and most people do almost anything to avoid chores.

Purpose provides that context. Purpose is very general—it's a direction, a theme. You can never actually complete a purpose; it's an ongoing process. Take a moment and think about what is really meaningful to you. Are there any common threads: one statement that encompasses your ideals, values and dreams? You may have a purpose for your life and purposes for every major area of your life.

Overall Life Purpose Examples

I make a positive difference.
I am happy.
My life is an expression of love and joy.

You may find your life purpose shifting over time, becoming more refined. Remember, it isn't written in stone, though in most instances your priorities and goals are more likely to change, and not your life purpose. One of the most significant features of having a distinct life purpose is that it becomes easier to resolve any conflicting goals when you know the direction for your life.

If you have built castles in the air, your work need not be lost; that is where they should be. Now put foundations under them.
— Henry David Thoreau

The purpose of life is a life of purpose.
— Robert Byrne

Career Purpose Examples

My career supports myself and others in being happy and healthy.
I make a healthy difference.
My career is a source of joy and prosperity.
I am innovative and successful in my career.
My career is a joyous expression of who I am.

 ## Life Purpose Exercise

Clarify your life purpose. You may want to begin by reviewing your Personal Assessment Exercises from Chapter One. Think about your values, ideals and dreams. Create a statement that reflects the essence of your life. Then write a purpose for each spoke on the Wheel of Life: education; relationships; health; social life; joy; career; finances; spirituality; creativity; and home environment.

After you have clarified your general life purpose and written a purpose for each spoke on the Wheel of Life, the next step is to specify your major life priorities.

Priorities are general areas of concern. They are less vague and not so all-encompassing as purposes, yet not as specific as goals. Priorities are statements of intention that are connected with values.

General Life Priorities Examples

My relationships are nurturing and fun.
I am creative in all that I do.
Each and every day I learn something new.
My body is a manifestation of health and beauty.
My communications are open and honest.

Career Priorities Examples

My career is fulfilling and provides me with the income that I desire.
I enjoy my work.
I regularly participate with other colleagues.
I continually expand my knowledge and skills.
I am creative in my work.
My work environment is nurturing and professional.

Life Priorities Exercise

Take some time to think about the aspects of life that are meaningful to you and create priorities for those areas. Be sure to include all areas on the Wheel of Life. I suggest you have at least five priorities for every purpose.

Goals are very specific things, events or experiences that have a definite completion, and you are able to objectively know when you've achieved them. Effective goals have the characteristics found in the acronym of **SMARTER**: **S**pecific, **M**easurable, **A**ttainable, **R**ealistic, **T**imelined, **E**nthusiastic, **R**ewarding. When setting your goals, I recommend that you set at least four goals for every priority.

Career Goal Examples

I earn at least $40,000 per year.
I have a wonderful music system in my office.
I keep my client files current.
I invest at least five hours each week in marketing.
I review my business plan every three months.
I read at least one business-related book each month.
I am an active member of two business groups.

Goal Setting Techniques

1. Always state your goals in the positive PRESENT TENSE. If you write in the future, they may remain in the future—never attained.

2. Personalize your goals: use a pronoun (e.g., I, we, they, "your name") in every sentence.

3. Make your goals real: something you know you can accomplish on your own, without help or without someone waving a magic wand over you.

4. Do not use the terms "try," "will," "not," "never," "should," "would," "could" and "want."

5. Include deadline dates whenever possible.

6. Have fun!

If one advances confidently in the direction of his dreams, and endeavors to live the life which he has imagined, he will meet with a success unexpected in common hours.
— Henry David Thoreau

Effective goal setting is the groundwork for success. I advocate that you actually have written goals in addition to any other techniques you employ. The written word is so powerful! By inscribing your intentions, you say to yourself and the world that you know you deserve to have these things happen. Sometimes people are afraid to write down their goals because they don't think they can achieve them, and thus they don't want a written reminder of their failures. Failure, per se, doesn't really exist in goal setting. Usually when you don't accomplish a goal it's due to setting an inappropriate deadline, having inaccurate information, experiencing blocks, encountering conflicts, not really wanting the goal or being unwilling (or unable) to do what's required to accomplish the goal. Having written goals can only serve to support and teach you, enhancing your self-knowledge.

One of the ways to magnify the power of your goals is to involve as many of your senses as possible (particularly sight, touch and sound) in the process. In addition to writing, you may want to use a variety of methods from visual illustration to audio recordings to physical representations.

Collages are a wonderful way to visually create your goals. To make a collage, you need to first get a large piece of poster board (22" x 28" is available in many colors at art supply stores). Set aside a couple of hours, get comfortable, put on some nice music, make yourself a cup of tea, get a stack of magazines, a pair of scissors, some glue and prepare to have a fantastic experience! (By the way, this is a lot of fun to do with friends.) The next thing to do is to decide the purpose of your collage—be it a representation of your whole life, your career, the next six months or even just one major goal. Keeping your purpose in mind, go through the magazines and cut out pictures and words that appeal to you. Let your intuition be your guide. The items you choose may not be what you had anticipated. Don't worry about finding the "perfect" pictures or words. They may be very abstract or elicit a certain emotion. Remember, this is a representation of your dreams and goals.

Give yourself a time limit for cutting or else you may find yourself there for days. After you've cut out plenty of pictures and words, glue them onto the poster board. You also may want to write some goals or affirmations on the board. Then spend some time with your collage—allow yourself to experience the full impact. Finally, hang your collage in a place where you can see it every day.

Audiotape Recordings of your goals are also very effective. Write out your goals before you tape them, following the suggested Goal Setting Techniques. If possible, use a high quality recording system. The beauty of taping your goals is that you can listen to them at any time. It can be particularly beneficial to listen to your tape while sleeping for the subliminal effects. An interesting alternative is to tape some of your goals in your voice and have someone who is a positive authority figure, role model or mentor tape some of the goals. Experiment!

Picturebooks are also a great way to visually create your goals. The supplies needed are a large three-ring binder, a set of at least eight dividers, notebook paper, scissors, glue and magazines. Use the dividers to arrange the categories of your goals (e.g., health, finances, education, clients and marketing). Then follow the same directions for the collage, except glue the pictures and words by category onto notebook paper and then put the sheets in the binder. You may also want to write your goals next to the pictures. The advantages of a picturebook are that you can carry it with you and you can easily add more pages to it. The disadvantage is that you may not look at it as frequently as you would a collage. In any type of goal setting, the more frequently you review your goals, the more likely you are to achieve them.

The secret of success is constancy to purpose.
— Benjamin Disraeli

Pictureboards are a combination of a collage and a picturebook. Instead of gluing the pictures and words to paper or poster board, you pin them on a bulletin board. This technique makes it easy to literally shift your goals—put them in different perspective, add more goals and take them down once they've been achieved.

Physical Representations are excellent tools for depicting your goal(s). The idea is to create a three-dimensional object that you can see and touch. This can be very powerful. It makes you really "look" at what you say you want. Generally, it's a time-intensive endeavor but it can be well worth it, particularly for the goals that are very meaningful to you and the ones you've been having difficulty in achieving.

For example, if one of your goals is to remodel your office, you may want to build a miniature version of your office with all of the proposed changes. Get samples of the paint or wallpaper and put them on the walls. Make (or buy) miniature furniture. Create it as close as possible to your plans. If one of your goals is to exercise regularly, you may want to make a sculpture of yourself exercising. If you are unable to easily recognize yourself, you can always attach a photo of your face to the sculpture.

The inclusion of scent adds another potent dimension. For example, if you've been telling yourself for the last few years that you'd really like to take a winter vacation in the mountains, and you still haven't even left the city, it may be that you need to make that goal more tangible. You might want to design a model of the desired location. Start by making a mini-mountain. Then construct a little cabin and inside it put pictures of yourself and whomever else you want for company. (It needn't be as elaborate as in "Close Encounters of the Third Kind.") Make some pine trees (using real pine needles if possible), and put pine essence on the trees. Now, every time you walk by your mountain, you will be able to see it, touch it, and take in a deep breath and smell the pine trees....

Make your physical representation really effective by paying attention to details and making it as realistic as possible. Be inventive and have fun! Do not let a lack of artistic proficiency limit your creativity in visualizing and expressing your goals.

Written Goals are a powerful visual (and actually auditory) declaration of your intentions. The two most commonly used methods for goal setting are outline format and mind mapping. The outline technique is very effective for logical thinkers. When you use the outline format (see Figure 2.1) you write your purpose and your priorities, and list the specific goals under each priority.

The mind mapping approach is excellent for visually-oriented thinkers. In mind mapping (see Figure 2.2) you actually write the purpose in the center of a page, attach spokes to the circle onto which you list the priorities, and extend lines off of each spoke onto which you write the specific goals. Another mind mapping option is to draw an image in the middle of a page (such as an office filled with clients or a stack of money). Then add related images as well as written priorities and goals.

You may find it helpful to use a combination of these two goal setting methods. One of the benefits of having written goals is that it's much easier to track progress. The

Opportunity is missed by most people because it is dressed in overalls and looks like work.
— Thomas Edison

other major advantage of writing your goals is you can cross them out when they are completed—this contributes to a feeling of accomplishment, reward and acknowledgment.

Figure 2.1

Outline Format Example

Purpose: *My career is an expression of who I am.*

Priority 1:   *I continually expand my knowledge and skills.*
Priority 1 Goals: *Each month I meet with colleagues to share business experiences.*
                    I read at least two business magazines each month.
                    I take a public speaking course before my second year in business.

Priority 2:   *My work environment is professional and nurturing.*
Priority 2 Goals: *I paint my office by July 1.*
                    I have a wonderful music system in my office by August 15.
                    I clean my office every week.

Priority 3:   *My career provides me with the income I desire.*
Priority 3 Goals: *I earn at least $40,000 this year.*
                    I take a three-week vacation this winter.
                    I increase my client retention rate by at least 20 percent.

Figure 2.2

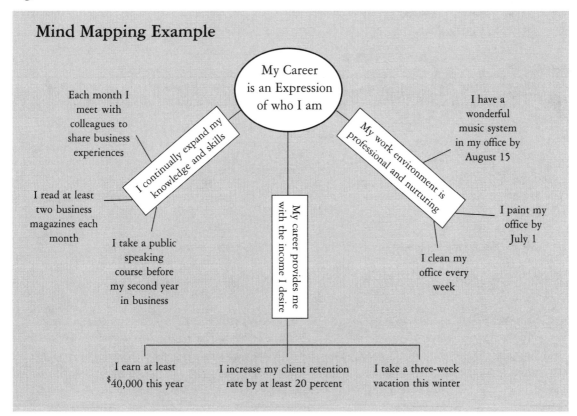

Mind Mapping Example

In goal setting, use the format with which you feel the most comfortable and proves the most effective, keeping in mind that it's important to have some type of written goals in addition to any other format, particularly for your career. You may want to use some of the other methods as a means of positive reinforcement and/or visualization. What is crucial is the way you actually state your goals and the individual steps necessary to accomplish them. Be sure to keep your goals **SMARTER** (**S**pecific, **M**easurable, **A**ttainable, **R**ealistic, **T**imelined, **E**nthusiastic, **R**ewarding), follow the suggested goal setting techniques and most importantly of all, be sure they are YOUR goals. Setting goals can be creative and exciting. If you tend to use mainly one method, experiment with other techniques. Use as many of your senses as possible. Goal setting is a necessary component of success, but it doesn't have to be a burden. Remember, the purpose of setting goals is to make your dreams become reality.

Clarifying Purpose, Priorities and Goals ⁓

Before you even begin to consider developing or enhancing your business, it's imperative to set a strong foundation by clarifying your life's purpose, priorities and goals. Then you can more effectively create your other plans. The following exercise guides you in writing your purpose, priorities and goals for your overall life and (then with a focus on your career) for the next five years, three years, one year and six months. Your Wheel of Life and the previous exercises in this chapter can serve as guides.

Take a few deep breaths, relax and let your dreams and goals express themselves. Let them guide your mind, heart and hands. For now, don't worry about "how" you write them. Let your creativity flow. You can always go back later and rephrase your goals.

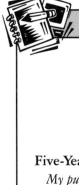 **Life Planning Exercise**

Overall Life Plan
My purpose in life is...
My major priorities in life are...
My major goals in life are...

Five-Year Plan
My purpose for the next five years is...
My major priorities for the next five years are...
My major goals for the next five years are...

One-Year Plan
My purpose for the next year is...
My major priorities for the next year are...
My major goals for the next year are...

Three-Year Plan
My purpose for the next three years is...
My major priorities for the next three years are...
My major goals for the next three years are...

Six-Month Plan
My purpose for the next six months is...
My major priorities for the next six months are...
My major goals for the next six months are...

Ranking Goals ~~~

CONGRATULATIONS! You now have written your intentions for your life and created your purposes, priorities and goals for your career. Having built this foundation puts you miles ahead of the general public and well on your path to success. Just writing some of your goals may be all the planning you need to do—given that you actually do them.

There is no such thing as an inappropriate goal: just a faulty time frame.

Not all goals or activities carry the same ultimate value. Some goals have a higher intrinsic worth, while others require more immediate action. This holds true whether you are planning your life, month, week or day. Review your goal lists and rank them with an "A," "B" or "C." The "A" goals are the ones that are the most crucial for you to attain—the ones you can commit to right now. The "B" goals have importance to you, but are not as significant as the "A" goals. The "C" goals are ones that would be nice if they actualized, but you are not ready to commit to accomplishing them at this moment.

The next step in ranking your goals is to arrange them in terms of time priority. Start with your "A" goals. Make sure all goals have assigned target dates for completion. Then numerically rank each goal according to time priority (1 being the highest). Using the Sample Career Goals (see page 16), your time priority list might look like this:

> 7. *I earn at least $40,000 per year.*
> 5. *I have a wonderful music system in my office.*
> 2. *I keep my client files current.*
> 6. *I review my business plan every three months.*
> 1. *I invest at least five hours each week in marketing.*
> 4. *I read at least one business-related book each month.*
> 3. *I am an active member of two business groups.*

• Strategic Planning •

Some goals may be very complex and require numerous sub-steps in order to be accomplished. This process of "divide and conquer" (i.e., breaking down a difficult problem into manageable chunks), is what strategic planning is about. This is also the phase that many people neglect to do and wonder why they feel so overwhelmed. The steps involved in strategic planning are: list the purpose and priority from where the goal originates; describe the situation; define the major goal; list the benefits of achieving the goal; brainstorm possible courses of action; choose the best alternative; outline the action—include the advantage, potential conflicts and solutions; identify resources needed; and outline the specific steps (with target deadline dates) necessary to achieve the goal.

Let's say that your vision is to work with 25 clients each week; practice in an office space with other health care practitioners; share a secretary who handles all the

Strategic Planning
Blank copies of the Strategic Planning sheets are found in Appendix A.

paperwork, bookkeeping and scheduling; and net $40,000 per year. Of the many goals necessary to manifest this vision, the goal we will use to illustrate the strategic planning process is to increase weekly clientele bookings from 15 to 25 clients within six months.

Figure 2.3

Strategic Planning Example

Today's Date: *February 15*   **Target Date:** *August 15*

Situation Description: *I have been in practice for almost two years. I had a corporate account with ABC electronics, but the company relocated. Now I am averaging only 15 clients per week.*

Goal: *I work with at least 25 clients per week.*

Benefits of Achieving This Goal: *I can meet my lifestyle needs, pay off my school loans, take a vacation and start a savings account.*

Possible Courses of Action:

1. *Get a part-time job at a clinic.*
2. *Hire an agent.*
3. *Actively market my practice.*

Best Course: *The most appropriate long-term solution is to actively market my practice, which could also include securing another corporate account.*

Proposal Outline: *In order to have 25 clients per week, I need a base of 100 active clients: 5 weekly, 15 biweekly, 40 monthly and 40 occasional. I design a creative, fun marketing plan that includes increasing client retention.*

Advantages: *By augmenting my client list, I increase the odds of achieving my goal. Once my base is established, I won't have to put in as much effort into getting new clients because I will incorporate client retention techniques.*

Potential Conflicts/Disadvantages:

1. *I don't really like marketing.*
2. *I'm not sure what to do.*
3. *There's a new company in town (with four therapists) offering corporate massage.*

Solutions:

1. *Do clearing exercises. Remind myself that marketing is simply sharing who I am and what I do. Do some of my marketing activities with colleagues.*
2. *Read books and magazines. Take marketing classes. Work with a business coach. Invest five hours per week on marketing.*
3. *Affiliate myself with the corporate massage company or determine what my differential advantage is and pursue other accounts.*

Action Required to Begin: *Review my client files to determine massage frequency. Set aside at least two hours to outline my marketing plan.*

Resources Needed: *Time, paper, pencils and files. Ideally, samples of therapists' marketing plans.*

Specific Steps to Achieve This Goal

	Target Date
I receive weekly massages	*Starting 2/15*
I finalize my marketing plan (vision, goals and analysis)	*2/28*
I invest five hours per week to marketing for new clients	*Starting 3/1*
I attend at least two networking functions monthly	*Starting 3/1*
I do daily affirmations	*Starting 3/1*
I invest two hours per week in client retention	*Starting 3/1*
I do thorough intake interviews and treatment plans with all my clients	*Starting 3/1*
For each of the next six months I add 10 new clients to my client base	*Starting 3/1*
I distribute at least 150 business cards monthly	*Starting 3/1*
I do weekly client follow-up through calls and cards	*Starting 3/1*
I review and update my marketing plan monthly	*Starting 3/1*
I redesign my brochures	*3/20*
I sponsor a Massage-a-thon for my favorite charity	*3/20*
I join a business support group	*3/30*
I send a letter containing some type of incentive to non-current clients	*3/30*
I secure at least one corporate massage account	*4/30*
I distribute at least 100 brochures monthly	*Starting 4/1*
I make at least one corporate massage proposal/presentation monthly	*Starting 4/1*
I do at least two presentations/demonstrations monthly	*Starting 4/1*
I contact at least two allied health care providers monthly	*Starting 4/1*
I send a welcome packet to all new clients	*Starting 4/1*
I read at least three business books	*4/1, 6/1, 8/1*
I send a newsletter to my clients	*4/20, 7/20*
I participate in at least two cooperative marketing projects	*5/15, 7/15*
I have a booth at the Wellness Expo	*5/20*
I develop a summer special for current clients	*5/25*
I get interviewed by the local paper	*5/31*
I am a featured guest on two radio programs	*6/2*
I host a chair massage booth at the Annual Street Fair	*6/15*
I appear on four television programs	*6/30*
I continue to add four new clients each month	*Starting 9/1*

Strategic planning is a layered system: start with your major goal, analyze it and break it into smaller goals/steps. You may find that some of the smaller steps need to be refined further. I recommend that you make a master list of the activities required to achieve the major goal and separate sheets for each project. In the strategic planning illustration, several of the goals need to have their own project sheet because of the many steps required to attain the goal, (e.g., getting interviewed and doing the cooperative marketing projects). Other goals are more straightforward and self-explanatory, such as reading three business books and doing daily affirmations. If you experience any resistance or difficulty with any of your goals, I suggest that you break the goal down into as many specific steps as possible.

The most elaborate plan isn't going to create results if it isn't implemented. Transfer your goals and items from strategic planning sheets to a calendar (computers make planning much less cumbersome) and refer to it often. It takes time, but long-term planning is time well-invested. The clarity you acquire and the organization created always save you at least the amount of time spent in actual planning.

Strategic Planning Benefits

- You're less likely to forget a major step.
- Creative ideas and brainstorming comes easier.
- Goals become clarified and more "real."
- You gain a better overall picture.
- Realization that some steps may require immediate action over others.
- Knowledge of what is necessary to accomplish the goal.
- A more accurate time table is developed.
- A written description of your intentions is a self-motivational tool.

Planning helps renew enthusiasm, especially if a goal is tough to accomplish. Whenever you reduce a goal to its component parts, the small steps toward reaching it are less overwhelming and more possible. You gain confidence with each little step forward.

• Follow-Through •

Creating your life to be what you desire is an ongoing process. In terms of goal setting, the actual statement (written, verbal and pictorial) of the goals is only one step. In order to increase the potential of achieving the goals, it's important to incorporate clearing, strategic planning, activity prioritization, tracking, affirmations, visualization and self-acknowledgment.

So far we have covered clearing, goal setting and strategic planning. Tracking and activity prioritization are techniques to assist you in staying on target and are discussed in Chapter Three. The rest of this section is focused on visualization and affirmations.

Visualization ～

The concept of visualization is one that has inspired many people and accelerated their ability to change their lives, yet for others has been a source of frustration. A popular saying goes "If you can't see it, you'll never have it." That statement is true, but only in its purest sense.

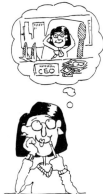

Not everyone "sees" the same way. Perhaps "experience" would be a better word. When some people envision a goal they don't actually see it, but they get a physical sensation or they hear the sounds associated with the goal. For example, let's say you have a goal of going on a hike this weekend. You may actually see yourself waking up in the morning, getting dressed and walking through the hills—fully seeing the surroundings. Another possibility is you might feel how it's to be hiking: the stretching of your muscles, the smell of the flowers and the emotional interaction you have with the environment. Finally, your "visualization" might be verbal. You may actually talk yourself through the day or even imagine the sounds of the animals, the wind and the conversation of the others on the hike. Your visualization may also include a combination of sight, sound, smell and sensation.

Indeed, the more senses you incorporate into your visualizations, the more powerful they become. You can visualize in your head, use the methods described under Goal Setting Techniques or create your own process. Another option using a visual representation is to carry a picture of the goal. For example, if you want a new car, have someone take a picture of you sitting in the exact model you desire or cut out a picture of the car from a brochure (and possibly glue on a picture of your face in the driver's seat). It isn't necessary to "visualize" in any specific way. Do what works best for you. The possibilities for creativity are abundant!

Affirmations ～

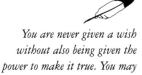

You are never given a wish without also being given the power to make it true. You may have to work for it however.
— Richard Bach

An affirmation is a positive declaration that something is already so. It can be general or very specific. It's a constructive thought that you deliberately choose to place in your consciousness to produce a desired result. The purpose of writing/saying affirmations is to support you in actualizing your dreams and goals by replacing negative self-talk with positive self-talk. When you create affirmations, you are in essence planting a seed for new beginnings. Avoid becoming attached to the specific details of "how" the affirmation will manifest. As with goal setting, always state your affirmations in the positive present tense and personalize them. Choose affirmations that feel good to you. What works for one person may not work for you.

Affirmations can be used in many ways to produce powerful results. Experiment with some of the following suggestions.

Affirmation Techniques

- Read your affirmations at least three times per day.
- Write each affirmation 10 to 20 times in succession.
- Write your affirmations while speaking them aloud to yourself.
- Write your affirmations in the first, second and third person.
  For example: *"I, Sue, am healthy." "You, Sue, are healthy." "She, Sue, is healthy."*
- Write your affirmations and tape them up (or use Post-it® notes) around your home, car and office. Put them on the telephone, the refrigerator, your desk, mirrors, doors, over your bed and on the dashboard.
- Make bookmarks with your affirmations on them.
- Record your affirmations on tape and listen to them as you drive, exercise and before you go to sleep.
- Meditate on your affirmations.
- Stand in front of a mirror and look at yourself while saying your affirmations.
- Take turns saying and accepting affirmations with a friend.
- Make flash cards with your affirmations and carry them with you.
- Design or buy clothes with affirmations on them.
- Sing or chant your affirmations.

Doubt, resistance and physical discomfort are a natural side effect of the affirming process. If you notice these feelings while you are creating an affirmation, do not fight them. Accept them, acknowledge them and allow their expression. Sometimes these feelings are signals of deep conflicts that may require more (or other types) of clearing. You may be able to discharge the negative energy by doing the following clearing exercise. Write down the affirmation on a piece of paper and then write the response that comes to mind. Then rewrite the affirmation and the next thought that comes to mind.

Affirmation Clearing Example

I, Bill, love my life!   *Sure bet.*
I, Bill, love my life!   *But not my job.*
I, Bill, love my life!   *Not right now I don't.*
I, Bill, love my life!   *Maybe someday—if I win the lottery.*
I, Bill, love my life!   *I just wish it wasn't so painful.*
I, Bill, love my life!   *Hmmmm.*
I, Bill, love my life!   *I see the possibilities.*

Continue writing the affirmation and your reactions until you no longer elicit negative responses. Do this for several days or until you feel you've discharged the negativity. Now you can return to working with the original affirmation. This exercise can be time consuming, but you are worth it! Affirmations are most effective when the path is clear of resistance.

Figure 2.4

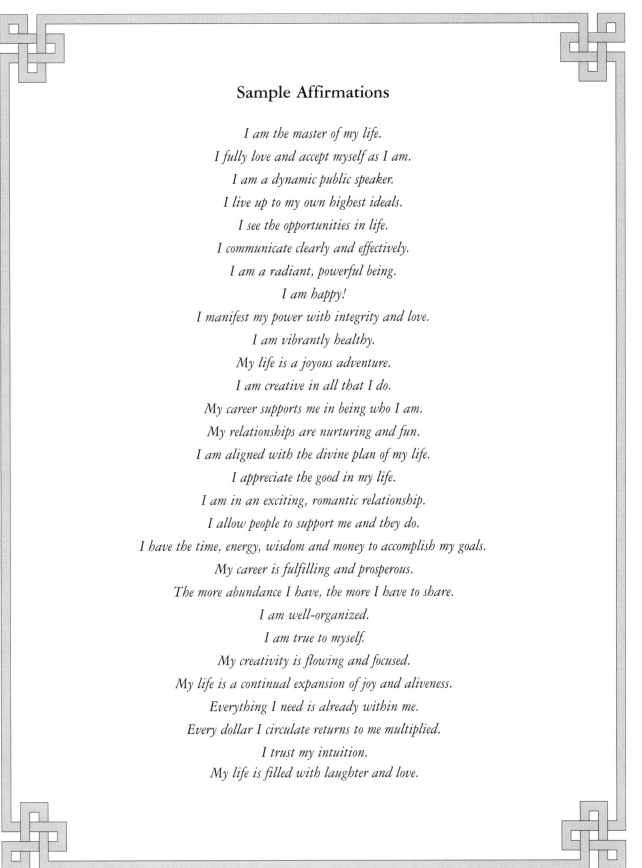

Sample Affirmations

I am the master of my life.

I fully love and accept myself as I am.

I am a dynamic public speaker.

I live up to my own highest ideals.

I see the opportunities in life.

I communicate clearly and effectively.

I am a radiant, powerful being.

I am happy!

I manifest my power with integrity and love.

I am vibrantly healthy.

My life is a joyous adventure.

I am creative in all that I do.

My career supports me in being who I am.

My relationships are nurturing and fun.

I am aligned with the divine plan of my life.

I appreciate the good in my life.

I am in an exciting, romantic relationship.

I allow people to support me and they do.

I have the time, energy, wisdom and money to accomplish my goals.

My career is fulfilling and prosperous.

The more abundance I have, the more I have to share.

I am well-organized.

I am true to myself.

My creativity is flowing and focused.

My life is a continual expansion of joy and aliveness.

Everything I need is already within me.

Every dollar I circulate returns to me multiplied.

I trust my intuition.

My life is filled with laughter and love.

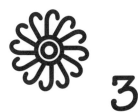

3

Success Strategies

• Self-Management •

"Thriving on chaos"—a phrase that Tom Peters has made common in the marketplace—is also an apt description how many of us lead our lives. But what is the price of our success through chaos? Have we excised ourselves (and our families) from our lives? It's easy to get enmeshed in our projects—telling ourselves that we will take time off next weekend, or maybe next month, well, at least sometime this year....

Quite often we have conflicting ideas of what it means to be successful and our requirements for success may vary greatly in the personal, business and social realms. Explore your values and how they relate to your success. Consider what it means to be successful: Are you successful only if you earn a certain amount of money, perform miracles in your work, look a particular way, are in a perfect relationship, drive a great car or live in the right neighborhood? In other words, what are your values? Is success a "thing" to be achieved or a way of being?

In the book *Lead, Follow or Get Out of the Way*, Jim Lundy describes success as the achievement of predetermined goals. This means any goal! The key word is "predetermined." For instance, you may have accomplished something (possibly even something major) that you hadn't really intended or even given much thought to, and somehow the victory seemed hollow. Most likely that feeling was because you hadn't previously claimed it as a goal. Achievements are so much more fulfilling when they are planned. Thus, success is really a process—one that involves setting and achieving goals.

Refer to Chapter Two

for specific information on goal setting techniques

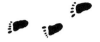

There is truly an art to being successful in the business world while staying balanced. It would be simple if our lives weren't filled with meaningful activities. That just isn't the case. Most of us have a career/business, a family, social activities and civic responsibilities. All of these are important. At times we may feel as though we're jugglers in a circus—keeping everything going, yet not being able to fully enjoy any one aspect. So, what can be done? We certainly can't create a 30-hour day.

The key lies in self-management. Self-management is the ability to artfully direct your life so that you easily and joyfully accomplish what you desire. It's about taking personal responsibility for every facet of your life and increasing personal productivity while staying true to yourself. Some of the components of effective self-management include: time management; assessing your values (Chapter One) and operating from them; clarifying your purpose, priorities and goals (Chapter Two); risk-taking; tracking; self-motivation; balancing personal and professional priorities; overcoming your barriers to success; flexibility; choosing appropriate advisors; and dedication to learning and self-improvement.

• Barriers to Success •

Most barriers to success have been forged by our own hands. Self-sabotage is a common occurrence. Sometimes we do this in little ways and other times it becomes a way of life. This usually stems from negative conditioning.

See Chapter One

for more information on negative conditioning.

Typical manifestations of self-sabotage are: possessing a poor self-image; blaming others for misfortunes; expecting failure; putting yourself down (negative self-talk); repeating errors (not learning from past mistakes); and surrounding yourself with inappropriate people. The most common symptom of self-sabotage with the small business owner is procrastination.

Nothing in life is to be feared. It is only to be understood.
— Marie Curie

"Never put off until tomorrow what you can do today!" is the cliché which makes every procrastinator cringe. Everyone has experienced putting off various duties, tasks and responsibilities until the last possible minute (or longer). If this becomes a habit, it can be detrimental to the success of a business.

Procrastination brings to mind words such as lazy, unproductive and inefficient, yet procrastination is not necessarily a negative state. In fact, it's simply a signal that it's time to evaluate the status of the task in question and discover the reason(s) it's staying at the bottom of the "to-do" pile.

The reasons for procrastination are numerous. Perhaps one of the most common is setting such high, perfectionistic expectations for performance that accomplishing the task appears overwhelming, if not impossible. It's easy to set yourself up in this manner—to never feel quite good enough, continually dissatisfied with your performance even though you got the job done. The put-off project then becomes a representation of your fear of failure and inadequacy.

Perfectionists believe that "adequate" or "sufficient" performance simply is not good enough. "Adequate" and "inadequate" come to mean the same thing. It's important to put these three words: perfection, adequate and inadequate—in their proper perspective. Nothing is inherently wrong in having high standards but they need to be evaluated to determine if they are realistic. Perfection is impossible. To do a job adequately is to do what is needed. Inadequate means not meeting minimal requirements. If you feel fear about some task that you have to do, it could be that you are setting perfectionistic standards for yourself that are difficult to meet.

Oftentimes people can convince themselves that a task is critical when it isn't. It's prudent to evaluate whether a task is actually necessary. You must evaluate and rank your tasks (this may take the assistance of a consultant). If the task is not something that you want to do and it isn't really necessary, then maybe you can take yourself off the hook.

Possibly you've agreed to do a certain task or activity that you really didn't want to do. If this is the case it may not be too late to renegotiate. If you frequently find yourself having difficulty saying "no!" and procrastinate as a result, learn how to set limits and boundaries.

Sometimes procrastination is brought on by a lack of information. If you expect yourself to do a task without having the necessary knowledge, even the most routine task can become overwhelming. Before you begin a project, map out the technical, informational and functional requirements. Once you have determined what supplies, information and other resources will be needed to complete the task—obtain them and begin your project. Being organized can make any task more palatable and run more smoothly. Additionally, give yourself permission to ask for the help you need. Asking for help can provide you with the energy and support to accomplish the task.

When procrastination simply comes down to having to do a task that must be done but is loathsome, there are some techniques to choose from that may help you move on. These techniques are reframing, task breakdown/simplification and delegation.

Reframing is finding an alternative way to view the project at hand. This may be done by creating a more pleasant environment to work on the task, such as listening to enjoyable music, sitting in a comfortable chair, sipping on a glass of iced tea or involving another person (preferably with a good sense of humor) in the task.

Task Breakdown involves clarifying the components and progression of a project by setting clear goals with target dates. This is basically taking things one step at a time and keeping them as simple as possible.

Procrastination is the fear of success. People procrastinate because they are afraid of the success that they know will result if they move ahead now. Because success is heavy, carries a responsibility with it, it is much easier to procrastinate and live on the "someday I'll" philosophy.
— Denis Waitley

Your attitude, not your aptitude, will determine your altitude.
— Zig Ziglar

Delegation (or sub-contracting) is often an alternative. Explore the possibilities. Determine if there are portions of the task (if not the whole thing) that can be done more easily and effectively by someone else. Consider trading tasks with a colleague. It's important to remember that when you delegate or trade, you are not handing over total responsibility for the finished product. You still need to oversee the tasks to assure their completion.

Procrastination is not only a personal issue, it also affects associates and staff as well. If you have discovered that you are a perfectionist, it can be extremely difficult to accurately gauge others' performance. You may be setting standards so high that not even you could attain them. Are you projecting your own perfectionism? Are you creating an atmosphere where people are afraid to take risks? Is it safe for your co-workers to make mistakes?

If this is indeed the situation, discuss it with your associates and staff. Let them know that you are aware of your tendencies and address methods to improve working conditions. You need to set new standards—they can still be high, but not out of reach. If you can come to an agreement, everyone wins—you are happy, the people you work with won't feel as pressured and the company gets higher quality work from the staff.

Procrastination in self and others is an issue that most people have to deal with at some point in their lives. Procrastination is a symptom. The important thing to remember is to listen to yourself. Find out what is behind the behavior. Evaluate the dynamics. Then you will be able to alleviate the procrastination by making the necessary changes—be they internal or external.

Creative minds have always been known to survive any kind of bad training.
— Anna Freud

What we sow or plant in the soil will come back to us in exact kind. It's impossible to sow corn and get a crop of wheat, but we entirely disregard this law when it comes to mental sowing.
— Orison Swett Marden

Strategies to Overcome Barriers

- Clarify your values and operate from them.
- Do clearing work or therapy.
- Set clear goals.
- Become a calculated risk taker.
- Work smarter—not harder.
- Be informed.
- Keep balanced.
- Learn from your past mistakes.
- Create a positive support system.
- Keep things in perspective.

• Time Management Principles •

One of the keystones to self-management (hence, success) is time management. What is time, really? The dictionary defines time as indefinite, unlimited duration in which things are considered as happening in the past, present or future. It's a system of measuring duration.

Time management isn't about which appointment book you use. It isn't creating a 30-hour day—everyone has the same amount of time. Time management is about your attitudes and perceptions. It's based on realizing how much your time is worth and choosing activities that are the highest priority for you to achieve your goals.

Time management is really a matter of how well you use your time. Time can either be an asset or a liability; it all depends on your attitudes. You can't alter time, only your attitudes and behaviors relating to time. Your attitudes toward time are influenced by conditioning and by your self-esteem.

There was a young lady named Bright, whose speed was far faster than light; She set out one day, in a relative way, and returned home the previous night.
— Arthur Bullery

Time Attitudes Exercise

What thoughts and feelings do you have concerning time?
How did your family relate to time?
Do you respect yourself by taking the time to take care of yourself?
Do you view time as your friend or your enemy?

In terms of behavior change, many possible ways exist for taking action. Learn (or enhance) the skills that are required to improve your productivity: goal setting and strategic planning; scheduling; dealing with interruptions; being able to decline offers; delegation; keeping current with your job skills; product knowledge; communication skills; management skills; and stress management.

Effective Time Management Benefits

- Doing the same work in less time.
- Accomplishing more work in the same number of hours.
- Increasing personal productivity.
- Getting more recognition.
- Earning more money.
- Decreasing frustration and stress.
- Having more time for planning.
- Devoting more time to your family.
- Spending more time with hobbies and recreation.
- Improving your health.
- Experiencing increased joy and satisfaction.

There is a fundamental difference between working harder and working smarter.

The fundamental basis of time management is the Pareto Principle: The Pareto principle states that 80 percent of your results are produced by 20 percent of your activities. And conversely, 20 percent of your results are produced by 80 percent of your activities. Time management techniques are effective because most people spend a lot of time in activities that are not an efficient use of their time. These percentages vary for individual cases, but the principle holds. The more you learn to focus on these 20 percent activities and turn them into 40 percent or even 60 percent, the more productive, prosperous and balanced you are.

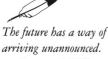

The future has a way of arriving unannounced.
— George F. Will

Time Management Tips

- Invest at least 10 minutes in planning daily.
- Focus on the "A" goals first.
- Review your master goal list at least once per week.
- Group similar activities together.
- Set specific times for taking and returning phone calls.
- Throughout the day ask yourself, "What is the best use of my time?"
- Discourage interruptions.
- Learn to say "no."
- Track important data and activities.
- Avoid procrastination.
- Respect your body's and mind's cycles.
- Do your most challenging work during your peak performance cycles.
- Delegate whenever possible.
- Take a quick stretch break every 20 minutes.
- Keep supplies stocked and accessible.
- Set a schedule and follow it.
- Review files regularly.
- At the end of the day, create the next day's goals and activities list.

He who every morning plans the transactions of the day, and follows out that plan, carries a thread that will guide him through the labyrinth of the most busy life.
— Victor Hugo

Types of Time Needed to Run a Business

In order to effectively run your business you must remember that there are many areas for which you need to allot time. You need time to plan, work with clients, manage the business, continue your education, market your practice, communicate, develop ideas, take care of yourself and have fun. Effective daily planning is crucial to time management. Many people create incredible to-do lists, but lack the motivation to complete them. When you have a clear purpose, priorities, goals and plans of action, you don't get so overwhelmed. You know what you have to do, the order in which to do it and when it needs to be done. Sometimes people imagine things to be far more complicated than they really are.

It's important to recognize that there are different types of time you need and the amount of time spent in each category may vary from day to day. Set a regular schedule for your business. Decide what days and what hours you will work. You may want to do this on a weekly or monthly basis. Once you've made your schedule, stick to it. Even if you don't have the time slots filled with clients, you can always do other business activities. It can be so tempting to look at your appointment book, not see anything scheduled for the afternoon, and decide to go play. Occasionally this is fine, and be careful it doesn't become a habit.

The time you spend in planning is always well-invested. When you have a clear plan for the day and a crisis does occur, you are then more flexible in handling it and making necessary adjustments. Your day flows easily and you stay on target.

The basis of productive planning is effective goal setting. The major element in planning (especially daily planning) is ranking. After you have written your daily plan, evaluate it. Decide which activities absolutely must get done today and rate them as Imperative. Review the other items and indicate the ones that need to be done very soon by labeling them as Important. Mark the rest of the activities (the ones that it would be nice if you accomplished them, but they're not of major significance) as being Desirable.

When you first start planning it may seem to take a long time; after doing it on a regular basis, you can plan your day very quickly. Remember, planning is to ultimately simplify your life—not make it more complicated.

Managing your business is covered from both philosophical and business skills perspectives in subsequent chapters. We often forget to schedule appropriate time for the day-to-day tasks such as doing laundry, making phone calls, supervising staff (if you have any), keeping files and purchasing supplies. All of these activities take time, often a lot more than anticipated.

Another aspect of managing your business has to do with respecting yourself and time in relation to bartering (or trading) services. Barter is usually a supplemental method of obtaining products and services that you prefer to not purchase with cash. The down side is that some people get so into bartering they never earn any money. Be very clear of your reasons for trading. Before you do any type of bartering, ask yourself if you would spend money on that product or service if you had the cash. If not, don't trade. Also, remember that barter is considered taxable income by the Internal Revenue Service.

Working with clients is the area where most of your time is spent. Your ability to effectively schedule your appointments greatly impacts your success and your stress level. It's important to allot sufficient time between clients and yet not have large blocks of unproductive time. You may discover that you need to schedule an extra half-hour for new clients and some ongoing clients who regularly need additional time. You may need a longer recuperation time after certain clients. The longer you are in practice, the more adept you become in judging how much time is necessary to spend with clients and between sessions.

Refer to Chapter Two for specific planning techniques.

See Appendix A, page 380 for a Daily Planning Form. The form is provided as an example for you to adapt to your specific needs.

See Chapter 7, pages 190-194 for more information on barter.

If you fill your mind with coins from your purse, your mind will fill your purse with coins.
— Benjamin Franklin

See Chapter Nine
for specific ideas on how to effectively market your practice.

See Chapter Eight
for tips on improving your therapeutic communications.

Continuing your education is necessary to your career. It's important to always be broadening your knowledge, particularly in the areas of interpersonal skills, product knowledge, technical skills and business skills. Some ways to do that are: reading magazines and books; taking classes; attending seminars; watching videos; and networking.

Developing ideas is one of the most exciting and creative aspects of any business. Always be open to new opportunities. Brainstorm ways to streamline your procedures. Find methods to reduce your effort by diversifying your practice (e.g., hire employees, sell products or subcontract out work to other practitioners and take a percentage of the fees). Create ways in which you work with more than one client at a time (e.g., offer group sessions, give seminars and publish articles and books). The possibilities are legion!

Marketing your practice is vital to your success. This is the aspect of business that most health care practitioners neglect. You can't rely on your clients to bring you more new clients. Marketing is necessary during all phases of your business. When you first start your practice, you may spend more hours marketing than actually working with clients. Then, even when your business seems to be established, you still need to actively market yourself. People move, change practitioners and try alternate methods of self-improvement. I have known several very successful practitioners whose businesses appeared to fall apart over night. They were not marketing themselves well; they hadn't noticed the changes that were occurring until it was too late. So, they had to "start all over again." You can avoid this through regular marketing. It's critical that you invest at least 15 percent of your work time in marketing.

Communicating is essential to your business. You need to be able to fully understand your clients and their needs. You spend most of your communication time listening—ironically most people have never been taught how to listen. When talking with your clients, focus on their message—not their method of delivery. Delay making any evaluations. Take responsibility for understanding what you are hearing. If you are not certain you understand what you have heard, ask questions or rephrase what you think you heard.

Having fun tends to be one of the least planned aspects of life. People are inclined to leave their enjoyment to chance. Remember to balance your professional goals with your personal goals. Be sure to include fun in your life EVERY DAY!

Taking care of yourself is imperative, yet many people put themselves last. It's so easy to get caught up in your business and being there for others, that literally no time is left for you. It's important to take care of yourself mentally, physically, emotionally and spiritually. Make sure that every day you do at least one thing just for yourself. Respect your needs and wants. Create a support system for your business and personal life. Caregivers have a tendency to not allow themselves to be care-receivers. Don't let yourself fall into that syndrome. Allot as much time as needed to take care of you.

One of the major factors that influences your time is stress. If you do not handle stress productively, you can waste hours of time each day—not to mention time lost due to stress-related illness. Make certain that you exercise regularly and follow a healthy eating plan.

Take a quick stretch break every 20 minutes. Allot a five-minute break every two hours to more thoroughly stretch your muscles, do some deep breathing, exercise your eyes and revitalize yourself.

Keeping balance in mind is the key to stress management. You need to keep things in perspective. Don't react to things that aren't your responsibility. Learn to deal with interruptions: internal and external. Learn how to say no.

Last, but most definitely not least, develop and maintain a positive self-image. You must be true to yourself. Make certain that your needs and wants are being met. Live your life (and run your business) according to your values and principles.

Time can be your enemy or your friend. It becomes your friend when you learn how to manage yourself.

High Priority Activities

High priority activities are the "20 percent" ones that produce 80 percent of your results. Before you can begin to increase the time spent in those important activities, you must identify them. The following exercise is designed to assist you in clarifying your high priority activities. You may be surprised at what you discover. The objective of this exercise is for you to take this list and begin concentrating your time and energy on items you've rated as being the most crucial to your success.

High Priority Activities Exercise

Make a copy of the High Priority Activities form found in Appendix A (page 379) or take out a piece of paper and draw three columns with the center column the widest. Label the left-hand column "Importance," the middle column "Activity" and the right-hand column "Time Spent." Think about the various activities involved in your business. List at least 10 of the most important things you do in the center column. Then in the left-hand column rate them in the order you think is most important to your success. In the right-hand column rate them in the order of how much time you spend in each activity.

The more you focus on your high priority activities, the more productive you will be. You may also discover some conflicts. If this happens, refer to your purpose, priorities and goals. They usually provide direction. Sometimes you have to make difficult decisions and either delegate the other activities, simplify them or eliminate them. It's also recommended that you show your list to a colleague. It's possible that you overlooked something or you need to switch some of your priorities—and it's usually easier for someone else to be objective.

• Tracking •

Frequently, in business, we have no idea why things are going the way they are; including when they are going well. Was it that last ad? Could it have been that interview in the newspaper? Maybe it was the new brochure? Or was it due to extending office hours on Thursday? Even though it isn't always possible to know for certain the exact action that did (or didn't) generate the desired results, you greatly increase your knowledge and optimize your efforts by tracking the important components.

Results! Why, man, I have gotten a lot of results. I know several thousand things that won't work.
— Thomas A. Edison

Tracking is a documentation of your progress used to illustrate trends. Your appointment book, checkbook and accounting journal don't really tell you the whole truth. A lot of critical data is not included in those books and if you use them as your major reference point for judging your success, you may find yourself in a predicament. Oftentimes things are not as they appear.

For example, imagine that you have been fairly well-booked and have had a satisfactory level of income for the last few months, so you haven't been putting much attention into marketing. Then the next month goes by and you discover (to your dismay) that your client load has decreased and your income level has significantly dropped. You don't quite understand how this could happen—after all, everything seemed to be going so well. You decide to carefully review your books and find that you've only had three new clients in the last two months, four clients have completed their work with you and the time between sessions for the rest of your clients has been substantially increasing. Had you been keeping track of that kind of information on a summary sheet or a graph, you could have noticed the trend earlier and taken action (e.g., done some type of marketing) to rebuild your clientele base. In any business, particularly one that's small, one slow month can be devastating.

Statistics are no substitute for judgment.
— Henry Clay

Tracking can help you anticipate potential problems so that you can take the appropriate steps to avoid or overcome the obstacles and modify the direction of the trend more to your liking. Tracking is dynamic in nature; it focuses on the way things change—the "motion" of business.

Another way tracking is helpful has to do with timing. You may notice that for the last three years, your business drops dramatically every October. Using that information you can decide to increase your advertising and promotion in August and September or you may just choose to take advantage of the slow period and plan a vacation for October. Conversely, it wouldn't be judicious for you to plan a vacation during your peak period.

Tracking is also quite beneficial in determining which advertising media and promotional events have been most effective.

Tracking Tools ⚹

The methods for tracking are varied. You might use graph paper, computerized spread sheets, custom-designed forms or simple notebook paper. Make the forms very clear and as straightforward as possible to fill out. Also, be certain to design your client forms so they provide you with information (e.g., how they heard about you), demographics and session notes for your tracking sheets. You may want to make charts and post them on the wall or put your tracking forms into a notebook.

Experiment with tracking activities on a daily, weekly, monthly or quarterly basis. Consistency is essential, particularly when tracking the results of marketing campaigns, since it often takes several months to discern those results. Additionally, you may discover that the results were due to a combination of factors. Thus the measurable benefits of tracking are derived from the knowledge you receive over the long run.

Even if you're on the right track, you'll get run over if you just sit there.
— Will Rogers

Useful Items To Track

- Client demographics
- Total number of clients
- Types of clients
- Session time spent per client
- Time spent per client in adjunct support
- Time between sessions
- Type of techniques utilized
- Number of sessions per client
- Average cost of total treatment plan
- How your clients heard about you
- Referrals generated by specific marketing campaigns
- Time spent in all business activities
- Total income (e.g., daily, weekly, monthly)
- Total expenses

Sample Tracking Forms ⚹

Tracking is an essential component in making a business plan work. First you must decide what you want to track. The above list, your business plan and your list of high priority activities are excellent places to begin. This data provides you with the information you need to assess the progress of your long-term goals and strategies, as well as enhances your decision-making abilities when it comes to planning your future marketing campaigns and general business direction.

Studies show that tracking in itself increases your productivity. It's an excellent way to keep yourself motivated, evaluate your status and help you determine the most appropriate areas in which to invest your time and money to build your practice.

Figure 3.1

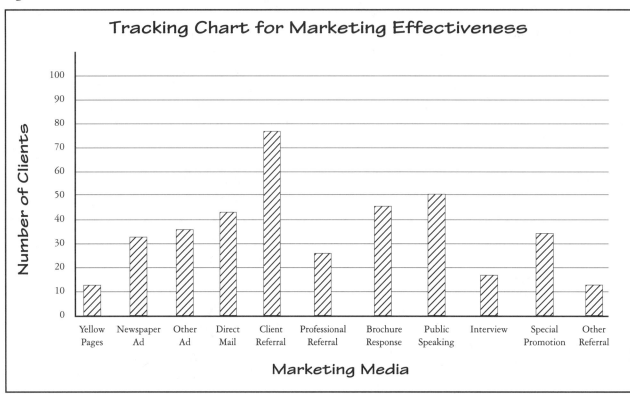

Tracking Chart for Marketing Effectiveness

Figure 3.2

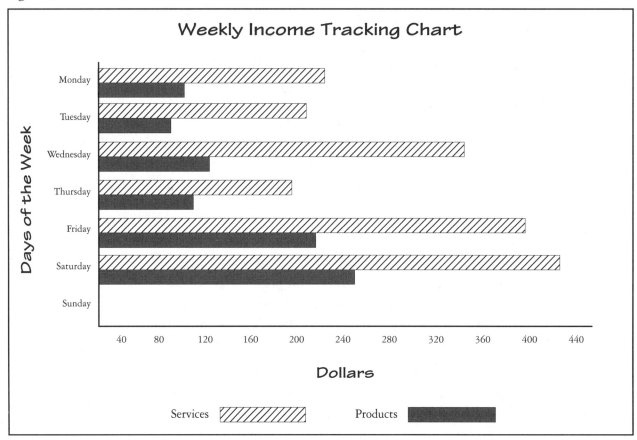

Weekly Income Tracking Chart

As with daily planning, it usually takes a little while to become adept at tracking. After you have experimented with various forms, you will discover the ones that are most appropriate for your needs and then it won't take you very much time at all to track (see Figures 3.1 and 3.2).

Invest the time required for tracking—it's an informational and inspirational tool to help you run a productive and profitable business.

• The Art of Risk Taking •

Ideals are like stars; you will not succeed in touching them with your hands. But like the seafaring man on the desert of waters, you choose them as your guides, and following them you will reach your destiny.
— Carl Schurz

Two commonly heard truisms are "nothing ventured, nothing gained" and "no guts, no glory." Taking risks is an integral part of life, especially true in business. It's the doorway to success; the art is knowing how to take **smart** risks. Some people consider themselves to be risk takers when in reality they are simply daredevils. Taking risks is not about blindly jumping into any situation. To become proficient in taking risks, it's vital that you understand the components of risk taking, learn how to minimize your potential losses and strengthen your risk-taking abilities.

The two major elements that influence your ability to successfully manage risks are the level of comfort you have in experiencing new or unusual situations, and your self-esteem. Think about the source of your self-confidence. To what degree do you base it upon your opinions and values? How much do you look to others for validation? Is your behavior mainly motivated by external factors such as social approval and material consequences, or by internal considerations such as your beliefs and feelings?

Don't play for safety; it's the most dangerous thing in the world.
— Hugh Walpole

In terms of self-esteem, the primary discomfort in taking risks stems from the fear of rejection. In considering your ability to feel confident in novel circumstances, the fundamental discomfort is usually due to inexperience. People take the safer routes so often that they haven't developed a bank of experiences from which to draw. Reflect upon your childhood. What messages were you given regarding the safety of your environment? How did your family deal with crises? What behaviors did you learn to adopt? You can alleviate a lot of anxiety by keeping your expectations realistic and embracing the opportunities for new experiences.

Risk takers are achievers. They are not content with the status quo. They prefer action to inaction and follow through on their goals with little hesitation. They are exhilarated by challenges rather than intimidated by them and proceed despite their fears. They also carefully evaluate risks and develop strategic plans of action. They distinguish facts from their emotions, which enables them to handle crises well and empowers their decision-making process. Risk-takers have a strong commitment to being and producing the best.

The Do's of Risk Taking

- Do have a life plan with clear goals.
- Do make sure the risk is aligned with your life plan.
- Do evaluate the potential gains and losses.
- Do ask questions and research the situation.
- Do know your strengths and limitations.
- Do brainstorm several alternatives.
- Do list potential conflicts and solutions.
- Do set a realistic timetable.
- Do be flexible.
- Do trust your intuition and instincts.
- Do follow through and give it your best.
- Do review and possibly revise your strategy.
- Do ask for support.
- Do acknowledge the people who give you support.

The Don'ts of Risk Taking

- Don't be unrealistic.
- Don't be a perfectionist.
- Don't deny your feelings.
- Don't ignore or minimize problems.
- Don't mistake emotions for facts.
- Don't rush.
- Don't procrastinate.
- Don't blame others for your mistakes.
- Don't give up too soon.
- Don't be afraid to cut your losses and move on.
- Don't trust blindly.
- Don't risk just to prove yourself to others.
- Don't combine too many risks at once.

Developing your skill in taking risks is a lifelong process. As you go through life, the stakes just seem to get higher. Build your repertoire of risk-taking experiences so that you are able to successfully manage risks. By drawing upon your past experiences to see the similarities to the current situation, you can better determine an effective solution. Put yourself in situations that require you to exercise your creative problem-solving abilities. Start with low-risk situations—gradually increasing your confidence level so you feel more comfortable taking greater risks.

The continual enhancement of your self-image is vital in cultivating risk-taking behaviors. Begin with positive self-talk. Fill your mind with thoughts about your potential. Become grounded in the knowledge that you are your own source of power and that this power is honorable. Expect to succeed. Release some of your conditioned apprehension and fear by doing the following clearing exercise.

Risk-Taking Exercise

Think about a situation that makes you feel uneasy. Imagine what is the very worst thing that could possibly happen. Then evaluate the situation. Is it really that bad? Are your fears justified? Finally, visualize yourself being comfortable and confident while in that risky situation.

Your attitudes about the world can greatly influence your facility in taking risks. Be enthusiastic about the present and future. Expand your view of life. Focus on the prospects for success and joy. Don't become immersed in the potentials for disaster. Accurately evaluate what would really happen if you were to take a risk and not succeed. Remember that success lies in taking action.

The last factor that impacts people's freedom to take chances is finances. Most people are overly concerned with money. The truth is that most successful business owners have failed at least once before finally making it. Again, you are the best judge of what's appropriate. You are the only one who can determine whether or not a risk is worth it. One step you can take now is to reduce your debt as much as possible. If you are considering taking a risk that has monetary ramifications, take the time to thoroughly evaluate the possibilities. Often what is more scary than the possibility of losing money is the potential for losing face.

There's only one corner of the universe you can be certain of improving, and that's your own self.
— Aldous Huxley

• Motivation •

Motivation is about satisfying desires and needs. Abraham Maslow's hierarchy of needs are physiological (satisfaction of hunger, thirst and sex), safety (security and stability), social (belongingness and love), esteem (self-respect and ego) and self-actualization. It's extraordinarily difficult to be motivated toward self-actualization if your safety or ego needs aren't met.

So, if you find that you just can't motivate yourself to do a particular task, find out what other needs you have that are not being met. You must appeal to the needs and desires that are the strongest at any given moment. Once you have satisfied those other needs, it's easier to complete the specific task.

The two most common motivators are fear and incentive, both of which have serious shortcomings. Fear motivation is the oldest, easiest and universally least effective means of motivation. It forces you to act out of fear of the consequences. Parents frequently use this technique with young children. The primary limitation of this style of motivation is that most people (particularly children) can quickly build up a tolerance to fear, and since the repercussions are rarely enforced, they usually aren't taken seriously.

Ability is what you're capable of doing. Motivation determines what you do. Attitude determines how well you do it.
— Lou Holtz

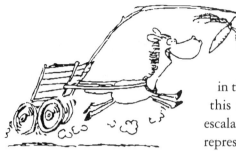

Incentive motivation promises a reward for behavior. This method is often used in business as a way to increase productivity. It's also frequently used by people in the process of altering habits. The problems associated with this motivation system are that the rewards have to keep escalating to merit the same impact, and withholding the reward represents a punishment. Incentive motivation won't satisfy your desire for achievement.

The most effective motivation is self-motivation, being inspired by the pure joy of accomplishment. Approaching life from this point of view is extremely empowering to yourself and to those around you. It can be very freeing to not need outside stimulus to induce action. This can be difficult because the results of your actions are often intangible or may not be realized for a long time. Sometimes people don't feel motivated to accomplish certain goals because they really don't care about the goals in the first place. Be honest with yourself. If you really don't want to do something, don't try to convince yourself that you do want to achieve it.

Self-motivation is an attitude that takes time to develop and fully integrate into your life. It may take longer to master motivation in some areas of your life than in others. The clearer you are about your purposes, priorities and goals, the easier and more natural it will be to become motivated by the sheer act of attaining your goals.

Your history plays a major role in attitude development. Throughout your life you have been influenced to some degree by your environment and the people around you. Your cumulative experiences and feelings impact your perception. For example, you may view a certain task as boring while someone else might find the same task exciting. One technique for altering your feelings about an activity (and thus making it easier to accomplish) is to remove any negative descriptive terms associated with it.

The principal factor in motivation is goals. Without goals, motivation has no direction. You can even create goals about motivation. Your mind is a powerful tool that is ready and waiting for you to utilize it more effectively.

If your motivation is still blocked, do some clearing exercises as described in Chapter One. Oftentimes people lack inspiration and determination because of negative thought patterns and conditioning. Sentence completions exercises are an excellent method for releasing energy associated with negative conditioning. If you are having difficulties with a specific problem, first take an honest look to see if you are truly willing to resolve the problem. If you are, put aside approximately two hours and do the following clearing exercise.

The future belongs to those who believe in the beauty of their dreams.
— Eleanor Roosevelt

Dissolving Problems

Take some notebook paper and write the following questions on the top of each sheet of paper, putting one question per piece of paper and keeping them in the order given. Spend at least five minutes per page actually doing the exercise. (Please refer to Chapter One for detailed instructions on Sentence Completions.)

- What is the area you are having difficulty with? Describe in detail.
- What are your fears and attitudes regarding your problem?
- What aren't you getting?
- What are you getting that you don't want?
- What are you getting that you do want?
- Regarding this problem, how have you been trying to resolve it?
- Regarding this problem, what do you think you should be doing?
- What is it that you want?
- What is it that you should want?
- What are the benefits of not resolving this problem?
- What would you have to give up to resolve this problem?
- What would you have to realize to resolve this problem?
- What are you holding on to or protecting in regards to your problem?
- Who or what is limiting you?
- By solving this problem, what new problems will be created?
- What is it that you really want?
- What are the specific things you will do to resolve this problem?

• Balance •

One of the most disturbing things to encounter is burnout. It's ironic how most people in the health care field are wonderful givers but are often terrible receivers. This is most often caused by not keeping balance physically, emotionally, mentally and spiritually.

The essence of balance is proper thinking. We need to be very careful how we think about things and hold them in our minds. Being overwhelmed and losing our balance can easily happen. When it does we don't see things clearly, become confused, draw inaccurate conclusions or don't give ourselves enough options.

Keeping a realistic frame of reference is crucial. Many people operate with a "go with the flow" philosophy in most areas of their lives, but when it comes to their business their perspective often changes to one of scarcity. Poverty thinking burns you out faster than anything else.

Human beings can alter their lives by altering their attitudes.
— William James

I remember attending a party where a woman mentioned that although her three-year old practice was okay, she was considering getting a part-time job to help out. I was appalled! It wasn't as though she was just starting out and needed to transition into her career. If you figure that it takes approximately three hours of marketing to get a new client—why settle for a $6 an hour temporary job when you can spend these three hours to earn at least $40 instead of $18 (and that's if the client only comes in once). Her shortsightedness was staggering. This is a classic example of poverty thinking.

Hoarding ideas is another example of acting from scarcity. All too often people say they don't want to share their ideas because they are afraid someone else will take them and become successful. This type of thinking is very skewed. First of all, has this ever happened or is it just a fear? It's extremely rare for someone to come up with a truly unique marketing idea. Second, this thinking implies a shortage of ideas. The most innovative and successful marketing ideas I've encountered were formulated in brainstorming sessions involving several people. Finally, consider how much more fun and economically feasible it is to share your marketing ventures with other people.

A major area of faulty logic centers on education. Practitioners save their pennies so they can take some new modality workshop, desperate in the hope that this will bring them more clients or more security in their business. They take classes believing that "this will be the magic formula to make me successful." If they aren't able to market themselves well now, it's unlikely that the addition of a new modality will be the panacea. Some modality workshop facilitators offer advice on marketing the new skills; most do not. Furthering your knowledge base is important but don't confuse your ability to be good at your hands-on work with the ability to market yourself well. They are different skills. If you need to learn more about business, take a business course. If you want to expand your technical repertoire, take a modality training. Do each for the right reason.

Disrespect of time also contributes significantly to burnout and imbalance. Oftentimes people don't set appointments at accurate intervals, don't pace themselves well to accommodate breaks for clearing and centering, don't allow sufficient preparation time for clients, or don't schedule time just for themselves. Thus they're not serving themselves or their clients well. Pay attention to how you're working smarter—not harder. Take the time for your self-care: do stretches, take breaks, make adjustments in your body mechanics, use proper equipment, exercise, eat properly and get some type of touch therapy weekly. Walk your talk: If you are a massage therapist, get weekly massages; if you are an esthetician, get weekly facials; if you are a dentist, make sure your teeth are in great condition. How can you realistically expect clients to be convinced to regularly incorporate your services into their lives if you are not practicing what you preach?

Also, be sure to set aside time for planning and thinking—whether it's about your business agreements, goals, marketing, client relations or evaluating what is working and what's not. In other words, think before you leap. Life is much more enjoyable and successful when one is coming from a proactive position than one of reaction.

If you learn only methods you'll be forever tied to those methods. However, if you learn the principles behind those methods, you'll be free to devise your own methods.
— Ralph Waldo Emerson

I am convinced that it's of primordial importance to learn more every year than the year before. After all, what is education but a process by which a person begins to learn how to learn?
— Peter Ustinov

It's easy to forget about ourselves, yet as caregivers we must make certain we are also care-receivers. This is why I love being a rebirther and maintain a rebirthing practice. Rebirthing is all about letting breath (and everything else) flow in and out, seeing things as they really are and being present. By doing this work I am constantly reminded to stay balanced.

In any career, you experience ups and downs. The key is to recognize the difference between a natural phase and a downward spiral. Step back and objectively (as possible) evaluate the situation. Determine what is really happening. Ask yourself the following questions: What goals aren't being met? Why? What can be done about them? Is it too late? How can this situation be avoided in the future? After you have assessed the situation and brainstormed ideas for managing the predicament, discuss the issue with an advisor. Get some feedback from a different perspective.

Practitioners who have been in business many years may find themselves falling prey to boredom. Sometimes a great rhythm turns into a deep rut. Here are some ideas to prevent this burnout: diversify your practice; alter your work environment; join forces with other health care providers; start a whole new business; take a sabbatical; learn new skills; volunteer your services; and revamp your business plan.

I advocate you do whatever is necessary to take care of yourself, whether that means creating a support system, setting a schedule that includes YOU, getting weekly body therapy treatments, eating well, exercising, laughing or just appreciating the bounty of life.

Luck is a matter of preparation meeting opportunity.
— Oprah Winfrey

See Appendix A, page 378 for The Wheel of Life exercise. Make plenty of copies of the wheel and use it regularly.

Self-Assessment Exercise

You already have been doing a lot of soul-searching and clearing throughout the process of "working" this book. Now it's time to evaluate yourself in order to determine the skills you need to learn or enhance. Be honest.

- What are your strengths?
- What are your challenges?
- How do you intend to alleviate those challenges?

The following chart is a summation of the principles and techniques covered in this book. Refer to it often.

Be Your Own Best Manager

Identify your values and operate from them.
Clarify your purpose, priorities and goals.
Design and implement an effective business plan.
Create strategic plans of action.
Learn to work smarter—not harder.
Track important components.
Eliminate time wasters.
Plan your days.
Set a schedule and keep it.
Take a stretch break every 20 minutes.
Be dressed for "work."
Get feedback from colleagues and experts.
Collect information: quotes, articles, statistics.
Keep your work space organized.
Enhance your telephone skills.
Follow through with clients.
Market your business consistently.
Join at least one professional association.
Develop powerful networking abilities.
Keep accurate records.
Be a calculated risk taker.
Be willing to move on.
Make sure your needs are being met.
Exercise regularly.
Create a support system.
Continue your education.
Get out of the house/office EVERY DAY!!!
Take responsibility for yourself.
Choose appropriate advisors.
Keep things in perspective.
For tasks you hate—delegate (or subcontract).
Respect your mind's and body's cycles.
Balance your personal and professional life.
Remember, we're all human—we make mistakes.
Acknowledge your accomplishments every day.

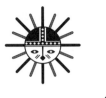

4

Conscious Business

• Are You Open For Business? •

Studies continue to show that the primary reasons most businesses fail are due to improper management or undercapitalization, not because the owners are underskilled in the performance of their profession.

Most health care providers have little training in business and are even reluctant to acknowledge themselves as business people. Many practitioners, and even industry leaders, view business as inherently evil. They see business practices, particularly marketing, as anti-caring and against what they stand for. Visions of ogres and used car salesmen lurk in their minds. Yet the best-run and most effectively marketed practices are not based on a hard-core approach at all, but are founded on personalized customer service.

Whether in private practice or working for someone else, you are part of the business world. Being successful in the business world need not be in conflict with one's values.

At best, business is downplayed in this field, and to complicate matters providers are deluged with information on new modalities by companies making claims that their added technique (or product) will ensure success. Just because you may

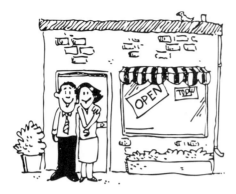

have these techniques or products doesn't mean that you'll use them. Additional modalities can make you a better service provider but won't guarantee a full practice. After all, you need clients first. If you are unable to build your practice given your current skills, it's unlikely that more skills will do it—unless, of course, your repertoire is severely limited.

However, it's wise to learn new techniques for your own well-being as well as to offer a wider array of services for your clients. Being current with the specific skills in your field is crucial to developing and maintaining a thriving practice. Stay up to date with the trends, read all of the new literature, attend seminars and learn new techniques.

In addition to your treatment skills you need to know how to obtain new clients, retain current clients, communicate effectively, keep proper documentation, do bookkeeping and manage your time well. Most schools haven't allotted sufficient time in their curriculum to adequately provide practice management skills so you need to learn these on your own.

Being a good practitioner involves far more than just your hands-on work. It's also about who you are, how you manage your practice and how you relate to your clients. The more you can make business a natural expression of who you are, the more successful you will be in your practice.

Many options are available for advancing your business acumen. Read books, take classes and consult with other professionals. It's important to keep balance in your pursuit of knowledge between hands-on modalities, product information, business skills and personal development. Take classes on marketing, bookkeeping, body mechanics, public speaking, assertiveness training, time management, insurance documentation, case management, taxes, self-care, telephone skills, financial management and general communication skills.

One of the most effective methods of expanding knowledge on different techniques is experiencing sessions by others in your particular profession on a regular basis, preferably at least once per week (although this can be difficult if you are a dentist, for instance). Even if you have a favorite person to go to, try out others. Remember you are getting these sessions not only for the direct benefits but also as a means of experiencing other techniques. You may discover a technique that is absolutely wonderful and then you can take the necessary steps to learn it and incorporate it into your practice. In addition, receiving these treatments on a regular basis assists you in being more attuned to your clients' needs.

It's also helpful to be assessed periodically. This can be done by your clients and by colleagues. Some practitioners have every client fill out a form for every session and others go through this process only once or twice per year. Feedback is essential for your professional growth. This concept can seem a bit scary—the idea of being

Education should prepare people not just to earn a living but to live a life—a creative, humane and sensitive life.
— Charles Silberman

Most businesses fail from lack of imagination.
— Paul Hawken

evaluated does have some ego risk involved, but how are you going to know which areas to enhance if no one tells you? Remember, knowledge is power. Since most work in this field is very individualized, it's recommended that you obtain as many evaluations as possible in order to get broader, more objective feedback. These evaluations are for your benefit. They are also a good way to get your clients involved in their treatment.

See Chapter Eight
for tips on client retention.

Getting assessed by your colleagues is essential. They can give you the kind of technical feedback that a client probably would not know. Again, it isn't necessary to be evaluated every time you work with your peers, but do it regularly. You can also make it fun. Your purpose is not to "find fault" but to support each other in achieving excellence.

In order to continue doing the work you love, it's imperative that you take responsibility for your business' health. Often it's our fear and lack of knowledge that makes situations appear deceptive. Being a good businessperson does not mean being cold, ruthless or totally profit-oriented. A good businessperson is one who manages her/his company well and offers a quality service for a fair price.

The universe pays every man in his own coin; if you smile, it smiles on you in return; if you frown, you will be frowned at; if you sing, you will be invited into cheerful company; if you think, you will be entertained by thinkers; if you love the world, and earnestly look for the good therein, you will be surrounded by loving friends, and nature will pour into your lap the treasurers of the earth.
— Mike Lea

Always remember why you chose your profession and stay grounded in the experience of the difference you make. Rachel Naomi Remen wrote an inspiring article in the Spring 1996 issue of *Noetic Sciences Review*, titled "In the Service of Life." She states,
> "Service rests on the basic premise that the nature of life is sacred, that life is a holy mystery which has an unknown purpose. When we serve, we know that we belong to life and to that purpose. Fundamentally, helping, fixing and service are ways of seeing life. When you help, you see life as weak, when you fix, you see life as broken. When you serve, you see life as whole. Lastly, fixing and helping are the basis of curing, but not healing. Only service heals."

• Social Responsibility •

As an individual and business owner, you can make a difference socially, economically, environmentally and politically. Running your practice from a place of love, integrity, compassion and personal values creates a sense of empowerment and fulfillment. Many businesses are learning how to be profitable *and* heed their social missions. As the concept of "quality of life" evolves, time and freedom become the dominant concerns (although financial security is clearly important). In addition, companies are becoming more ecologically aware; reducing the number of consumables, choosing "environment-friendly" products and instituting recycling programs. As more numbers of small and large businesses incorporate values for the overall benefit of humankind into their everyday practices, political pressure comes to bear upon governments to create policies and laws along the same lines.

*Do all the good you can,
By all the means you can,
In all the ways you can,
In all the places you can,
At all the times you can,
To all the people you can,
As long as ever you can.*
— John Wesley

As a result of the changes in business philosophy, new operating procedures have developed. Purchasing products and services is no longer based only on price and quality. Companies that embrace the philosophy of social responsibility often offer discounts to businesses that belong to specific political, professional, social or networking organizations. Company support of volunteerism and tithing is on the rise. Many individuals and companies are donating their time, money and expertise to their favorite charities. Also groups of individuals are joining together to form organizations expressly committed to responding to emergency conditions.

New Traditions in Business
edited by John Renesch
Berrett Koehler

Profiles 〰

The Body Shop, Ben & Jerry's and Tom's of Maine are great examples of companies that demonstrate the feasibility of being financially successful while doing good in the community. All of these companies are known for treating their employees well, providing excellent customer service and donating a percentage of their profits to those in need.

Ben & Jerry's premium ice cream and frozen yogurt manufacturing company believes in what they call Caring Capitalism: a business that makes top quality, all-natural products, is a force for social change and is financially successful. Some of its initiatives include: buying products from family farmers and cooperatives; buying milk and cream from dairy farmers who do not use rBGH (a bovine growth hormone); starting a legal fight to require a national rBGH label; using space on the ice cream containers to talk about issues they believe in; launching an innovative program to convert dairy waste to compost; treating employees well by offering profit-sharing, a stock purchase plan, and a full range of benefits (including domestic partner health insurance and a 15-minute massage about every six weeks); and being a prominent force in the long distance phone company called Working Assets, which donates a hefty percentage of profits to charitable causes.

I don't know what your destiny will be, but one thing I do know: the only ones among you who will be really happy are those who have sought and found how to serve.
— Albert Schweitzer

Ben & Jerry's social mission incorporates making the world a better place by empowering its employees to use available resources to support and encourage organizations that are working toward eliminating the underlying causes of environmental and social problems. It donates 7.5 percent of pre-tax profits to the Ben & Jerry's Foundation, employee Community Action Teams and corporate grants.

Tom's of Maine is a body-care product manufacturer whose mission includes: to serve customers by providing safe, effective, innovative, natural products of high quality—using only pure, simple ingredients nature provides and packaged in ways which respect nature; build relationships with customers that include responsiveness to feedback and information exchange; respect, value and serve customers, co-workers, owners, agents, suppliers and community, to be concerned about and contribute to their well-being, and to grow with integrity so as to be deserving of their trust.

The company is guided by a Statement of Beliefs: *"We believe our company can be financially successful while behaving in a socially responsible and environmentally sensitive manner."*

Some of the ways Tom's of Maine demonstrates its commitment are: donating 10 percent of pre-tax profits to charity and worthy causes; encouraging employees to use up to five percent of paid time doing volunteer work; and providing employee benefits such as child care subsidies.

The Body Shop is a body-care products retailer that takes a strong political stand. Its mission is to make and sell high quality, economical skin and hair care products that satisfy real needs without making false promises. It takes pride in being successful without resorting to sex, glamour and hype. The Body Shop is committed to the following: banning animal testing; ingredient sourcing; addressing the needs of ethnically diverse customers; working for change within the industry (e.g., managing waste); and pursuing social and environmental change for the better. It seeks to understand and help improve the self-image and self-esteem of people everywhere.

The company contributed to the call for an end to the practice of testing products and ingredients on animals and started a campaign to find out the hidden facts about animal testing. One of its major projects is community trade. This program helps create a long-term, global economic sustainability by purchasing ingredients and accessories directly from socially and economically developing communities.

Companies of all sizes are taking action. For instance, The Bodywork Emporium has always maintained an active social and charitable giving philosophy. In 1996 it started The Touch Foundation, whose mission is: "It's time to touch the untouched." Dubbed "The Massage Peace Corps" by its founder, Shane Watson, the Touch Foundation reaches out to  those who can't normally afford a massage or a helping hand. It coordinates a network of bodyworkers who provide healing touch to the orphaned, the needy, the elderly, the dying, the neglected, and people with disabilities. The Bodywork Emporium demonstrates commitment to the volunteer therapists in the following ways: furnishing the coordinators, training, equipment and supplies; providing money to help cover therapists' basic expenses; recognizing therapists' participation; and creating a fun and rewarding environment.

Gadabout, a salon and day spa with five locations in Tucson, Arizona, started the IMAGE UP™ Campaign for Kids in 1995. The salons and their employees "adopted" 15 children from a local elementary school. They provide 100 percent of their school clothes, shoes and haircuts for six years. The IMAGE UP concept is based on research that shows that a child's appearance is directly related to academic achievement, behavior, peer relationships and teacher expectations. The students, parents or guardians, and school representatives sign a compact with the salon. Gadabout sponsors three shopping trips per year, four haircuts per year, books as holiday gifts and participation in a summer camping program. To stay in the program, students must meet specific goals (e.g., attendance, tardy rate and reading progress) and the parents or guardians are required to participate in one school event per quarter.

You do not need to be a corporate giant to take an active stand toward social responsibility. All great movements spring from small individual actions. For example,

The goodwill and heightened visibility generated by being a socially responsible business can greatly impact your success.

I firmly believe that any organization, in order to survive and achieve success, must have a sound set of beliefs on which it premises all its policies and actions. Next, I believe that the most important single factor in corporate success is faithful adherence to those beliefs. And, finally, I believe if an organization is to meet the challenge of a changing world, it must be prepared to change everything about itself except those beliefs as it moves through corporate life.
— Thomas Watson, IBM

When strangers start acting like neighbors...communitiies are reinvigorated.
— Ralph Nader

Robert Toporek, a Rolfing® practitioner in Philadelphia had a mission to make a positive impact on the children who live in the "Badlands," one of the worst neighborhoods in Philadelphia. He founded The Children's Project, where every summer since 1993, volunteers go to the neighborhoods on a weekly basis, offering Rolfing structural integration, massage, music, books and computers. Currently the community is now computerized! The city of Philadelphia has given him an old building (a former crack house) which he plans to develop into a community center.

Efforts to create a Massage Emergency Response Team began in California after the Loma Prieta earthquake struck in October 1989. People at the National Holistic Institute (NHI) got involved to help heal the community—8,000 massages were given by 300 massage therapists. It has evolved since then to become the National AMTA Massage Emergency Response Team™ (AMTA-MERT). There are eligibility requirements to join—although being a member of the American Massage Therapy Association is not mandatory—and members all receive standardized training in providing massage at an emergency response scene. MERT teams will be established in each state and be prepared to offer massage to emergency response personnel and others. Other examples of where massage emergency response teams have served the needy are the Oakland (California) Hills fire, Hurricane Andrew in Florida and the Oklahoma bombing.

Steps You Can Take Now

As an individual and a business owner, you can make a difference, socially, economically, environmentally and politically. The five major ways are to act responsibly, volunteer, fund projects, use your purchasing power and be respectful.

Act Responsibly

You are not limited to contributing your specific vocational services. You can stuff envelopes, organize events and even build homes.

Acting responsibly is predicated upon being aware of your environment. In addition to embracing the slogan of Reduce, Re-use, Recycle and buy Recycled, it requires being knowledgeable about the world. Expand your horizons: read your industry trade journals and alternative magazines, such as *Mother Jones* or the *Utne Reader*. In your waiting room post brochures, fliers and announcements on community events and ways your clients can make a difference.

Be an advocate: vote; write letters and place phone calls to politicians about issues that concern you; and join a progressive campaigning group like Friends of the Earth, Amnesty International or an animal rights organization, such as People for the Ethical Treatment of Animals.

Volunteer

Donate your time and expertise to your favorite charities: join an industry group such as the AMTA-MERT or The Touch Foundation; do community service work with organizations such as Habitat for Humanity or the Literacy Foundation; donate blood; be a mentor for a child; pick a population of people who can't afford your services and "adopt" them; form a local community group; volunteer to walk a dog at your local animal shelter (there's often not enough staff to take animals for walks and this gives the animals attention and you get to be a virtual pet owner—no muss, no fuss); give presentations in public schools (e.g., career day, health education week); take part in special events such as Make A Difference Day; and sponsor an activity such as "Adopt a Highway."

Make A Difference Day

This annual day of doing good was created by USA WEEKEND in partnership with the Points of Light Foundation. Held on the fourth Saturday in October, Make A Difference Day is the largest, annual national day of helping others. Projects can be personal (e.g., helping an elderly relative with their chores), neighborly (e.g., organize a neighborhood beautification day) or major productions such as refurbishing a children's recreational center.

Join in with more than 1 million volunteers as they contribute to millions of others. The organizers request that if you currently volunteer regularly, make an extra effort in your volunteer activity. If you need more than one day for your project, still do a significant part of your volunteering on the fourth Saturday. If you can't participate on Saturday for religious reasons, do your project Friday or Sunday. Contact the organizers so they can include your volunteer activities as part of the DAYtaBANK.

Phone: 800-416-3824   Website: www.usaweekend.com

Fund Projects

In addition to donating money to worthwhile causes, you can grant scholarships and help coordinate fund raising activities. You can donate your services as prizes or raise money by sponsoring an event such as a "massage-a-thon." You can designate a charity and donate a day's revenues or run a promotion where for every specified dollar amount (e.g., $50) that a client donates to your favorite charity, they get a free treatment (such as a half-hour session or an adjunct service).

Random Acts of Kindness
by Conari Press

One of the most common ways to fund causes is through tithing. Tithing is contributing a set amount (usually 10 percent) of time or money to charitable causes. It's important to give back to your community. People often associate tithing with religion, but that is only one arena. Some popular forms of tithing include donating a specific amount of profits to an organization, doing pro bono work (providing services free of charge) and offering a sliding fee scale.

Use Your Purchasing Power

The greatest pleasure I know is to do a good action by stealth, and to have it found out by accident.
— Charles Lamb

Let your voice be heard through your acquisitions. Purchase ecologically sound products (e.g., natural fiber linens), use environmentally friendly detergent for linens as well as clothes and print your promotional materials on recycled stock. Invest wisely. Actively support businesses that are aligned with your values and boycott companies that oppose them.

Be Respectful

Respect is the foundation of a socially responsible business: Respecting yourself, the environment and your clients. Caregivers get into this field because they want to be of service. Clients are looking for practitioners with whom they share similar values. Be true to your beliefs, and express them in ways that respect differing viewpoints. While it isn't appropriate to foist your beliefs on your clients, you can encourage them to explore alternatives. Better yet, make sure your marketing attracts clients with similar beliefs.

CivicSource

CivicSource is a wonderful resource for social responsibility. The following information is reprinted with permission from the CivicSource website: "The Academy of Leadership at the University of Maryland has established a project titled CivicSource to link individuals, businesses, communities and movements with resources to meet the needs of a new century of civic activism and transforming leadership. CivicSource consists of a unique site on the World Wide Web, plus a political collection of leadership resources and a national outreach campaign. Through CivicSource and its link to the nation's most prominent leadership scholars, the Academy of Leadership is developing a national database of leadership development programs and resources, and providing information to support citizen action on public issues. The goal of CivicSource is to multiply these successes by recording, retelling and sharing the ideas, tools and resources that are leading the way in the ongoing project of democracy."

Phone: 301-504-5751   Website: http://civicsource.org

• Goodwill •

Goodwill is an integral component for success in any service industry, and especially so in the health care field. Goodwill is defined as benevolence, friendly disposition, cheerful consent, willingness and readiness. In regards to business it's the commercial advantage of any professional practice due to its established popularity, reputation, patronage, advertising and location, over and above its tangible assets. In other words goodwill is an abstract impression, the "positive feelings" you inspire in others. It's based upon the supposition that you are doing the best you can and will be fair and ethical in your dealings and behavior. It implies warmth, congeniality and trust.

You can't build a reputation on what you are going to do.
— Henry Ford

Take a moment to think about the businesses and people that you respect. Why do you hold them in such regard? What have they done to encourage these feelings of goodwill? How have they demonstrated their concern? Your responses are the key to understanding the concept of goodwill.

It's essential to cultivate alliances. Many branches of health care (particularly "alternative" ones) have substantial distances to cover before they achieve the recognition they deserve from the general public and the health industry. Chiropractic is a prime example of a profession that has demonstrated its validity and is still not covered by all insurance carriers. Massage and other touch therapies are just beginning to gain mainstream endorsement. A major part of this guarded acceptance of touch therapies stems from a lack of standardization. The general public doesn't know what to expect. The variety of educational levels, styles, modalities, philosophies and fee structures are as diverse as those who practice them.

To gain further headway for recognition it's imperative to enhance the public image of your specific industry—in other words, promote more goodwill.

The health care field tends to rely on attraction (e.g., word-of-mouth, reputation and client referrals) rather than traditional methods of promotion. The downside is that word-of-mouth often revolves around "who" you know more than "what" you know. And even then, it isn't enough to just know the "right" people. To obtain their support you need to nurture those associations. You must have good people skills. For example, you could be the most brilliant practitioner in your area, yet if you don't promote goodwill with your clients, centers of influence, colleagues and the community, you still may not do well financially. One of the most important habits to develop is prompt and gracious acknowledgment of all of the people who support you. A little recognition goes a long way!

It takes time, thought, creativity and some money to foster goodwill. Being good at what you do is only one aspect of it. Make certain that your actions reflect that you are proud of your profession and are sincerely concerned about people's well-being.

You can't buy goodwill, particularly if it's an attempt to repair a bad reputation (although corporations have spent millions of dollars attempting to do just that). You can bolster the general public's opinion of you and your profession by donating your services and knowledge to charitable organizations and events—especially if you get media coverage.

You cannot do a kindness too soon, for you will never know how soon it will be too late.
— Ralph Waldo Emerson

If you help others, you will be helped, perhaps not tomorrow, perhaps in one hundred years, but you will be helped. Nature must pay off the debt... It is a mathematical law and all life is mathematics.
— Gurdjieff

• Professionalism •

Professionalism stems from your attitudes and is manifested through the image you portray, your technical skill level, your communication abilities and your business practices.

No matter how many hours you work, this is your profession. There is a major distinction between part-time and spare time. You may have other facets to your career besides being a health care practitioner, but it's important to be clear about the roles each facet plays and be committed to excellence in each one. *Quantity does not determine quality.*

See Appendix B, pages 416-422
for directories of professional associations business organizations and independent living resources.

You are a health care professional, and you are a business person—even if you only work three hours a week. The more you treat your practice as a business, the more professional you appear and the more successful you become. Sometimes this can be difficult, particularly if you don't have a modicum of technical business experience. Your attitudes toward yourself and your business are communicated directly and indirectly to your clients, colleagues and potential clients. You need to respect yourself and your abilities.

The basis for true professionalism lies in integrity. Someone may talk, walk and appear the part, but if that person doesn't come from a base of integrity, the facade wears thin quickly. Your work is intimate on many levels: if you don't treat your clients with the utmost respect, you won't have many clients. Integrity is the quality or state of being complete; unbroken condition; wholeness; honesty; and sincerity. Integrity is often considered as a thing to have—people have integrity if they are ethical, can keep confidences and keep their word. But there is more to it than that.

Integrity can be divided into three major levels: the first level is keeping your agreements; the second is being true to your principles; and the third level is being true to yourself. Integrity is a state of being and if that is where you are really coming from, you are professional.

We rarely find caregivers who put on an air of professionalism without the integrity behind it. More often we have people who love what they do and are genuinely concerned about the well-being of their clients, but they neglect to develop a professional demeanor.

Professional affiliations are an important part of the business world and the development of a professional image (in addition to educational, social and networking benefits). I highly recommend belonging to at least two organizations: one that specifically relates to your profession and one that supports your visibility in the local community. Numerous associations exist for the health care professions ranging from modality-specific associations to more general health and well-being organizations. An excellent source for these groups is the Encyclopedia of Associations (at your library). Looking under the "Health and Medical" section you will find thousands of listings of specialized, auxiliary and local branches of associations. Membership in a professional association makes a statement of your commitment to your career field.

Involvement in business organizations also demonstrates belief in yourself as a professional. Many groups exist on a national level. Locate them by referring to the "Business" section of the Encyclopedia of Associations (available at most public libraries). Locally, groups such as the Chamber of Commerce and business leads/ support groups can be found by looking through the phone book, talking with other business owners and checking the newspaper's Money and Calendar sections.

Take a few moments to do the following professionalism visualization exercises. Make notes in your journal.

Professional Characteristics

Think about someone you regard as being very professional.

- What is this person's occupation?
- What is his/her philosophy of life?
- How does s/he feel about her/his career?
- What does s/he look like?
- Where is his/her place of business?
- What does the business look like from the outside?
- Can you easily see the office from the street?
- Is parking easily accessible?
- What does the office look like?
- How does this person greet you?
- What does s/he say and do?
- How do you feel when you are with this person?

Professionalism Inventory

- Think about what professionalism really means to you.
- Describe yourself in terms of professionalism.
- Describe how you imagine others see you in terms of professionalism.
- List any of the changes you would like to make.

• Image •

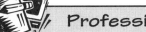

The image you portray influences how people react to you. Your public image is determined by the way you present yourself, your office, your business practices and the manner in which you treat your clients. I'm not advocating being someone other than yourself; I am suggesting you take the time to make certain your "outward" image supports your vision of success. The following lists are guidelines to bolster your image and reputation.

You are Your Business. Exude Confidence, Competence and Compassion:

- Dress stylishly yet neatly, and keep jewelry to a minimum: your attire isn't meant to be a distraction or a loud statement.
- Keep good personal hygiene and don't wear heavy perfume or cologne: you don't want to bring tears to your clients' eyes or make them choke.
- Keep your technical skills excellent and current: do not pretend to be an expert in what you're not.
- Be punctual and prepared: make your clients feel important and respected.
- Know how to introduce yourself and others: it can be very embarrassing if you stumble over your own tongue.
- Get involved in your community: become active in civic, social and political groups.

Your Office Needs to Generate a Comfortable, Professional Ambiance:

- Be aware of the noise level and make any necessary adjustments: turn off the phone bell and soundproof thin walls.
- Keep the interior clean: particularly the bathroom.
- Make sure that the building and address is visible from the street: this may mean investing in signage.
- Maintain the area outside your office: this may include landscaping.
- Keep the temperature comfortable for the client: if you don't have easy access to the temperature control, put a portable heater and fan in the room.
- Create a sense of privacy: you may have to be very inventive.
- Make certain that all equipment and furniture is comfortable and sturdy: you do not want a table to squeak and groan with every movement or to collapse under a client!
- Provide closet space or a shelf (at the very least, a hook) for your clients' belongings: most people don't like to throw their possessions in a corner.
- Keep supplies stocked and handy: you don't want your clients searching for a tissue while they're sneezing.
- Post your business license, policies, continuing education certificates and awards in a conspicuous place: these items represent the time and effort you've invested in your career.
- Have your business cards and literature available: make it easy for your clients to take what they need to help promote your business.

Your Treatment of Clients Determines if They Become Regulars:

- Be empathetic and understanding: keep in mind that not everyone shares your particular beliefs about health and well-being.
- Greet your clients appropriately: some people may not be up to a bear hug, while others may welcome it.
- Keep what happens during a session confidential: this can be tricky when your clients know each other and ask about the other's appointment. Be noncommittal and recommend they speak to the person directly. Even a casual remark can damage your trust factor.
- Remember that you are here to serve your clients: it isn't their job to counsel you during their sessions.
- Observe your clients' likes and dislikes: make the effort to do those "extra little things."

The Manner in Which You Run the "Business" Part of Your Practice Directly Affects Your Long-Term Success:

- Answer your phone professionally: you don't have to be overly formal, but remember you are a business. If you don't have a receptionist, I advocate hiring a *reliable* appointment service. They can significantly increase your bookings.
- Return calls within 24 hours: you never know the influence and connections that a potential client may have; promptness is always appreciated.
- Answer important mail within four days and nonessential mail within two weeks: don't wait until you have the time to write a brilliant letter. I always keep a supply of postcards handy. This way I can quickly acknowledge correspondence without worrying about having to fill up the page or making sure my typewriter is working.
- Send newspaper clippings, articles and items of interest to clients and colleagues: this lets people know that you are thinking about them and are genuinely concerned.
- Acknowledge in writing any item or gift sent to you: thanking people over the phone is okay, but people usually keep cards for several days. Every time they look at your card, it reinforces their feelings of goodwill.
- Send thank-you notes for referrals: it's vital to show your appreciation, particularly since many people aren't totally comfortable telling others about their health care methods.
- Set clear boundaries: don't let your personal life interfere or intrude with business.
- Return borrowed property promptly and in good condition: never borrow anything that you are unable to replace (in case you damage or lose it).
- Never repeat a rumor that could hurt someone's reputation: it's wise to stay neutral. Gossip never reflects well on any of the parties.
- Keep accurate client files: review them before you see each client. Don't rely on your memory for all the details of your last session.

Your level of integrity, professionalism and grace determine how you are perceived. Taking the time to project a professional image is always worth the investment. It isn't necessary to have a huge budget either—just creativity. Most of the above guidelines don't involve any financial outlay. The desired result is that your image is professional, and it's vital that you don't lose yourself in this process. Who you are is what makes you good at what you do. It distinguishes you from the others. Keep your style and personality intact.

• Ethics •

Conscious businesses incorporate a strong code of ethics. The definition of ethics is: A system or code of morals and conduct of a person or group; the discipline dealing with what is good and bad or right and wrong.

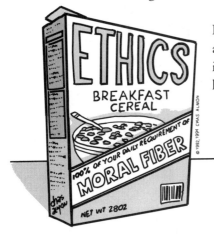

Ethics have been debated and postulated by philosophers great and small for millennia. It's extremely difficult to agree upon what is good and bad—so much depends on the situation. Tom Peters has a wonderful definition for it: *"High ethical standards—business or otherwise—are, above all, about treating people decently. To me (as a person, business person and business owner) that means respect for a person's privacy, dignity, opinions and natural desire to grow; and people's respect for (and by) co-workers."* In general, typical business ethics cover adhering to prevailing laws, upholding the dignity of the profession, being service oriented, staying committed to quality and demonstrating loyalty to staff.

We are continually faced with ethical concerns. Most of them are easily reconciled, though occasionally we encounter a major conflict. Examples of common ethical dilemmas in the health care professions are: practicing beyond your scope; breaking confidentiality; sexual misconduct; misrepresentation of educational status; financial impropriety; exploiting the power differential; misleading claims of curative abilities; dual relationships; bigotry; dishonesty; inappropriate advertising; and violation of state/city laws or regulations.

Ethics are different from morals and laws. Morals relate to character. Laws are codified rules of conduct that are based on ethical or moral principles. Laws often set the minimum standard necessary to protect the public's welfare, while ethics epitomize the ideal standards embraced by a profession.

Most ethical dilemmas involve situations where you are unclear what is the best or right course of action. At times you may find that you have several viable options, each with merit and are not clear as to the most appropriate choice. You may also find yourself in a position where your values are in conflict. One method of resolving an ethical dilemma is the following four-part process.

Resolving Ethical Dilemmas

1. *Identify the problem.* This is the point where you would determine whether it's truly an ethical problem.

2. *Clarify the problem:* gather relevant information; talk to the parties involved; define the specific type of ethical breach (e.g., personal, professional, business); consider the consequences if someone doesn't intervene; and ascertain the potential dangers to the individual or the profession.

3. *Describe what action should be taken.* Map out the best way to resolve the problem (e.g., who should be contacted first if multiple parties are involved? Do you need outside support?). Then consider who, if anyone, should know about the problem (such as a supervisor, friend, client, doctor, police, professional association, school or colleague).

4. *Identify who should take action.* Sometimes a breach of conduct is difficult to discern. It takes diligent personal reflection to run an ethical practice. Discussing this topic with your colleagues and engaging in peer supervision are two excellent methods for clarifying your feelings and identifying questionable behaviors.

The Ethics of Touch
by Cherie Sohnen-Moe and
Ben E. Benjamin Ph.D.

Let's analyze the following scenario using the above resolution model:

Ethics Scenario

On Monday your session with Sally was very intense. She was experiencing significant pain in her legs and lower back. During the session she also released a lot of emotions and briefly shared about the issues she was confronting. Sally's partner, Terry, shows up for his weekly treatment on Tuesday afternoon. He mentions that Sally was exhausted and a bit withdrawn after her session. He jokingly makes a comment about how powerful it must have been and asks you what happened.

1. **Identify the problem:** This is a common occurrence when working with clients who know each other. They often ask how the other person is doing, how the session went. This is usually done out of genuine concern and not a need for gossip. Yet, even just saying, "Oh, it was a good session" is not appropriate and most likely feels awkward. You determine this is an ethical problem.

2. **Clarify the problem:** By telling Terry about Sally's session, you would be committing a breach of confidentiality. Yet you know that it would be helpful to Sally if Terry was aware of what occurred. The potential hazards of sharing this information with Terry are: Sally may become upset with you and decide not to return; you may lose your credibility with both Terry and Sally; and you may lose potential clients due to the bad-will generated by this incident. You decide not to breach confidentiality by disclosing nothing about Sally's session.

3. **Describe the action to be taken:** You have several options. First you need to decide what to say to Terry. You can shrug your shoulders and say "Well, I guess it was rather intense" and then continue on with your session. Or you can say, "I highly value my commitment to client confidentiality. It would be best if you ask Sally directly about her session." You decide to tell Terry the latter.

   You will be able to determine if you should pursue this any further at all (remind Terry to talk to Sally, or recommend to Sally that she talk with Terry), depending upon how Terry responded to your reply about the session and your sense of the benefits resulting from Sally sharing the information with Terry.

4. **Identify who should take action:** You decide to take the action. You restate your confidentiality policy to both Terry and Sally and encourage them to share their experiences with each other.

He who walks in truth and is devoted to his thinking, and furthermore reveres the worthy, is blessed by heaven.
— Confucius

A code of ethics simplifies the problem-solving process when confronted with an ethical dilemma. A code of ethics is a document that outlines the duties, rights, responsibilities and conditions of justice that are appropriate in client/practitioner interactions. Many of the individual professional associations have their own specific code of ethics. Among the components of a Health Care Provider's Code of Ethics are a statement of basic concerns (e.g., honesty, integrity, respect, compassion and making a difference); standards of service; a description of how the treatment/session will be delivered (condition, place); when the treatments are given and by whom; the quality of materials used; and service guarantees.

I believe that it is advisable to develop a general code of ethics that all health care professionals can endorse with provisos for specific industries. Such a document could serve as a tool to educate the public about the basic conduct and level of professionalism they can expect from any health care provider. I realize that once this code of ethics is adopted we also face other exciting challenges such as: how to implement it, determining the consequences of breaches, resolving the manner of enforcement and educating the public. This calls for much introspection and dialogue.

Sample Code of Ethics

We, as health care providers, have the responsibility to guide our actions to serve the best interests of the client. As members of this profession we realize this responsibility can only be upheld by maintaining the highest degree of personal and professional integrity. As a health care practitioner, I make the commitment to provide personalized care and knowledgeable techniques, in a clean, comfortable atmosphere, thereby ensuring the client's safety and well-being. Therefore, I agree to the following:

1. Maintain a professional appearance and demeanor by keeping good hygiene and wearing attire that is appropriate for the client setting.

2. Respect all clients regardless of their age, gender, race, national origin, sexual orientation, religion, socio-economic status, body type, political affiliation, state of health and personal habits.

3. Demonstrate my respect by honoring a client's process, being present, listening, asking only pertinent questions, keeping my agreements, being on time, draping properly, and maintaining professionalism.

4. Maintain confidentiality of information concerning clients, and refrain from discussing client care details except under appropriate circumstances.

5. Provide a safe, comfortable, clean environment that is stocked with quality equipment and supplies.

6. Perform only those services for which I am qualified and (physically and emotionally) able to do, and refer to appropriate specialists when work is not within my scope of practice or not in the client's best interest.

7. Be honest in all marketing endeavors.

8. Customize my treatments to meet the client's needs.

9. Charge a fair price for my services and offer a sliding scale when appropriate.

10. Keep accurate records and review charts before each session.

11. Educate clients by providing them with feedback and resources (e.g., literature and exercises).

12. Make return and follow-up calls when appropriate and in a timely manner.

13. Post my credentials and policies.

14. Undergo peer review bi-annually.

15. Never engage in any sexual activity with clients.

16. Refrain from the use of alcohol or mind-altering substances before or during sessions.

17. Stay current with information and techniques by reading, receiving weekly treatments and taking at least one workshop per year.

18. Continue membership in at least one professional association.

19. Adhere to city, county, state, national and international requirements.

20. Educate the public about my services and benefits through activities such as: giving presentations, workshops and demonstrations; holding open houses and writing articles.

5

Business Start-Up

• Overview •

At this point, let's say that you have what it takes to be successful in your business: the required energy, conviction, talent and skill. The next steps are to: determine the feasibility of your business; decide whether you want to start your own practice or purchase one; choose a business structure; name the business; obtain financing; find a location; determine regulations; procure appropriate insurance coverage; and set fees.

Proper business start-up makes a tremendous difference in your practice. If you are aware of the local and national requirements of your particular business (e.g., zoning, licensing, federal identification number), then you can make appropriate choices and structure your business (before opening your doors) so that you comply with these rules and regulations.

The final step before opening your business is to develop a business plan. A business plan (see Chapter Ten) is a written summary of what you aim to accomplish and how you intend to organize your resources to attain those goals.

• Initial Research •

Explore your career field. Find out the number of other businesses that are the same as or similar to yours. Start by looking at listings and advertisements in phone books, newspapers, journals and other local publications. Interview the owners of these businesses, ask them how they got started, the services they offer, what trends they see happening that will affect the success of this field and then ask them for any advice. Read trade journals, industry magazines and books related to your field. Attend professional association meetings. Meet with people whose businesses service health care providers (e.g., product suppliers, equipment manufacturers, bankers, accountants and consultants) and ask them for their viewpoints and advice.

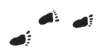

See Chapter Nine, pages 271-280 for additional information on target market research.

Research your potential markets. You may do an informal survey or hire a consultant to do the research. Discuss the industry with other people who service your potential clients. Let's take athletes as a sample target market. The professions and companies that service athletes with care and products include massage therapists, medical doctors, sports psychologists, chiropractors, trainers, sporting goods stores, nutritionists, equipment manufacturers and hypnotherapists. These people may be able to give you a broader view than someone who does your type of work.

Ascertain the economic capacity of the community to support your business. You may find you need to expand your target markets or diversify your practice to increase your business viability.

This information gathering process is also crucial when expanding or revamping a current business. "It's never too late to start over" is a common saying, although one not normally associated with business. Yet in many ways you really can "start over" regardless of how long you have been in practice. Although it can be more difficult to make changes after you are established, it's often worth the time and energy.

Initial Exploration Questionnaire

- How well does your educational and career experience fit this industry?
- How soon will you need advanced training?
- Are you familiar with running this type of practice?
- Did they teach practice management at school?
- Have you interviewed colleagues and industry experts?
- Do you feel comfortable with the "business" aspects?
- Does this business provide sufficient opportunities?
- Are you aware of industry trends and regulations?
- Have you assessed your strengths and challenges?
- Do you have adequate financial resources to start your business?
- Is the time commitment compatible with the rest of your life?
- Are your friends and family supportive?
- Can you identify at least two target markets that will eagerly embrace your practice?
- Have you identified your differential advantage?
- Do you have the personality to market your services?
- Do you have a support system of colleagues and advisors?

• Financing •

Financing your business (whether for start-up or expansion) can be frustrating. Even though a lot of venture capital is available, it's extremely difficult to procure investment money for a service business. Be extremely wary of any company that guarantees (for an up-front fee) to find you venture capital. There are a lot of scam operations being perpetrated against the naive small business owner. To find reputable sources of funding check out the resource guides at your local Small Business Administration office.

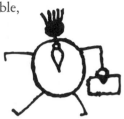

A bank may be willing to give you a loan, and the amount is usually based upon your assets. Applying for a loan (or venture investment) takes a lot of work: research, correspondence, proposals, refining your business plan—including financial statements and cash flow forecasts (they want to see numbers) and putting together an impressive presentation.

Most small business owners finance their company with money from personal savings or through loans from close friends and relatives. If you decide to borrow money from friends or family, treat them with the same consideration that you would give to a formal lending institution. Make an official presentation and submit a loan proposal and a business plan. Clearly delineate the terms of the loan and the repayment schedule. We've all heard horror stories about borrowing money from loved ones; if you do it correctly and set your boundaries, it can be a rewarding experience—one in which everyone benefits personally and financially.

When starting a business, you may need to be creative in obtaining services and supplies. For example, if you think that a brochure will attract potential clients, don't wait until you have the money. Talk to graphic designers and printers until you find someone who will do your brochure in trade for your services. You must be willing to take the initiative. You don't need to know the people ahead of time. When you are attempting to set up a trade, talk to the person face to face, if at all possible. If you are determined to find people to barter with, you will eventually find them. Don't let imagined limitations prevent you from pursuing this kind of arrangement. Your creativity, talent and persistence are the qualities that will help balance out the shortage of start-up resources.

The most valuable of all capital is that invested in human beings.
— Alfred Marshall

A health care practice is one of the easiest to set up, particularly since the initial costs tend to be minimal (unless you require expensive equipment). In many instances you can operate out of your home. People often build their private practices slowly while working for another company. This is an acceptable route to take as long as you develop an action plan for attracting clients and actively market your practice. Otherwise you may find yourself with a permanent part-time practice.

• Buying a Practice •

The idea of buying an existing practice may seem very appealing. After all, you avoid all that's entailed in building a strong business foundation. Although it may be easier and faster to buy an established practice, you also inherit the previous owner's problems, along with no guarantee the clients will stay on with you.

There are many advantages and disadvantages to buying an existing practice. Before you jump into a purchase, it's wise to assess your reasons for taking this route.

Self-Assessment Exercise

Ask yourself the following questions:

- Why do I want to buy an existing business?
- What are the potential risks versus the perceived benefits?
- What are my other options?
- What conditions need to be present to make it worthwhile?
- Why might this be inappropriate?

If after answering these questions, you decide to pursue purchasing an existing practice, ask yourself those same questions for each business you consider. All businesses are not created equally. Clarify exactly what it is you are buying. Are you purchasing one or more of the following: rights to use a well-known business name; a client list; established contracts; goodwill and reputation; an office location; or equipment.

The most common instance of a health care provider buying another practice is when that practitioner is just starting out (or moving to a new location) and buying a practice may essentially be a way to secure a "job." An established practitioner might consider purchasing a practice if she is interested in expanding her current target markets or wants to branch out into another area.

Steps to Buying a Practice

- Evaluate your reasons for buying.
- Determine the "fit."
- Conduct a preliminary evaluation.
- Offer a letter of intent.
- Analyze documentation.
- Clarify legal agreements.
- Open negotiations.
- Purchase the business.
- Begin the transition stage.

Determine the Fit ∼

When meeting with a specific seller, attempt to discover the true reason for the sale. This could dramatically influence your decision. For instance, if the seller is moving to another state or even retiring that's one thing, but if the move is within 30 miles, you may not be buying anything because the majority of the clients may still continue to see the therapist at the new location.

The seller may not be versed in the protocol for selling a business. Usually sellers view their practices in terms of the work they've invested in making it successful. It may not be set up for someone to easily take over. It's rare to just step in and retain all the clients. They may not like you or you them. More than anything else, assess the "fit" you would have with the business. Your chances for success are much greater if your knowledge, training, personality, modalities and style are similar to that of the seller. One way to determine this is by receiving a session from the seller. Ask to be treated as though you were a typical new client. Although the seller will most likely be on her best behavior, this experience gives you insight into her style as well as what the current clients are accustomed to receiving. If the company's policies and procedures don't suit you, or the types of treatments offered are outside your desired scope of practice, it most likely isn't in your best interest to buy the practice.

Conduct A Preliminary Evaluation ∼

Many factors come into play in judging the viability of a business. The seller should have a fact sheet including the company history, mission statement, business description (including the number of clients, the services offered, the equipment and products used, location description, items for sale to clients, fee structure, client profile, position statement, competition analysis and differential advantage), assets, financial history, reason for sale and pricing terms. Insist on this fact sheet so you both know exactly what is being sold.

Obtain this fact sheet as well as samples of promotional materials before making an offer. Ask to view the current appointment book. Check to see how many appointments are scheduled each week and how far in advance the practitioner is booked. After reviewing these materials and receiving a session, you will be in a better position to decide whether to make an offer.

Analyze Documentation ∼

When you make a written offer, be sure to state that it's contingent upon verification of the detailed documentation. This documentation should include the following: a detailed business description; a copy of the lease; names of all owners, associates, and staff members; profit and loss statements for the past three years; tax returns for the past three years; copies of current contracts; a listing of accounts payable and receivable; a list of fixtures, equipment and inventory with their replacement value noted; and a "portfolio" of promotional materials about the company and owner.

Evaluate the Business Premises ～～

One of the most beneficial aspects of buying a practice can be obtaining a lease on a "prime" location. Sometimes this is more important than the actual number of clients the current owner has. Let's say a massage therapist has a concession in a very busy, upscale gym, but this therapist has not been marketing his practice very well. If you are willing to invest the time in marketing, you could probably do quite well and it would be worth a reasonable selling price. But, before you allow a location to inflate the selling price of a business, do the proper research.

First, verify the building is zoned for your particular profession. Don't assume that because someone is currently running the same type of business in that location, it's therefore legal. Zoning may have changed or the current business might have somehow slipped through without anyone noticing (yet).

See pages 79-85
for more information on location assessment.

Next, find out if the current lease can be subleased or assigned, or if a new lease needs to be negotiated. Ascertain the particulars about the lease.

Determining the worth of a lease during the negotiations of a selling price is a rather subjective process. After researching the property, weigh your findings with the perceived importance of the space to the current clients.

Clarify Legal Agreements ～～

Another positive consideration is whether the business has outside contracts. Continuing the massage practice example, find out if the company has any corporate massage accounts. Two common types are holding contracts with businesses to furnish on-site corporate massage, and a contract with the local convention bureau (or major hotels) to supply therapists for chair massage during conferences.

The International Business
Brokers Association
P.O. Box 704
Concord, MA 01742
508-369-2490

The Institute of Certified
Business Counselors
P.O. Box 70326
Eugene, OR 70326
503-345-8064

Open Negotiations ～～

Determining a fair price for a practice is difficult at best. The seller will set what he feels is a realistic price. You must do the math. Calculate how much time, energy and money it would cost you to build your practice to the same point as the seller's. Remember that there is no guarantee the current clients will stay with you.

Most buyers take out loans (from friends, a bank or the seller) to finance the purchase of a business. When a service business is sold, the seller often becomes the loan holder. I highly recommend using a business broker to negotiate the purchase of a business.

Practice Sale Scenario

A seller is asking for $10,000 for her practice. She has been in business for five years and during that time her clientele has steadily increased. She sees an average of 15 clients per week and charges $40 per session. Her office is in a small professional building. Her monthly operating expenses run approximately $1,000. She is making a major life change and has decided to move to a tropical island. She is including her equipment and supplies as part of the package.

If the assets are items you want and you could retain the majority of her clients, this would be a reasonable price. Unfortunately, this scenario isn't typical. You can minimize your risks by requiring that in addition to the hard assets, the remainder of the selling price be based on the actual number of clients that stay with the business. Two examples are: making payments only if the business meets certain client retention requirements (e.g., at least 50 percent of the clients stay); or you only have to pay the seller a set percentage of the fees received from the current clientele (e.g., 40 percent of fees collected until the original loan is repaid).

Many brokers work on either an hourly consultation rate or a flat transaction fee. A qualified broker knows what questions to ask and can identify potential problems. If for no other reason, it's wise to get objective feedback. You can locate one through the resources listed here or in your local telephone book. In your initial interview, ask if the broker has ever negotiated a sale for the type of practice you desire (or a similar type of sale). The most important factor is that the two of you communicate well with each other. Also have your accountant interview a potential broker. Your accountant already knows your business, has your best interests at heart and would be able to determine if the broker is qualified. After the sales contract has been negotiated, have an attorney review it before you sign.

Final Stages

The final two stages are the completion of the purchase and the transition time after the sale. The ideal situation would be to work as an associate for several months before actually purchasing the business. This way the current clients would get to know you, you could assess whether you like working in that environment (particularly if an office space or working with other practitioners is part of the sales agreement), you would discover the little nuances of the business, you would be able to familiarize yourself with the logistics of running the business, and it would make the actual transition much smoother.

As a buyer, it's wise to understand the process a seller goes through, so please refer to the section on selling a practice. Buying an existing practice is very risky, yet the potential benefits can be rewarding. Keep in mind that even if the practice is a strong one, you will need to continue nurturing it through marketing and an active client retention program.

See Chapter Seven, pages 201-210 for information on how to sell a practice.

• Legal Structure •

See page 424
IRS Publication 334: *Tax Guide for Small Business,* and IRS Publication 542: *Tax Information for Corporations*.

The most common legal entity choices for your practice include sole proprietorship, partnership, corporation and Limited Liability Company (LLC). The majority of new businesses open as sole proprietorships, mainly because this is the simplest, fastest and least expensive structure. The decision to opt for a different structure is usually based on tax and liability considerations. It's vital to consult with an accountant or tax attorney because each person's situation and needs are unique, tax laws frequently change and requirements vary by locale.

This section provides a basic description of each type of business structure along with some thoughts on the advantages and disadvantages.

Sole Proprietorship

See Chapter Seven
for more detailed tax information.

If you don't incorporate, create a partnership or form an LLC, your business is automatically considered a sole proprietorship. The Internal Revenue Service (IRS) usually allows a married couple to operate as a sole proprietorship. In all other cases where two or more people co-own a business they must choose an entity other than sole proprietorship.

The major disadvantages of sole proprietorship are having to be responsible for all business aspects, relative difficulty in obtaining financing and unlimited liability. All business debts and liabilities are the *personal* responsibility of the owner. Damages from lawsuits brought against the business can be taken from your personal assets.

The main advantages of sole proprietorship are the ease of formation (minimal governmental regulations on how the business is operated), possession of profits, control of all decisions and relatively simple financial record keeping.

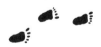

See page 95
for information on municipal licensing requirements.

The type of business license required for a sole proprietor who is a health care provider varies from state to state. You may even need more than one license.

From a legal standpoint as a sole proprietor you and your business are one entity. You can't be treated as an employee of the business. You may withdraw money from your business, but it isn't considered a wage and can't be deducted as a business expense. Although you don't pay payroll taxes on "draw" you pay self-employment taxes and income taxes. The business doesn't file income tax returns or pay income taxes. You file a Schedule C with your 1040 form, and pay personal income taxes on the profits.

Partnerships ~

Having an associate or partner can be quite beneficial. It can help ease the loneliness of being self-employed, allow you to take time off, add diversity of services and approaches, infuse capital, decrease overhead expenses, enable you to share the activities involved in running a business and provide you with another person with whom you can brainstorm ideas. It could also be a nightmare. A written partnership agreement is crucial.

An association is when two or more people get together to share some resources and expenses, yet keep separate business identities. A partnership is when two or more people contribute assets to carry on a jointly-owned business and share in the profits or losses. To be considered a partnership you do not have to use the term "partners," or have a written partnership agreement or equally share ownership. The operative phrase is "jointly-owned."

A partnership is similar to a sole proprietorship in that governmental regulations are still fairly minimal. The financial record keeping is a bit more involved, although insignificant compared to a corporation. You must obtain a federal identification number (contact the IRS and request Form SS-4). Partnerships file a Schedule K-1 (Form 1065, partnership informational tax return), but the partnership itself pays no taxes. Each partner submits a copy of the K-1 to report their share of profits or losses on their individual tax returns (Form 1040).

You can be held personally responsible for debts and legal obligations incurred by the partnership, even those made without your knowledge or consent. Incorporation or forming an LLC is the best way to protect yourself against this kind of liability.

Corporations ~

The major categories of business corporations are C Corporations, S Corporations and Professional Corporations. The type of business you operate and your tax requirements determine which structure is the best for you. Many people incorporate because they think it will give them an air of legitimacy—without considering all the legal implications.

A corporation provides a business entity that is separate from the owner as an individual. That distinction assists in creating clear boundaries between your work and the rest of your life, an important consideration since health care providers have a tendency to become so enmeshed in their work that it becomes difficult to "switch off." Owners who work in an incorporated business are considered employees and are paid as such. My relationship to my work dramatically shifted when I incorporated my business: I became more detached (which is good); the ups and downs of business are a bit easier to take; and I pay myself regularly. Now there is Cherie the person and Sohnen-Moe Associates, Inc., a company which I happen to own. Of course, I always knew there was a difference between me and my company, but I hadn't really experienced the separation on an emotional level.

See Chapter Six, pages 157-162 for more information on partnership agreements.

Consult with appropriate advisors before deciding which structure best suits your needs.

The Company Corporation will incorporate you for as low as $45.
800-542-2677
www.incorporate.com

A corporation tends to be the most costly legal structure to form and dissolve in terms of finances and time. There are required filings with the IRS as well as the state in which the corporation is formed. Though there are no federal fees involved, the state may require an initial filing fee and annual report filing fees. Contact your state Corporation Commission or Secretary of State to ascertain the specific requirements and fees for incorporation. In general, the minimal components of the incorporation process are: Adopting and filing the Articles of Incorporation; developing the Bylaws; having the First Directors and Shareholders Meeting and writing the Minutes; issuing Stock Certificates; filing for an IRS Employer Identification Number (EIN, Form SS-4); Filing Subchapter S status if so adopted within 75 days of incorporating or start of business (IRS Form 2553 which requires your new EIN); and setting up your corporate book which will contain all corporate documents. There are a myriad of other details involved for each step. The incorporation process varies from state to state according to their regulations. Therefore, so will the requirements for the content of your bylaws. Now that we have entered the age of telecommunications, be sure your bylaws include the approval of telephonic meetings for shareholders and directors. This saves time and travel.

The general minimal requirements for maintaining a corporation are conducting annual meetings and filing the minutes in your corporate book, as well as filing required documentation with the state on an annual basis. In the event your corporate status is questioned by the IRS or the state, the first thing they will do is inspect your corporate book to make sure you have followed all the requirements. If you have not, your status as a corporation can be nullified which could result in severe tax consequences. Keeping your corporate book up to date is essential. Even though there are do-it-yourself incorporation kits, it's strongly recommended that you consult with an accountant and an attorney.

One of the primary motivations for incorporating is to limit liability. If your business is a sole proprietorship, you could lose your personal assets (e.g., your home or car) if your business is sued. Health care providers in partnerships often incorporate to shield individual owners from possible losses and lawsuits stemming from actions (e.g., a malpractice suit) of the other partners. In most cases incorporation protects your personal assets from being taken by creditors; but it doesn't shelter you from lawsuits.

Other popular reasons for incorporating include the ease in which the business can be transferred, the ability to raise capital by selling shares of stock, potential tax advantages and fringe benefits such as health and life insurance premiums, tuition reimbursement and tax-sheltered retirement plans that can be deducted partially (and often fully!) as business expenses.

C Corporations

C Corporations are subject to a corporate income tax on the net business profits. Although there is the potential for double taxation (the corporation as well as you as an individual), most small businesses use all the profits as tax-deductible salaries and fringe benefits, or retain money to expand the business. Income can be divided

Success seems to be largely a matter of hanging on after others have let go.
— William Feather

between paying money to shareholders (salaries and dividends) and keeping the rest of the profits in the business. This process is called income-splitting. The retained earnings are taxed at the initial rate of 15 percent, which is usually lower than the individual income tax rates of the owners.

C Corporations must file annual returns (Form 1120) by the 15th day of the third month after the close of their fiscal year and make quarterly estimated tax payments.

S Corporations

S Corporations are taxed like partnerships but retain the liability protection of C Corporations. They have the same basic structure as C Corporations and file corporate tax returns, but the corporation doesn't pay federal income tax as the profits are passed on to the owners who pay the taxes at their individual rates. Losses are treated in the same manner.

A primary tax advantage of an S Corporation is reducing the potential for double taxation. Another financial consideration is that start-up businesses often show a loss in the first year or two. Given those circumstances, an S Corporation might be the most appropriate choice because it allows the owners/shareholders to directly declare business losses on their individual tax returns.

One of the prime eligibility requirements for S Corporations is that the number of stockholders be 75 or less. To form an S Corporation, fill out IRS Form 2553 (Election by a Small Business Corporation) within 75 days after incorporating. S Corporations must file annual returns (Form 1120-S).

Professional Corporations

Professional Corporations are also known as Personal Service Corporations (PSCs). Health care providers as well as other service professionals (e.g., accountants, attorneys, engineers, business consultants and performance artists) often opt for this status. In some states these types of service providers are *required* to choose this incorporation designation.

The benefits include the separation of the owners from the business entity (which also makes it easier to carry on the business should one shareholder withdraw), fringe benefits similar to those under C Corporations and limited liability protection. If you are a sole business owner, a PSC might not be advantageous. This designation is more common with group practices, particularly given that most states require all owners of a PSC to be licensed to render the same type of service. Again, I caution you to consult with an accountant or attorney before making any legal status decisions.

Professional corporations lost their popularity in the late 1980s when tax laws changed. Now they are taxed at a higher rate than other corporations and income-splitting is not allowed. Limited Liability Companies are preferred.

Limited Liability Companies ~~~

Limited Liability Companies (LLCs) are the newest form of legal entity. They are a hybrid of a partnership and a corporation. Most states require a minimum of two owners (they can be spouses) and these owners are generally called members (membership title and status changes depending on the type of LLC chosen).

LLCs offer many of the benefits as S Corporations with fewer drawbacks. This designation gives the individual owners a separate entity from the actual business and provides them with a limited personal liability shield. The profits from an LLC flow through to the owners (as in a sole proprietorship or partnership).

The paperwork isn't as complicated as with other types of corporations. You must file Articles of a Limited Liability Company, develop an Organizational Agreement, and file for an IRS Employee Identification Number. There may not be any requirement for annual meetings or additional filings with the state. Since regulations vary, contact your Corporation Commission or Secretary of State. Currently LLCs file an IRS Form 1065 and issue each member Form K-1 at the end of each year. Then each member reports their share of the profits or losses on their individual income tax returns.

• Business Name •

Choosing an appropriate name for your business takes some contemplation. Most health care practitioners are their business and thus need not go further. If you choose this route, I recommend that you also include a title such as: Tracy Jones, D.C.; Steve Smith, L.M.T.; or Terry Richards, Licensed Esthetician.

See Chapter Nine for ideas on clarifying your image and differential advantage.

You may want a separate business identity, particularly if you have a group practice. If so, choose your name carefully and avoid anything gimmicky. Select a name that conveys the essence of your business in a manner that inspires people to find out more about your services. Names such as Riverside Wellness Clinic are okay, but they lack oomph. One of the best named massage centers is in Tucson—The Right Touch. The Relaxation Center, Just Feet, Transformations Day Spa and The Athletic Edge are examples of names that convey a company's mission or identify target markets.

When you have selected a potential company name, say the name out loud several times to be sure it's easy to pronounce and understand. Test the name out on your friends and potential clients. Make sure your business name doesn't mean something derogatory in another language.

Naming a business can be an arduous process. In two decades, I still haven't found a name that encompasses the many facets of my business. If I decide to change my company's name, the transition will be a bit bumpy because Sohnen-Moe Associates is well-known (even though it's extremely difficult to understand over the phone). If you choose a business name other than your own, request a name search with the Corporation Commission or Secretary of State. They will usually do this by phone and let you know if the name is available for use. Regulations and fees vary, as do forms. For example, in Arizona, there is a difference between a "trade name" and a "trademark." Each has its own form and fees. With the trade name, you are registering the actual name of your company (e.g., Hands That Heal). A trademark is the registration of your logo and its description which can be a design or set of words. If you plan to use a company name, specific word(s) or logo in interstate commerce, consider obtaining a national trademark. This is a somewhat complex process which needs to be carefully done. Current fees are $325 per mark per classification. Should the application be rejected, the fee is non-refundable. Contact the U.S. Patent and Trademark Office (703-308-4317 or 800-786-9199) to obtain an application packet.

Whenever your business name is different from your personal name, most states require that you publish a DBA "Doing Business As" (also referred to as a Fictitious Name Certificate) in the classified section of at least one newspaper in the county where you operate. Contact your county clerk for forms and procedures.

As a sole proprietor health care provider, you don't need an employer identification number (EIN) unless you have employees or a Keogh plan. (See IRS Publication 583 for specifics.) Otherwise, you can use your social security number. To get an EIN, file form SS-4 with your local IRS. You can also mail or, in some regions, fax the completed and signed form. Contact the IRS for the fax number for your region. If you include your fax number on the form, the IRS will fax the EIN to you as well as send you a notification. It generally takes seven to 14 business days to obtain a number once the request is received by the IRS.

Trademark: How to Name a Business & Product
by K. McGrath and S. Elias
Nolo Press

Internet Trademark Search Companies:
Thomson & Thomson
www.thomson-thomson.com
Corsearch
www.corsearch.com

• Location •

You spend a lot of time in your office, so it's critical to choose a location that you like and that also attracts clients, fits your business image, accommodates your business needs (and potential expansion) in terms of size and layout, is properly zoned and priced within your budget.

A large number of practitioners have home offices as their main business site. Even those with commercial office space still see some clients at home. A home office yields many advantages such as low overhead (a home office is less expensive than most commercial offices), you can more easily accomplish household tasks (e.g., do laundry between sessions), it allows you more time to be with your family and the commute is within walking distance. The flip side is that some people are not productive at home. They are too easily distracted and lack discipline. Other problems arise from family members not respecting their boundaries. Plus zoning restrictions often restrict or prohibit home businesses.

See page 81
for details on zoning.

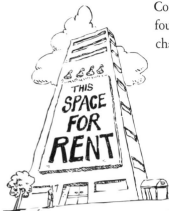

Commercial office space conveys an image of professionalism that is rarely found in a home office, no matter how nice it is. Although this perception is changing as more and more people in diverse professions are working at home.

Most people want their offices close to home, yet that choice can be disadvantageous. The main question to ask is, "Will your clients want to come there?"

The building in which your office is located impacts the atmosphere you wish to create. Your room (or office suite) doesn't exist independent of its surroundings. Your clients are affected by the totality: including the lobby, restroom facilities, the parking area and even the building itself.

Consider the Following Questions

- Is the building in an area that is easily accessible to your target markets?
- Does the location and the building itself fit your image?
- Is the building in a safe neighborhood?
- Do the premises provide space to expand your business?
- Are you able to alter the layout?
- Do the premises need major improvements or remodeling in order to be appropriate for your practice?
- Once you have furnished and organized the space, will it blend in with the style and decor of the rest of the building?
- Is there adequate parking, storage and space for signs?
- Is it accessible to the physically challenged?
- Does the space provide privacy and security?
- Are the utilities sufficient (e.g., do the air conditioning and heating units have adequate capacity)?
- Do you have direct access to the temperature controls?
- Are the other businesses in the building compatible with your practice?
- Is the noise level suitable? (It's difficult to mask the sounds and vibrations if an aerobics class is in the adjacent room or if someone leads primal-scream therapy groups next door.)
- Do other allied professionals work nearby?
- Will your clients feel comfortable transitioning from your office to the outside—or will it be culture shock?
- What are the terms of the lease?
- Who is responsible for the repairs and maintenance of the premises?
- Who is responsible for upkeep or possible replacement of major items such as the roof or air conditioning unit?
- What type of insurance coverage is provided?
- Who pays the utilities, taxes and insurance?
- What are the sales options or renewal provisions?
- By what formula are lease increases determined?
- Can you sublease, and if so, will the terms be the same as the original lease?

Most practitioners do not generally have a large walk-in clientele—although locating a business in a high traffic area can provide exposure. They tend to choose office buildings where the tenants are health care practitioners or other service providers.

Office prices vary greatly depending on the actual location and the local economics. Check out the going rates on other comparable office space. "Comparable" is the key word. Read the fine print. The quoted price might not include such things as utilities, parking, leasehold improvements (lighting, decorations and structural changes to the floors and walls), maintenance and signage.

Safety Note:
If you work at night, make sure other tenants also keep evening office hours.

Make sure the office space is right for you before signing a lease. Research the office's historical information: find out why the space is vacant; ascertain the number of tenants who have held the space in the past 10 years; and get a listing of other current tenants (including their types of businesses, office hours and schedule of lease expiration dates). Visit the area at different times of the day and night to get a sense of the traffic flow. Ask the landlord (or leasing agent) for a copy of the operating rules and regulations to ensure they are compatible with your practice. Determine if the building is properly zoned for your type of work.

Inspect the physical structure; make sure the roof is sound, the heating and cooling system is in good condition, and the building is secure (e.g., appropriate exterior lighting, stable stairs, lockable lobby door). Check with building and fire inspectors to see if the space has been cited.

The last step before finalizing a lease agreement is to review all legal documents with an attorney. The relatively few dollars spent in counsel can save you thousands later on should disputes arise.

Zoning: Your Rights and Responsibilities

Now that you have found an excellent site, can you practice there? Zoning ordinances can be a potential source of frustration and financial cost. It's imperative that you are knowledgeable of the local zoning requirements before opening up a business, buying an existing practice or even remodeling your current office space. Health care providers are often required to obtain several types of licenses and permits. It can be difficult to ascertain the requirements because each locale has different zoning laws and it isn't always clear which departments issue the various permits.

The two main purposes for licenses and permits are raising revenue and protecting the health and safety of the public. Zoning ordinances essentially divide an area into sections in which various activities/businesses are allowed or prohibited. The four major types of zoning are residential, commercial, industrial and agricultural. Within these categories are subsections which define the types of allowable activities. For example, a commercial area might be zoned for professional businesses only, retail, a combination of professional and retail, light industry or major manufacturing. Some residential areas allow certain types of businesses (mainly professionals such as health care practitioners or artists) but not others.

The level of enforcement varies widely. Some areas have negligible standards of operation and others are strict. Often it becomes important only if someone complains. In some cities, you are required to meet certain codes before you open your business (e.g., building, health and safety). Health practice items commonly regulated in zoning ordinances are off-street parking, signage, wheelchair accessibility, shower facilities and types of business activities. For example, hydrotherapy is an area in which many practitioners encounter restrictions. A touch therapist in the Southwest was told that he could not do light steam treatments (even though he was using professional equipment) unless his office had a shower. Before investing money in adjunct equipment, make certain that the zoning regulations allow its use. If it doesn't, do your best to get a variance (see below).

Keep in mind that ordinances are amended frequently and just because a similar business is in operation, it doesn't mean that yours will be allowed. The other business could have been in place *before* a zoning change was made, and as such is allowed to stay in operation. But any new business or one that changes hands would have to meet the new requirements. Consider this case in point.

Warning!
Get your information in writing. It isn't unusual for two different people in the same office to give conflicting information.

Zoning Scenario

Susan Smith, L.M.T., decides to open an office in a well-established professional building. The tenants are a mixture of accountants, attorneys, doctors, counselors and a reflexologist. The office she wants formerly belonged to a massage therapist. She assumes that she won't encounter any problems since the businesses are similar and a therapist already was in the office. She proceeds to sign a lease, decorate the office and within a month Susan opens the doors of her practice, only to be served with a cease-and-desist order. She wonders how this could possibly happen. If she had researched the zoning ordinances, she would have discovered that two years ago, the regulations had changed. Since the previous therapist had already been there before the new regulations, he did not have to comply with the changes. But the moment Susan applied for an occupation license, it set off a chain of events that resulted in the zoning board discovering that she did not make the necessary changes to legally operate a massage practice in that building. Any time you apply for a business permit, license or building permit it tags your business for scrutiny.

To find out which ordinances pertain to your practice, first talk with the licensing bureau. The staff should be able to provide a list of the types of permits you need or at least the names of appropriate contacts. Next talk with people at city/county hall. Then meet with the planning department and the health department. If you are experiencing any difficulties in obtaining the necessary information, go to the library, the office of economic development or the state office of industrial development.

Home Offices

Home office requirements are often more stringent than those for commercial office space. Check your deed covenants for any specific limitations. Residential offices are often restricted to the amount of vehicular traffic generated, parking, the numbers of clients allowed in the home at any one time, signage, hours of operation, the percentage of floor space devoted to business and storage facilities. Many permits require a separate office entrance with an attached bathroom. In some locations home businesses are not allowed to have employees or sell products.

Now that more than 44 percent of American households have members who work at least part time in their homes, city officials are beginning to ease up on home office restrictions.

Still, it's risky to open a practice in a location where zoning is questionable. If possible, get the zoning changed before it's a necessity. If you are operating a home business, you may opt to take a "let's wait and see attitude" and not worry about the zoning ordinances. This can put you in a precarious position, particularly if you are investing a lot of money in remodeling your home office.

Variances

If you are found in violation of a zoning ordinance, you are sent a notice ordering you to cease your business. You must file an appeal immediately or cease operations, because every day you continue to operate can be considered a separate violation. Remember that a decision from a zoning official isn't necessarily written in stone. You can often appeal that decision, get a conditional use permit or even obtain a zoning variance.

When meeting with any official, it's best to have garnered support from adjacent business owners, your neighbors (for home offices) and other members of the community. (This is an example of why it's important to be involved in your chamber of commerce, business networking organizations and local trade associations.)

If you need to alter the current zoning requirements to legally run your business, begin by meeting with city officials to ask for a zoning variance or "special exemption" permit. This requires the cooperation of neighbors or nearby businesses. Get letters or have them sign a petition that says they support your business use. If your business is already established, bring photographs that illustrate the scope of your business.

If this doesn't work, take your request to the zoning board. It will be very helpful if you can get your neighbors/adjoining business owners to go with you and speak on your behalf. The next step would be appealing to the city council. And if all else fails, you can take your case to court.

Health care providers are often required to meet very stringent conditions founded upon antiquated regulations. I recommend that practitioners in each city get together and decide what requirements they feel are reasonable and submit them to the zoning board. Start a lobbying campaign now. Create a structure that you want, not one that's dictated by officials who may not understand your profession.

The Legal Guide for Starting & Running A Small Business
by Fred S. Steingold
Nolo Press

Home Office Association
of America, Inc.
909 Third Ave, New York,
NY 10022-4731
800-908-4622
212-980-4622
E-mail: HOAA@aol.com

Figure 5.1

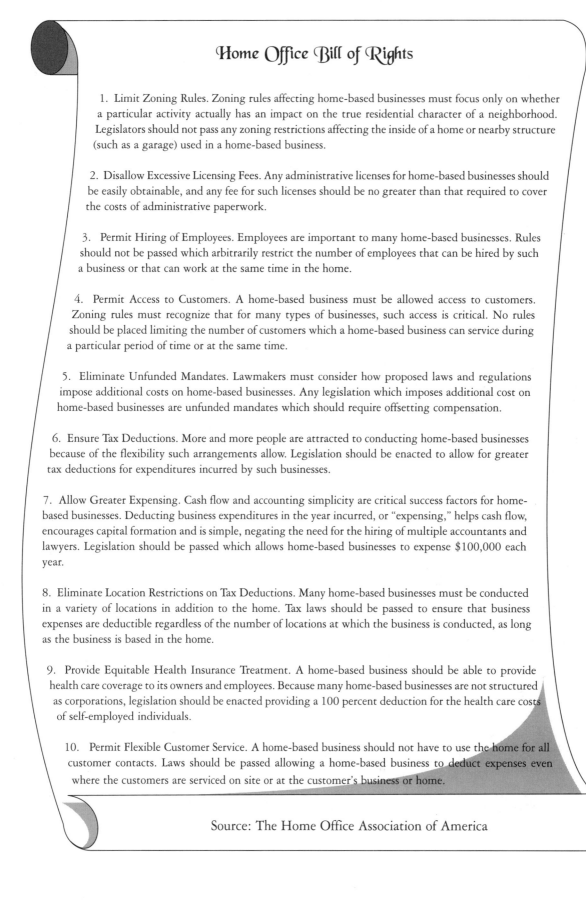

Home Office Bill of Rights

1. Limit Zoning Rules. Zoning rules affecting home-based businesses must focus only on whether a particular activity actually has an impact on the true residential character of a neighborhood. Legislators should not pass any zoning restrictions affecting the inside of a home or nearby structure (such as a garage) used in a home-based business.

2. Disallow Excessive Licensing Fees. Any administrative licenses for home-based businesses should be easily obtainable, and any fee for such licenses should be no greater than that required to cover the costs of administrative paperwork.

3. Permit Hiring of Employees. Employees are important to many home-based businesses. Rules should not be passed which arbitrarily restrict the number of employees that can be hired by such a business or that can work at the same time in the home.

4. Permit Access to Customers. A home-based business must be allowed access to customers. Zoning rules must recognize that for many types of businesses, such access is critical. No rules should be placed limiting the number of customers which a home-based business can service during a particular period of time or at the same time.

5. Eliminate Unfunded Mandates. Lawmakers must consider how proposed laws and regulations impose additional costs on home-based businesses. Any legislation which imposes additional cost on home-based businesses are unfunded mandates which should require offsetting compensation.

6. Ensure Tax Deductions. More and more people are attracted to conducting home-based businesses because of the flexibility such arrangements allow. Legislation should be enacted to allow for greater tax deductions for expenditures incurred by such businesses.

7. Allow Greater Expensing. Cash flow and accounting simplicity are critical success factors for home-based businesses. Deducting business expenditures in the year incurred, or "expensing," helps cash flow, encourages capital formation and is simple, negating the need for the hiring of multiple accountants and lawyers. Legislation should be passed which allows home-based businesses to expense $100,000 each year.

8. Eliminate Location Restrictions on Tax Deductions. Many home-based businesses must be conducted in a variety of locations in addition to the home. Tax laws should be passed to ensure that business expenses are deductible regardless of the number of locations at which the business is conducted, as long as the business is based in the home.

9. Provide Equitable Health Insurance Treatment. A home-based business should be able to provide health care coverage to its owners and employees. Because many home-based businesses are not structured as corporations, legislation should be enacted providing a 100 percent deduction for the health care costs of self-employed individuals.

10. Permit Flexible Customer Service. A home-based business should not have to use the home for all customer contacts. Laws should be passed allowing a home-based business to deduct expenses even where the customers are serviced on site or at the customer's business or home.

Source: The Home Office Association of America

A large percentage of touch therapists and rural health care practitioners work out of their homes (at least part time). In some cities the strict restrictions placed on home practices make it cost prohibitive to legally operate. The Home Office Association of America has developed a "Home Office Bill of Rights" for members who face restrictive zoning rules (refer back to Figure 5.1). They want this information disseminated so please feel free to make copies of it and pass it along to other home business owners as well as your city officials (as it is or as part of a specific proposal to change the health care practice zoning laws). The first five "rights" pertain to local ordinances and the second five are geared to the national government level.

Office Design ~~~

The major elements involved in office design are ambiance, professionalism, visual stimuli, sensations (scent, touch and sound) and layout. Make this a space that is mutually healing to yourself and others. The basic tenet is: Appeal to the majority of your clients while being inoffensive to all. The main sources of offense are forcing your personal or professional beliefs on others and invading people's sense of smell, sight, sound and touch. Oftentimes, people are affronted by things we don't even consider as potential problems.

60 percent of healing is environment.

For instance, you may hold strong spiritual or religious beliefs that are not shared by everyone. Most people would be fine with seeing one or two symbols in your office, but would probably feel ill at ease if they walked into a room filled with icons and artifacts. Your clients will be much more comfortable if your office space is client-centered. In other words, create a space that is comfortable for your *client*. This might not be your personal favorite decor; be sure to find some way to balance both your clients' needs and yours—after all, you are there day in and day out.

The first thing to do is review your client base and identify your major target markets. Next consider what would be an ideal space for them. You can also survey your clients and representatives of future target markets for direct feedback. After you've completed your research, the next stage is the actual creation of the session room. If you find the office atmosphere so abrades your natural tendencies, perhaps you should change your target market.

See Chapter Nine, pages 271-280 for information on target markets.

Your office design may need to be developed in stages. Begin by identifying the "must have" items and elements and include them as soon as possible. You don't have to own top-of-the-line equipment. Bigger, brighter, shinier isn't always better. Just make certain you have appropriate items in good condition for your specific target markets.

Consider hiring a feng shui consultant to help the session room's energy to flow and to create an overall sense of well-being throughout the office.

Keep in mind that the foremost reason your clients come to you is for your services; until you can establish your "ideal" office, make sure your space doesn't detract from your desired image.

Ambiance

Ambiance is a rather amorphous concept; it's a special atmosphere created by your environment. It arises from all of the previously covered factors and impacts your image and the mood you set. Establishing the appropriate ambiance isn't always an easy feat; although an unlimited budget would certainly help.

You always create a mood—intentional or not. Consider the image you wish to portray and the characteristics associated with it. Do you want your office to project a clinical feeling (which would be appropriate if many of your clients are insurance referrals)? Do you want a calm, quiet, soothing atmosphere to appeal to those wanting stress reduction? Do you want a cheery room with toys and lots of color for infants? Do you want a high-tech look for executives?

Professionalism

A professional office establishes credibility and demonstrates concern for the client. You validate your credibility by conspicuously posting your business license, policies, educational certificates, awards, interview clippings, business cards, brochures and letters of appreciation and recommendation. These items represent the time you've invested in your career and the goodwill you've generated in your community.

You express your concern for your clients by the ways in which you design your office to assist them in feeling comfortable, appreciated, and the center of attention. One of the most important factors is to create a sense of privacy. You may need to be inventive to accomplish this. For instance, some massage therapists and estheticians work in beauty salons. Often the walls don't even reach the ceiling or are paper thin, making a sense of privacy difficult to achieve. If remodeling isn't an option, perhaps padding the walls or enclosing the room with a false ceiling or canopy would help.

Several ideas to make your clients feel important are: provide a special area for your client's belongings such as a small closet, a shelf, a chair behind a screen, or at the very least a hook with hangers; keep supplies such as linens, tissues, blankets, and bolsters stocked and handy; and maintain a temperature that's comfortable for your client. If you don't have easy access to the temperature controls, place a portable heater and fan in the room. Keep notes about clients' preferences in their files: refer to the file before the session so you can properly prepare the room.

Nothing detracts more from a pleasant atmosphere than a dirty office space, especially the bathroom. Keep your room clean and free of clutter. In other words, make sure there are no product spills, no trash cans overflowing with garbage, no sinks filled with dirty dishes, no soiled linens piled in a corner and no dust-bunnies hiding under the furniture, on fan blades, in vents and around moldings.

Home offices present a few challenges. The main things to consider in conveying professionalism are privacy, sounds, cleanliness and environment. First of all, make sure you have a separate work space in your home. Ideally, this room would have a private entrance from the main house. The next best option would be to have a

Beware of "theme" rooms. They often have limited appeal and in time can become boring to both you and your clients.

separate room. If you must meet with clients in the main living quarters, do your best to set up a private area. Room screens work well for this.

Sounds are a major concern. Make sure you can silence the telephone ringer. Be certain that when receiving phone calls from potential clients you have surroundings that are free of outside noise. I highly recommend a separate business line from the home line, especially if you have children. You always want your phone to be answered in a professional manner.

Also, figure out a way to let others who may come to the door know that you cannot be interrupted. Be aware of ambient sounds such as children playing. A major problem could arise when you have family members in your home during a session. Set clear boundaries and rules with family members on noise and not disturbing you during a session. Pets are not always cooperative in honoring the silence rule. Extra steps may need to be taken to ensure quiet.

Cleanliness is imperative to your professional image. Pets can present a potential problem because no matter how well you vacuum, dander is always present if they are allowed in the session area. Also take into consideration that many people are allergic to animals. Any area in your home that your clients may see needs to be kept clean and tidy.

Visual Stimuli

Designing the physical appearance of your treatment room is where you can really be creative and have fun. Most people are visually oriented and are affected by the colors, textures and artistry of your room.

Creativity specialists contend that the key to creativity is to get out of your normal frame of reference, which in this profession is mainly standing upright. One technique is to lie on your table or sit on your chair and notice what you see. Include all positions: face up, face down and side to side. This is how your clients view your room. You just might be surprised at what they can see at those angles. For example, if you have a bookshelf, note which shelves are at eye level and be sure to place appropriate books in that line of vision.

Simple changes to alter the visual impact of your ideal session room include painting the walls, texturizing the ceiling, suspending a mobile, patterning the walls/ceiling with color or brush strokes, hanging artwork and charts, furnishing the room stylishly and installing unique window coverings.

Make sure the floor covering is constructed of high-quality materials. You may want to avoid light colors as they get dirty very quickly. If the office flooring is less than ideal, you can use throw rugs or an area carpet—just be certain they are skid-proof.

Lighting is another important element in the design of a session room. Ideally, you would have a source of natural light from a window or a skylight. If not, place lamps in different areas of the room to give balanced, indirect illumination.

If people knew how hard I worked to get my mastery, it wouldn't seem so wonderful after all.
— Michelangelo

Sensations

We are all sensual beings. Incorporate as many of the senses as possible—particularly touch, smell and sound—into your design plans.

In terms of scent, a clean, crisp, barely discernible fragrance is usually preferred. If your office is in a salon, you must eliminate or conceal the harsh chemical odors from nail polish and hair treatment applications such as dyes and permanents. Some solutions to these types of problems are to insulate your room or mask the odors with incense, potpourri or essential oils. Be careful with fragrances because your clients may suffer from allergies or your next client may want the opposite results of the aromatherapy essence used by the current client.

Physical sensation plays an important role—especially in touch therapy practices. In addition to the actual hands-on treatment are the tactile sensations from your equipment and linens. For many health care providers, a treatment table is one of the most important pieces of office equipment. Does it inspire feelings of safety and comfort? Can you make necessary adjustments in the unit? Is it wide enough? Is it long enough? Is it well padded? Does it squeak? Do your clients need to pole vault to get on it? Use a secure, well-padded table or futon and make sure your sheets, towels and gowns are soft. Linens may need to be washed several times before becoming adequately soft. You might also cover bolsters with a towel or sheet.

Most people like to touch things, so have items available for your clients to play with such as a skeleton, a replica of the foot with reflexology points, a model of a muscle, samples of products you sell and books they can peruse.

Sound, or the absence thereof, is the most commonly used means of creating a mood. Invest in a good system that's programmable or has an auto-reverse function. Purchase a wide variety of music and make sure you can easily adjust volume or change selection. Some settings might have piped-in music, but still you can often access the controls. I used to go to a dentist who played a style of music which I abhorred. I was always apprehensive about check-ups; not because I feared he might discover cavities, but because I dreaded listening to the music.

Regardless of the atmosphere you desire, it can be undermined if you don't block out external noise, so be sure you turn off the phone bell and soundproof thin walls. You can also create other auditory experiences with chimes, an aquarium, or even a specially designed indoor water fountain.

Layout

The most comfortable and inviting offices are organized, clean and free of clutter. Decorate the room with appropriate furniture and equipment. Don't put your favorite recliner in the corner if it takes up so much room that clients have to walk sideways to get to the table. Consider the ways in which you interact with your clients and design your office accordingly. For instance, if you like to teach clients how to stretch, make sure there's adequate, obstruction-free floor space.

My Ideal Session Room

As a receiver of many types of health care services, my vision of the ideal session room is one in which I feel comfortable and pampered.

I envision the room being located in a small professional building that is nicely landscaped. After walking through a small, lush courtyard, I enter through the front door and find myself in the lobby/waiting room. It's painted with pastel colors and the floors are tiled. There are several stuffed chairs, a couch, a magazine table and end tables with lamps on them and vases of fresh flowers.

Directly to my left is a desk where the receptionist works. Next to the desk is a beautiful ficus tree. Against one wall is a bookshelf with brochures about the various practitioners and literature on well-being. Along an adjacent wall is a display case filled with unique health-related items such as books, essential oils, diffusers, hot and cold therapy packs, relaxation tools, ergonomic support devices and tapes. In the corner is a water dispenser and a stand with cups and a pot of herbal tea.

The actual session room inspires a sense of deep relaxation the moment I enter. The lighting is diffused, the temperature moderate, the walls are painted a soothing color, the ceilings are vaulted, and I can feel a soft breeze from an overhead fan. I experience a sense of total privacy—no outside noises whatsoever.

The therapist guides me to a little alcove where I can get ready for my session. This dressing area has hangers for clothes, a shelf for belongings, a mirror and a chair. The natural sunlight gently streams through a skylight.

I proceed to get on the extremely comfortable table that is thickly padded and hydraulic with adjustable angles. I notice how good the soft linens feel, and appreciate that they're also fragrance-free. The table has a shelf that I can easily reach and on it I find tissues and a glass of water. I look around the room and see certificates on one wall, artwork on another and anatomical charts on the third wall. The window is covered with wooden shutters and several large potted plants are positioned in the corners. The room is uncluttered, clean and exudes professionalism. Then I hear faint sounds emanating from the stereo, lulling me into a state of deep relaxation....

Relocation ∼

At some point over the course of your business you will most likely need to relocate. Regardless of whether it's down the street, to the other side of town or across the country, moving can be an extremely stressful event. Before you actually relocate, set a foundation for success and ease your stress level by establishing a network, discerning the prevailing attitudes, ascertaining the regulations and becoming well informed about the amenities and limitations of the city. Any move provides you with an opportunity to re-evaluate your life and business, implement changes, meet new people and revitalize your practice.

Moving Within the Same City

One of the most important factors to consider in choosing a new location is the impact it will have on your clients. Whenever you move more than several blocks from your current location, you risk losing clients. This chance is heightened if a large portion of your clientele is based on geography. Let's say your office is in a downtown skyscraper and the majority of your clients are attorneys who work in that building. Attorneys tend to keep chaotic schedules and, most likely, one of the reasons they utilize your services is that you are convenient. If they can't simply take the elevator to your office (or at the most, walk across the street), they may not see you as frequently—if at all.

Regardless of how good a practitioner you are, many people won't travel far to see you, especially on a regular basis. Who wants to drive 45 minutes through traffic *after* getting relaxed? Other people may only have a limited amount of time they can take from work and thus need to schedule after hours or find another practitioner.

Figure 5.2

Moving Checklist

❑ Send moving notification (three weeks prior to moving date).

❑ Review files.

❑ Organize paperwork into active and archival boxes.

❑ Make an inventory list.

❑ Hire movers.

❑ Clean and organize new office before moving.

❑ Schedule an Open House.

❑ Send a second announcement (one week prior to move).

❑ Call current clients.

❑ Introduce yourself to your new neighbors.

❑ Forge alliances with businesses.

❑ Gain visibility in the local community.

❑ Post new address at previous location.

Retain Clients by Communicating Benefits

Most people generally do not embrace change. You need to find a way to communicate the benefits of your relocation to your clients. Some of those advantages may include: more space; improved ambiance; a location adjacent to other health care providers; proximity to public transportation; an office away from the hustle and bustle of the city or closer to the center of town; a more intimate, relaxed, private space (good way to describe downsizing); a safer location; an increased number or variety of practitioners in the same office; additional services; space for classes; better and safer parking; quieter neighborhood; and lower overhead to keep prices down.

Revitalize Your Practice

Moving provides you with an excellent opportunity to reconnect with your clients, particularly those you haven't seen lately. Many health care providers avoid contacting inactive clients due to the time involved in reviewing their files and writing individualized letters. A form letter without something specific to each client is usually ineffective in generating interest. But moving announcements don't require personalization! You can even offer an incentive for them to come back.

Take the time to go through your files as you are boxing them. Note who hasn't been in for a while and send them a special letter (if they don't attend your open house). Think about what you could do to provide further service to each client. For instance, a client has been diagnosed with fibromyalgia. You haven't worked with her in more than a year. Several months ago you read an excellent book on the subject and could share some information with her. Place a reminder in your tickler file to send her a note about the book and invite her to your new facilities.

After you have relocated, go through your client files and send out one letter or postcard each day.

Notification

Notify all of your clients, colleagues and associates as soon as possible. Send out announcements or fliers at least three weeks before the move. Include the date of the move, your new address and phone numbers, any changes in hours and a map detailing directions to get to your new facilities. Consider sending your active contacts another notice closer to the moving date. If your office accepts last-minute appointments or walk-in clients, call your current client list one week before the actual move to inform them of your new address.

Once you have relocated, post a note on the door of your previous office with the address, phone number and directions to your new location. If that option isn't available, perhaps you can leave a stack of fliers with the new tenants. Be sure to confirm all appointments and remind clients of the address change. To keep track of who has been reminded about the new location, code your clients' files with colored dots (or if you are computerized, create a special field).

Most phone companies wait from three months to one year before reassigning business numbers. Right before that time comes, call your old number and tell the new holder your phone number and address. Send a thank-you card and a gift (flowers, plant or gift certificate) to thank them in advance for forwarding your calls. Deliver additional thank-you notes as long as they continue to forward your information.

Figure 5.3

STRESS**Busters**

We're moving!

StressBusters is moving to larger facilities
on November 1st.
Our new location will be at:

**123 Breeze Court
Sea City, NJ 07094
908-555-5555**

Come celebrate with us at our grand opening on Saturday, November 1st from
10 a.m. to 2 p.m. We will be serving refreshments, providing mini-workshops on
stress reduction techniques and offering complimentary chair massages.
Please join in the fun. Bring a friend.

Redeem this invitation for $10 off your next massage!

Sally Smith

Generating New Clientele

Relocation furnishes you with a splendid opportunity to generate new clientele. Survey the surrounding area for other businesses that could be a source of referrals (mutual referrals are even better). Get to know your neighbors. Hand-deliver fliers or brochures to adjacent businesses, hold a special open house just for the people nearby and make yourself visible in the community. Get involved in local business association meetings (e.g., the Downtown Business Owners Alliance). If there's a local publication, advertise in it or offer to write a health column.

Forge alliances with other business owners for the purpose of cooperative marketing. Let's go back to the attorney example. You are a massage therapist who wants to increase the number of attorneys in your client pool. To heighten your differential advantage you decide to relocate to a building that is populated mainly with attorneys. A restaurant down the block offers free delivery service to tenants in your building. Together, you could do several marketing activities that would increase the range of people you reach and reduce the cost of reaching them:

1. Share the cost of hiring someone to hand-deliver your brochures and her menus to each office.
2. Offer a joint special such as "Receive a certificate for a free 15-minute chair massage with your 10th delivery" and "Receive a 10 percent food purchase discount coupon with every massage."
3. Keep a stack of menus by your office door. At the restaurant, place your cards and brochures (in a plastic holder) near the cash register.
4. Get the restaurant to cater your open houses (at cost or for free). Offer free massages for special events hosted by the restaurant.

5. Have monthly drawings at the restaurant for a free massage and at your office for a free dinner for two.

Most large buildings have news/candy stands in the lobby. You can ask to place your cards and flyers near the counter. Perhaps you can leave a container in which tenants place their business cards to win a free massage. In addition to generating visibility, this provides a means to obtaining the tenants' names for future marketing ventures. Offer the stand owner a free weekly 15-minute chair massage (preferably right in the stand area) in exchange for displaying your materials.

Moving to a New City

For most people, moving to a new city means starting a business from scratch. You can create a smoother transition and actually develop a strong referral base and network by doing legwork before the actual move.

Research

Research your new location to determine what it has to offer economically, socially, politically, culturally and climatically. Start by asking the Chamber of Commerce to send you a relocation packet with information on the city, population, demographics and major industries. Request that they send you the following: the Yellow Pages on your specific service, health, stress; holistic health care providers; listings of business and professional associations; and anything else that piques your interest. Not all chambers are so accommodating—you may need to order a phone book from the telephone company. You can also do some of this research at the library and over the Internet.

Another method for gathering information about the community and your specific profession is talking with people in that city. If you are a member of any professional association, contact other members in the area. If you aren't a member or if no other members live there, contact the officers or directors of allied professional associations. Send letters or call several people in your same profession. Request information from any local allied health care provider schools.

Some questions to ask are: What position does your type of service hold in this community? What are the attitudes toward the profession and the practitioners? How much publicity does this profession garner? What is the range of fees charged and what is the scope of practice? What is the average annual yearly income for a practitioner in your specific profession?

Call the relevant business, zoning and health licensing agencies to ascertain their requirements and obtain the number of licensed (or registered) health care providers in the area. You may need to contact state agencies to learn the specific regulations for health care providers. Get in touch with a commercial real estate agent to obtain information on the types of available office space and the going rates. Order copies of the local newspapers(s), holistic magazines and special interest publications—all of which provide valuable information about your new city.

There is nothing permanent except change.
Heraclitus

Librarians are good at searching for information and it's usually the favorite aspect of their job.

Network

See Chapter Eight, pages 260-261 for more introduction letters.

Begin to network even before you move. Ask your friends, relatives and colleagues if they know anyone in that city. Send a letter of introduction to allied professionals such as physicians, counselors, chiropractors, massage therapists and other health care providers (see Figure 5.4). Let them know who you are and what you do, including your abilities and qualifications. Address the potential mutual benefits of your association. Close the letter by telling them how to contact you and inform them that you will be calling them within the next few weeks. When you do, ask for any advice, suggestions or contacts they might recommend. Be sure to thank them for their time and consideration with a follow-up note.

Figure 5.4 Sample Letter of Introduction

Tracy Jones

974 Silverton Avenue • Tucson, AZ 85741 • 520-555-5555

27 June 2001

Dr. Terry Smith, M.D.
3000 Oak Knoll Road
Seattle, WA 98111

Dear Dr. Smith,
My name is Tracy Jones and I am considering relocating my practice to Seattle. This letter is a brief introduction of the services I offer, as well as my interest in networking with other health care professionals like you.

I have been in practice for three years after graduating from a 1,000 hour program at the Desert Institute of the Healing Arts in Tucson, Arizona. I am a licensed massage therapist and my training includes shiatsu and craniosacral therapy. I also have six years of experience in hypnotherapy and a master's degree in psychology.

My approach to massage focuses on the body-mind relationship and specifically how massage enhances the healing process for those in psychotherapy and recovery work. For many involved in chemical and emotional recovery, massage is a new experience that offers safe, nurturing touch. Massage also enhances the chemical detoxification process as it speeds up metabolism by increasing circulation.

The information I received on your center indicates that we share a similar approach to wellness. Your brochure doesn't state whether you have any massage therapists on staff. Massage would complement your services and assist in accelerating the recovery process. I hope you will consider me as a potential resource for mutual referrals and services.

I plan to visit Seattle in November to further research the area, and I would like to introduce myself in person. I will call in two weeks to see if you have any time to meet with me. You can reach me at the above address and phone number if you would like to contact me sooner.

I have included my brochure and an article by Clyde W. Ford, D.C., that further elaborates on the body-mind relationship. Thank you for your time.

Sincerely,

Tracy Jones

Tracy Jones
Enclosures

Scouting Expedition

If you are considering a place for relocation and it isn't definite that you will actually move there, visit the city during the worst (hottest, coldest, wettest, driest, most crowded) part of the year to see whether you can tolerate it. This is also a good time to meet with colleagues and explore potential associations.

• Licenses and Permits •

Business owners need to know the local, state and federal requirements that influence the starting or relocating of a business. The following list is an overview of the basic required licenses and permits, and who to contact for specific information and forms. This list doesn't cover every possible situation as your business may have special site requirements or industry regulations. Contact the Secretary of State or the Consumer Affairs office to find out about additional state requirements.

Business License

Allows you the privilege of doing business. Contact your Business Licensing Bureau.

Occupational License

Allows you to work in a specific industry as long as you comply with that profession's regulations. Contact the State Agency of Consumer Affairs or the local Business Licensing Bureau.

Transaction Privilege Tax License

Allows you to collect (and remit) sales tax. Contact your State Department of Revenue.

Planning and Zoning Permits

These permits are issued after your location has been assessed and shows that the business operation conforms with area plans, has proper zoning and has adequate parking. Contact your City/County Hall Planning Department.

Building Safety Permit

This permit is issued after your location is inspected and is found safe for you and your clients, and complies with fire and building codes. Contact the Fire Department.

• Insurance Coverage •

Being properly insured is imperative for any small business. Discuss your specific needs with an insurance agent (or three) to determine the types and amount of insurance that is appropriate for you and your business. You may need to have more than one insurance carrier since very few companies offer all of the types of coverage. Check your office lease thoroughly. Your leaseholder may not be responsible for providing complete (if any) coverage. Also, if you work out of your home, be certain to review your homeowner's or apartment-dweller's policy. While the standard homeowner's policy protects you from personal liability, if a guest is injured at your home, it will not cover you if the visit is related to business.

Liability Insurance covers costs of injuries that occur to business-related visitors on your property. Don't assume that this is automatically covered in your office lease. Also, if you work out of your home, your homeowner's policy might not cover this either. Liability insurance doesn't cover you or employees.

General Liability Insurance covers negligence resulting in injury to clients, employees or the general public while you are on their premises. This is particularly important if you do office calls or teach classes.

Small Business Insurance offers umbrella coverage for business losses in terms of general liability, business interruption, errors and omissions, and product liability.

Malpractice Liability Insurance protects you from claims due to a loss incurred by your clients as a result of negligence or failure on your part to perform at a professional skill level.

Product Liability protects you from claims by clients who use products designed, manufactured or sold by you. Health care providers rarely need this coverage.

Automobile Insurance is very important, particularly if you use your car in your business. Be sure to carry full coverage including disability, business interruption and loss or damage to business-related items.

Fire and Theft Insurance covers business equipment, furniture, supplies and documents. If you work out of your home, you may need to purchase a rider to get adequate protection. You will most likely need a separate policy for an outside office.

Business Interruption Insurance covers you if your business closes due to fire or other insurable causes. It pays you approximately what you would have earned.

Personal Disability Insurance safeguards you from loss of income if you are unable to work due to illness or injury. You are paid a certain monthly amount if you are permanently disabled or a portion if you are partially disabled (can include long-term illness).

Determine which types of insurance are required by law and purchase those policies first. Then decide what additional coverage is most important and purchase it next.

Personal Disability and Medical Health Insurance are essential if you are the head of your household or don't have sufficient savings.

Medical Health Insurance helps cover medical bills, particularly for complicated illnesses, injuries and hospitalization.

Workers' Compensation is required by law if you have employees. It covers all of the costs that you as an employer would be required to pay for any injury to an employee. It also provides the employee with disability and death benefits if injured or killed on the job. The employer is responsible for the cost of the insurance premium.

Partnership Insurance protects you against lawsuits arising from actions or omissions by any of your business partners.

• Setting Your Fees •

Fee structures vary greatly depending on the type of work you do and where you are located. Setting an appropriate fee structure and increase strategy is necessary in any business. No matter which method you choose for determining your rates, be certain your fee structure promotes credibility.

Four Major Fee-Setting Strategies ⟶

1. You can set a very high price, thus targeting a small percentage of the population. This usually only works if your service is innovative, in demand and has no competition.

2. A competitive pricing strategy is simply setting your price with the going rate for the industry.

3. If you want to get a larger share of the market, your strategy might be to set a significantly lower fee than the standard rate.

4. Finally, if you want to break into a new market, your strategy may include offering introductory (reduced or two-for-one) rates for a limited time, package deals or a sliding scale. Just beware of the ongoing-sale-syndrome.

Before you finalize your fee structure carefully consider all of the costs involved in running your business. This includes your fixed costs such as rent, utilities, phone, equipment, loan payments, maintenance, insurance, licenses, advertising and staffing, as well as the amenities that vary depending on the number and type of clients (e.g., providing free samples and educational materials, taxes, supplies, promotional costs and your time). Then there's your time: keeping client records, networking, planning, holding extended business hours, traveling, practice management, continuing your education and consultations.

Figure 5.5 illustrates how to determine your fees. It's based on a 40-hour work week, which leaves a maximum of 25 billable hours per week. Since overhead varies greatly from one business to another, it isn't included in this breakdown.

Figure 5.5

Time/Income Factor Analysis

One Year	= 365 days	-	104 days (weekends)
	= 261 days	-	8 days (holidays)
	= 253 days	-	10 days (health)
	= 243 days	-	10 days (vacation)
	= 233 days	x	8 hours per day
	= 1,864 hours per year		
	- 30% (promotion, operations, professional development)		
	= approximately 1,300 hours		
	= approximately 25 billable hours per week		

Annual Income*	50% 12.5 hrs/week (650 hrs)	70% 17.5 hrs/week (910 hrs)	90% 22.5 hrs/week (1170 hrs)	100% 25 hrs/week (1300 hrs)
$25,000	38.50	27.50	21.50	19.25
$30,000	46.00	33.00	25.75	23.00
$35,000	54.00	38.50	30.00	27.00
$40,000	61.50	44.00	34.00	31.00
$50,000	77.00	55.00	42.75	38.50
$60,000	92.00	66.00	51.25	46.00
$75,000	115.50	82.50	64.00	58.00
$100,000	154.00	110.00	85.50	77.00

* Does not include allowance for overhead and taxes

Let's say that you want to earn $35,000 this year before taxes. If you plan on working 50 percent (billing 12.5 hours per week), then you need to charge $54 per hour. If you think you will be able to work 90 percent (bill 22.5 hours per week), then you only need to charge $30 per hour. BUT, you also must include the costs in running your business.

Refer to Appendix A, page 393 for a Cash Flow Forecast.

Imagine that your fixed costs are $10,000 per year plus $6 per session. So, at a 50 percent workload, you need to cover $35,000 income, $10,000 fixed expenses, and $3,900 per session cost (650 sessions), which equals $48,900. Look at the chart and you will find that to bring in gross revenues of $50,000, you need to charge approximately $76 per hour. Yet, if you plan on billing 90 percent, then you need to cover $35,000 income, $10,000 fixed expenses, and $7,020 per session cost (1170 sessions), which equals $52,020 Check the chart and you will discover that you will only need to charge about $39 per hour.

This chart can have an unsettling effect. You may be wondering how you can possibly earn the income you desire while charging a fair and equitable price. Several possibilities exist for increasing your income potential. First of all, you can increase the number of billable weekly hours by working more than 40 hours per week (which isn't uncommon with small business owners). Another alternative is to reduce your overhead costs—but be certain this doesn't cause clients to experience a decrease in benefits. You can also diversify your practice by selling products, subcontracting work (or hiring other practitioners to work for you) and leading seminars. Finally, one of the most viable options is to delegate some of your business activities—which frees you to increase the number of hours of direct client contact.

Keep in mind that raising your hourly rates is not the only way to increase your income.

Determining your appropriate fee structure involves more than simply deciding what you want to charge per hour. You have to balance your desired income and requisite expenses with what's realistic. Your fees must be fair and instill trust. Even if you are considered to be the best practitioner in your field, it's futile to charge more than what the market will bear. Just because you desire a specific income level and feel you deserve to charge a certain rate, doesn't necessarily mean people will pay it. So, choose your market(s) carefully and strategize your fee structure.

Sliding Fee Scales

Sliding fee scales can be awkward. It's tough to set one up in advance of the first session unless a client has said something to you while booking the appointment. In general, I don't advocate advertising a sliding fee scale unless you know that your target market is going to need it (e.g., people on meager fixed incomes).

Usually what works best is to give parameters. A frequently used model that seems least offensive and fair is determining fees based on income level. For example, your sliding scale statement might look like this:

> *My standard rate is $5 per session. If this presents a hardship for you, then I will accept a sliding scale fee based on your combined family annual income level. If the total annual income earned is less than $15,000 annually the fee per session is $25, $15,000-20,000 = $35, $20,000+ = $45.*

Prepaid Package Plans

Prepaid package plans encourage people to book sessions more frequently and infuse extra income into your bank account. Some suggestions for prepaid incentives are: purchase three facials and receive a $5 savings per facial; seven counseling sessions qualifies for a 20 percent discount; and purchase five massages and receive the sixth one free. The most important thing is to keep it simple. Don't overwhelm yourself and your clients with a plethora of options.

See Chapter Eight, pages 246-247 for additional ideas on Client Incentives.

Raising Your Rates

Asking for more money can be an easy natural action, or it can be an excruciatingly painful process—regardless of whether you are self-employed or work as an employee.

Money is a myth. It's simply a medium of exchange for products, services and ideas. Your attitudes toward money in conjunction with your feelings about yourself greatly influence your affluence. A strong sense of self-esteem is vital to being able to ask for more money and get it. Self-esteem is a feeling—how you feel about yourself—who you are. It isn't based on what you look like, how much money you have or your position in the business world. If all your accomplishments, looks and material goods were taken away—how would you feel about yourself? You are not your accomplishments. You are not your possessions. You are not your looks—after all, in time that changes too. Who you are goes beyond the externals.

Money will not add to your self-esteem, it works the other way around.
— Phil Laut

When asking for more money, remember that who you are as a person doesn't necessarily correlate with your value to an employer or client. You may be dedicated, outgoing and honest—yet you still may not be able to live up to external performance standards. The better you are able to distinguish "you" from your actions, the easier it becomes for you to analyze your strengths and create a powerful negotiating base.

Assess The Worth of Your Services

In analyzing your worth to an employer or client consider these self-analysis questions:

- Am I achieving my goals?
- Am I performing at my peak level in quality and quantity?
- How have I improved my business skills?
- How have I improved my technical skills and knowledge?
- Am I reliable and consistent?
- Do I get my work done on or before deadline?
- Are my clients achieving their desired treatment goals?
- In what ways have I taken initiative?
- How have I contributed to the success of the company?
- Are my relationships with co-workers pleasant and productive?
- How have I improved my leadership abilities?
- In what ways have I given better/more service than I was paid to give?
- If I was my employer/client, would I be satisfied with my performance?

First of all you must be sure that your services are worth more than you now receive. Your financial desires and needs have nothing to do with your worth as an employee or provider of services. Sometimes this can be a very confusing area. You as a person deserve to have all the things you want in life. But, your skills may not be as valuable in the eyes of your company or clients as you would like them to be.

If, when you've finished answering these questions you aren't certain about being qualified to ask for more money—don't worry. Think about the areas you want to improve and set goals to improve your performance. Strengthen the areas that are weak. Take a seminar, read a book—do whatever is necessary for you to grow and improve your skills. Keep track of your accomplishments. Regularly review your accomplishments and ask yourself the self-analysis questions. Then when you feel more confident about your results, proceed with your strategy to create more money.

One of the first steps to preparing your strategy is to determine why you want more money. How long has it been since you received a raise or increased your fees? Find out if your income is comparable to your peers. Review your performance record. Note the times that you have performed well beyond what you were hired to do. Is your desire for more money based upon your needs or your performance? Or do you feel you have logged in enough hours and that alone should justify more money?

The difference between the top money winners on the PGA golf tour and the bottom money winners can be as little as one stroke a day.
— Steve Miller, former PGA tour player

Self-Employed Practitioners ⚞

As a self-employed health care practitioner, you have ultimate control over when and how much to raise your fees. When you have determined a fee increase is required, be certain the amount is appropriate. You will probably lose credibility (and clients) if you raise your rates more than once per year. Do a one-year financial forecast. Ascertain the amount of money you need to charge per session should you experience no growth in your business. Raise your fees accordingly, with a caveat against an increase of greater than 15 percent.

Inform your clients of your rate changes at least two weeks in advance. Springing a higher charge on them at the last moment—particularly right AFTER a session—is very disrespectful. If you offer series discounts, promote goodwill by allowing your clients the opportunity to sign up for a series at the "old" rates. Of course, they need to make this commitment before the new fee structure goes into effect.

Employees ⚞

Getting a raise as an employee requires additional consideration and negotiation. After evaluating yourself and following the preceding guidelines, take stock of the employee benefits you already have. Sometimes employers may not be willing or able to give you more money, but they may be able to increase benefits. Alternatives to cash include: an expense account; a company car; stock options; profit sharing; pension and retirement plans; insurance; paid travel; vacations; use of corporate lodge/resort; professional association dues; educational expenses; memberships to health clubs; tickets to sporting events and theatrical productions; company discount on products or services, nursery and day care centers; and flexible working hours.

Think about how you would spend the extra money you want. Be prepared with alternatives to cash. It's quite likely that right now some of your money is already going toward these items. When negotiating it's always advisable to have options.

The next step in planning your strategy is to research your company's history—how often it has given raises, what is the average percentage increase and what are some of the available perks. Determine your company's, supervisor's and clients' standards for excellence and compare them with your standards. Make certain your perceived priorities are the same as theirs.

The next stage is to compile a list of your accomplishments. Refer back to the self-analysis questions. Write a summary of your accomplishments. Whenever possible, include numbers. Be specific.

Accomplishment Examples

"Clients are completing their treatment courses on or before projected date."
"The number of clients on maintenance programs has increased by 40 percent."
"My department's productivity increased 20 percent."
"My promotion idea garnered us a $15,000 corporate contract."
"Turnover rate has decreased by 50 percent."
"Product sales have increased by 42 percent."
"We were $500 under budget this year."

Also include some of the less tangible results. For example, "Morale has improved," "Case management is more effective" and "I am more organized." Actually, you could figure out how much money you were saving the company even with the intangible results by analyzing the amount of time saved and multiplying that by the average salary per minute. Unfortunately, many people do not understand the financial value of time.

The next step in formulating your strategy is to imagine asking for an increase. Brainstorm the possible objections you might be given and have responses to each one. Include "why" questions—why don't you feel this job is worth $40,000 per year—why don't you think I deserve $35 per hour? We would all hope the discussion wouldn't get to this point, but it's best to be fully prepared. This may seem like a lot of work, but remember, asking for more money is sales—you are selling your talents and abilities.

Here is where the fine art of negotiation comes in. Tailor your presentation to the employer's personality. Be grounded in your capabilities and accomplishments. Remember, timing is very critical. What is a good time for you may not be the right time for the other person. Also, style often wins over substance. Your attitude can make a tremendous impact in negotiating. Before you ask for more money, role-play it. Have it be a win-win experience. Imagine everyone getting what he or she wants. Have a positive mental attitude. You know you and your services are worthy of earning more and you've prepared an excellent presentation. You are now ready to ask for that raise!

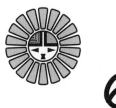

6

Business Management

• Overview •

Wouldn't it be wonderful if you could spend your days working with clients and not bother with the business aspects of your practice? Indeed, if you did that, you might not stay in business for very long—unless you hire others to take care of these aspects—which may be a superb solution. While effective management requires commitment and creativity, it needn't consume a major amount of time or energy.

One of the strangest phenomena is that most corporations spend too much time in planning and managing (thus not enough "doing"), while most small businesses invest little or no time in planning and managing themselves (thus are reactive rather than proactive).

Success strategies for managing a business include staying balanced, aligning your personal growth with your business development, having a written business plan, managing finances (including forecasting, accurate bookkeeping, cash flow management and investments), developing excellent self-management skills, writing goals, creating strategic plans of action, having a business support system, networking, refining communication skills, periodically reviewing all of your goals and plans and most important of all—making sure you have fun!

This chapter on business management focuses on providing you with practical information, forms and techniques to enhance your effectiveness in the actual day-to-day running of your business. Business management is the area most people neglect or avoid, yet it can mean the difference between having a smooth, joyful business and one that's operated by crisis management.

• Choosing Advisors •

Every business has management, legal and accounting aspects. It's important to know people you trust to advise you, particularly in areas where you lack knowledge, interest or skill. Selecting the most appropriate advisors directly affects the success of your business. Before you make any major decisions, discuss them with at least one other person—regardless of your expertise in the area. All too often the tendency is to do it all on your own, and it's almost impossible to be truly objective, especially with something as significant as your business/career. Your primary advisors are your lawyer, accountant, banker and business consultant/coach.

Reliable, affordable and trustworthy counsel is crucial to your business health. Pick the members of your advisory team before you NEED them. Don't wait for an emergency when you may not have ample time to find an appropriate advisor to assist in dealing with the situation at hand. Begin to build your relationships now (particularly with a banker) so you can establish your credibility and develop rapport.

The process for selecting trustworthy advisors begins by getting personal recommendations from friends and colleagues. In addition to the names, get specific information about them. Find out why they recommend these people and what types of dealings they have had with them. Whatever you do, don't stop at this point. You must also make your own assessments. The first thing is to trust your intuition. If you don't feel comfortable with someone—keep looking. Even if you feel good about the person, do further research. She may be an excellent advisor and not appropriate for you.

Check into the potential advisor's credentials and competency. If she has the required expertise and experience, the next phase is to discover if you are compatible. Find out the type of clientele she works with. Has she had many clients in your profession?

Interview potential advisors (make certain this initial consultation is free of charge). See if your personalities and styles mesh. This is someone you are going to work with for a long time. It's important that you share a similar philosophy and manner in which you like to get things done.

Assess your level of confidence and trust in this person—professionally and personally. How well you are able to communicate with each other is one of the most critical factors in choosing an advisor. This person may be totally qualified, works with many others in your profession, has an impeccable character and shares many of the

Experience is a good teacher, but her fees are very high.
— W.R. Inge

Accepting good advice increases one's own ability.
— Goethe

same beliefs as you, but it seems as though whenever you talk, you are speaking in two different languages. You have to decide whether or not it's worth the time (and money) it takes to work through the communication barriers to have this person be an advisor.

Finally, you have to determine if this person desires to have *you* as a client. Does she demonstrate a sense of commitment to you and your business? Is she available to answer questions when you need them? Finding appropriate advisors isn't always an easy task, but it can mean the difference between business difficulties (or even failure) and success.

• Policies and Procedures •

Lots of folks confuse bad management with destiny.
— Kin Hubbard

With respect to business operations, it's almost an imperative to have written policies and procedures (particularly if you are in a group practice or if you have employees). A Policy and Procedure Manual sets the tone for your business and helps you avoid potential conflicts. Policies are built on your philosophy regarding your practice; procedures are specific steps based on how you want to run the day-to-day details of the business.

Take the time to formulate your policies and create a written manual—even if you are the only person in your business. By going through this process, you may discover conflicts or potential risky situations, and thus be able to address and resolve these issues before they actually arise. Also, if you decide to expand your practice and hire staff (or bring in an associate), the transition will be easier if the operational guidelines are already established.

If you work for someone else, discuss the current policies and procedures with your employer. You may find that you can add to or alter them.

Policy Manual

Policies are generally divided into two branches—internal company policies and client interaction policies. In designing a policy manual, begin with a statement of your company's purpose, priorities and goals. Describe your qualifications, requirements and expectations of your staff. Be certain to explain exactly how you want these policies manifested. Include general personality requirements, educational standards, chain of command, work hours and schedule, salary, raises, overtime, pay dates, leaves of absence, tardiness, sick leave, bonuses, benefits package, reviews and evaluations, personnel records, grievance procedures, phone use, dress code and hygiene, smoking, medication, parking, employee purchasing procedures and discounts (of services and products), actions requiring discipline and specific consequences, disciplinary procedures, grounds for termination and (most importantly) customer relations.

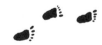

See Chapter Eight, pages 221-226 for additional information on client policies.

Procedure Manual ～

A procedure manual defines the methods you have chosen to operate your business. In creating your procedure manual, begin by describing how you want to commence each working day (what needs to be done the moment the first person arrives to open the facility). Delineate the important daily activities. Include how the phone should be answered, the handling of paperwork and client files (particularly crucial if you are billing insurance), the care and operation of equipment, how to write up sales, safety procedures and what to do in case of an emergency, bookkeeping, the desired manner for carrying out routine business activities, the stages of client interaction (the way you want clients to be greeted, the forms they need to fill out, financial arrangements, rescheduling, dispensing educational materials) and the procedures for closing the business at the end of the day.

Risk Management

The concept behind Risk Management is to minimize the risk a company has for physical, emotional and mental liability toward its employees, product liability, client and visitor liability, and as insurance liabilities for loss due to circumstances such as theft, fire and chemical hazards, neglect and misuse. Many large companies have separate Risk Management Departments, whose sole purpose is to analyze the physical layout of buildings, prepare ergonomically designed work space, assist employees in being comfortable (therefore more productive) in their working conditions, look for various hazards, make sure comprehensive and liability insurance coverages are adequate, and assess and develop plans for any other problems that put the company "at risk."

Within the realm of a small business, the concept of risk management (managing and therefore minimizing any risk you may be open to) is nonetheless important.

For further information, contact the Occupational Safety and Health Administration (OSHA) which may be listed in the state government section of the phone book under the heading "Industrial Commission" or "State Compensation Fund, Legal Division."

Risk Management Factors

- The condition of the building you are in.
- The escape routes in case of fire.
- How you position yourself as you work.
- Developing methods to mitigate repetitive use syndrome.
- Making sure you have adequate malpractice, liability and medical coverage.
- Ample lighting (particularly if people work at night).
- Potential hazards for clients as they use your facilities.
- Employee stress levels.
- Proper use of equipment.

After analyzing your working and client conditions at all levels, take care of any problems which can be eliminated and make plans to minimize any that you cannot completely resolve. In a nutshell, manage your risks before they become problems that manage you.

- Describe your philosophy toward your profession in general.
- Describe your philosophy and attitude toward your business in particular.
- Describe how you want to run your business.
- Sketch your procedure manual.
- List your policies for staff.

• Embracing Technology •

Many people avoid technology out of fear or misconceptions about the knowledge needed to operate the equipment and the cost. Time is the most important commodity business owners possess. Despite the learning curve and expenditures, the time saved, increased productivity and enhanced service provided more than compensates. Utilizing various combinations of communication techniques and devices enables you to stay connected at local, regional, national and international levels—which can improve and expand your business as well as yourself.

As with everything you purchase, check the warranties and keep all documentation.

Streamlining your business with the proper equipment choices is essential to efficient business practice and development. First, you must identify your needs.

Technology Needs Questions

- Will it reduce my expenses?
- Will it increase my income?
- Will it save me time?
- How much will maintenance and supplies cost?
- How long will it take me or how much will it cost to install?
- Am I willing to make the effort to learn how to properly use and maintain the equipment and software I need?

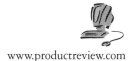

www.productreview.com

Even though there appears to be a lot of information here, it's only the tip of the iceberg. Yes, there is more technology out there than you can imagine, but when you define your needs and begin your research, you will find that it's indeed manageable. You can be its master and have it serve you well professionally and personally. One word of caution: with today's ability to be in contact at all times, it's necessary to establish boundaries for yourself and your clients. You are entitled to your personal life, as are others. It's way too easy to misuse high-tech equipment and the people it serves.

The following is a brief overview of some of the current technology and ideas on how to best utilize them.

Telephones ～～～

What could possibly be said about a telephone besides the obvious: every business needs one. They've come a long way from the rotary dial, single line phone of only a few years ago. Today we have different styles of phones to accommodate various services that are available such as caller ID, call waiting, call forwarding, voice messaging, and computer links.

See Chapter Eight, pages 222-228 for ideas on phone etiquette.

Phones come with features such as LCD panels, conference calling capabilities, multiple lines, redial, mute buttons and on and on. They can be desktop models (with and without answering machines), cordless and cellular.

The telephone is your primary link with clients, associates and vendors—in effect, all aspects of your business. Choosing the services and appropriate phone system is paramount. Research the different models and contact a phone representative to assist you in making the best choices for your circumstances.

Popular Telephone Services

Not all services are available for desktop, cordless and cellular phones; often the determining factor is the actual phone model (e.g., you can get caller ID with some cellular phones, but not others).

Caller ID: This can be used with either an LCD panel or a separate box that can be purchased. When a call comes in, the caller's name and number are displayed (unless they have blocked that capability or the number is outside the phone company's tracking area). Sometimes clients call and don't leave a message. Caller ID informs you who was trying to contact you and you can call them. Another interesting feature available in conjunction with Caller ID is Customized Messages. Phones with answering machines allow you to store personal messages keyed to play only when certain numbers come in. This allows you to make arrangements with clients or associates even though you may not be available to answer the phone.

Last Call Return (*69): This feature allows you to get the phone number of the last person who called. This service is available to most customers on a pay per use basis or a monthly subscription.

Call Waiting: While talking, you hear a tone and this service allows you to know when another call is coming in. By hitting the "flash" button on your phone or tapping the receiver button, you can put your current call on hold and answer the incoming call. This is especially convenient when you are expecting an important call or a client needs to speak to you urgently.

Call Forwarding: This feature re-directs ("forwards") your calls to another number where you may be or where someone can take messages for you.

Features and Accessories for Desktop Phones

Data Port: This reduces the clutter from wires around your desk by providing a jack on the phone for your modem line.

Headsets: When making several calls in a row, having a headset is far more comfortable than holding a phone. If you need to write while talking, a headset frees you from craning your neck to wedge a handset in place.

Message Lamp: Lets you know you have messages waiting with a blinking light.

Multiple Lines: In addition to allowing more than one person to place calls at the same time, multiple lines provide the capability to put one person on hold while you talk with someone else and enables you to do multiple tasks (e.g., talk on one line while sending a fax on another), and even connect the lines for conference calls.

Telephone Directory Memory: Some phones allow you to program in names and phone numbers for quick access.

Features and Accessories for Cordless Phones

While these phones give you the freedom to roam within a few hundred feet of the base station, they experience much more interference and static than desktop models. They also require batteries and recharging. Some manufacturers make multiple line cordless phones.

Antennae: Flexible or retractable antennae provide better reception and are less likely to be banged into and broken.

Bandwidth: For greater performance, it's suggested that you get a digital cordless phone with a bandwidth of 900 MHz. Reception is clearer and distance is farther than the analog 46-48 MHz models.

Channels: A multiple-channel phone gives you a better chance of finding a good signal path than a single-channel phone.

Features and Accessories for Cellular Phones

Not only are cellular phones important for emergencies while traveling, they can provide convenience in setting appointments, contacting clients and conducting business while in transit or in an area where a phone isn't available.

There are three types of cellular phones: mobile phones which mount in the car and include a booster battery in the trunk; hand-held phones that are one piece, self-contained phones that you can put in your briefcase or purse; and transportable phones—specifically designed for use in remote places, have heightened signal trackers and separate battery packs for use outside of your car.

Caution:
Be careful and attentive if you must drive, dial and talk. It's a distraction and can cause an accident. Consider pulling over to make calls.

Cellular phones also come in various power strengths so your choice is best determined by how you plan to use it. If you are going to be traveling a lot, a transportable phone with a higher range will provide greater access over longer distances. A mobile phone lacks the power, although you can purchase a car adaptor with a three-watt booster to reach remote cellular towers. I know someone who has a mobile unit for the car and a transportable not only for remote access, but to carry when hiking and away from the car.

Any-Button Answer: Lets you push any button to answer the phone.

Built-In Pager: This feature allows you to screen your calls by flashing the caller's number.

Computer or Fax Ability: Just plug a cellular fax/modem into the phone from your computer and transmit your data.

Dual-NAM or Multi-NAM (Number Assignment Module): Your phone can be linked to two or more cellular carriers.

Hands-Free Speakerphone: You can talk and drive more safely than grabbing and holding onto the phone. It really helps when making those turns.

Roam Alert: Your "roaming" charges are expensive and this feature beeps you when you've left your local area.

Voice-Activated Dialing: A safety feature that allows you to dial by voice thus keeping those hands on the wheel, or in the event of a medical emergency.

Pagers ~~~

These relatively inexpensive gadgets have low monthly fees and provide you with 24-hour access nationwide. You can now purchase pagers in colors, designs and even with Warner Bros.® characters on them. You can choose between numeric pagers and alphanumeric pagers that show you the phone number and a short message. There are two-way pagers that let you receive a message and respond directly from the unit. There are also voice pagers that serve as a portable answering machine/pager combination.

Message Systems ~~~

For those times in session or away from the office, there must be a system in place to receive your business calls. Some people use answering machines, others voice mail and some use a combination of both. Many practitioners utilize answering services so their business contacts can speak with a person.

Answering Machines

Answering machines vary in cost and capability. They provide a means to stay in communication with clients and business associates. Make sure you have a brief, warm, informational greeting (be aware of background noise) and that your machine works properly. There is nothing more annoying than a beep that is loud and shrill and goes on for what seems like forever. It's also helpful to be able to retrieve messages from remote phones by punching in an access code.

Answering Services

Answering services provides a human touch which is often lacking in the business world, but also leaves things open to human error. Find a service that has a track record for accuracy, dependability and timeliness. Make sure to provide all pertinent information regarding your practice so questions can be answered correctly, give your service up-to-date scheduling information if they are providing that service, and stay in communication with the service on a regular basis throughout your day.

See Chapter Eight, page 230 for ideas on how to effectively utilize an answering service.

Voice Mail

Voice mail is electronic messaging. I have found that voice mail is more dependable and more easily accessible than an answering machine. One of the prime benefits is that many people can call at the same time and not receive a busy signal. Most services can receive at least 15 simultaneous calls. The monthly service fee is well worth the uninterrupted service and ease of retrieving messages. Again, create a welcoming greeting providing necessary information.

Fax Machines ～

Fax machines come in two major styles; a stand-alone model or a hardware/ software combination you install on your computer. Even with the advent of the fax/modem, a stand-alone fax machine still comes in pretty handy. It's usually easier to put a document through the fax machine than to scan it into the computer, attach it to your fax and send it.

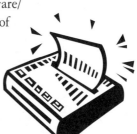

The biggest choice to make with fax machines is whether to use thermal paper or plain paper. Thermal paper units cost less and are smaller in size, but the paper itself is expensive. Also, thermal paper tends to fade within a short time which means you need to copy important information you wish to have for future use. Changing the paper rolls takes a little more time than putting paper into a paper tray and the paper cutter in the machine can jam. Plain paper faxes are more expensive, larger in size and need to have the ink cartridges replaced. However, the paper is less expensive, the print is sharper and it doesn't fade. Plain paper faxes are a wise option if you work with detailed or graphic information. And if you need to keep copies, it's easier on the environment and quickly pays for itself in time and money saved having to make copies.

Features

Auto-dial: Important feature if you frequently send faxes to the same numbers.

Broadcasting: The ability to send the same document to multiple destinations. This requires page memory.

Call sensing: The fax picks up on the incoming tone and bypasses voice calls by forwarding them to the handset or an extension (this feature is fairly standard now).

Delayed Transmission: Saves money by sending faxes after business hours when rates are lower.

Some fax machines have a simple copy feature.

Paper Capacity: As with printers, plain paper faxes can carry 100, 150 or 500 sheets. Thermal paper comes in two standard sizes of paper rolls. Getting a machine that uses the larger roll means not having to change it as often or having your faxes interrupted as much when the paper runs out.

Photocopiers ⁓

Photocopiers range from very simple, relatively inexpensive desktop units to machines that do everything except go to the post office for you. You can spend a couple hundred dollars or many thousands depending on what you need. Having quick access to a copier can save time (not having to run out to make a few copies) and provide clients with important information without having them wait.

Choosing a copier can be an adventure since there are so many that do different tasks at varying speeds. Again, deciding on your needs will narrow the field. Copier companies are willing to bring machines to you for a trial period. Pick out several brands and see how they work. Compare features, cost per copy, maintenance agreement coverages and costs, trade-in allowances for the future, speed and service availability. Over the years, having a full maintenance agreement covering all parts and labor has saved us time and money.

Word Processors and Desktop Computers ⁓

Until the 1980s, most office documentation was done on a typewriter. Then word processing typewriters arrived on the scene, offering the typewriter's ease of use, and additional features (such as the ability to make undetectable corrections) and limited memory (so you don't have to retype common passages). Now most offices use computer-based word processors for the majority of their written applications.

Choosing a computer is as individual a process as picking out your clothes. What suits one person may not suit another. The two most popular computers are IBM and Macintosh with various types of "clones" available. The IBM personal computer and its clones are often referred to as PCs—and all use an Intel® microprocessor, such as 386, 486 or Pentium®. PCs are most commonly supplied with Microsoft® Windows operating system; the Macintosh has the MacOS operating system.

Despite advertising claims, computers are not like toasters—they are more like automobiles. There is more to owning a computer than simply buying it and plugging it in the wall. You need to learn the special terminology (e.g., megabyte, RAM and hard disk), perform regular maintenance (e.g., file organization, cleaning and back-ups), buy accessories, and keep fueling it with additional memory and a faster processor (a bigger engine is always more fun).

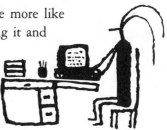

While Macintosh still rules when it comes to graphics and is extremely user-friendly, it isn't as popular as Windows. Windows dominates the market and the programs for PCs are generally less expensive than for Macintosh. The system power and speed requirements depend on how you plan to use your computer.

First determine what you want the computer to do. Then decide which software you want. Software choices often determine computer choice due to many factors such as the amount of disk space the programs will use and the speed you want. Some programs are only available for one platform.

Mail order is a source for saving on computer hardware and software costs. However, you need to be fairly computer literate to choose what you need, install additional hardware, load programs and learn how to use the software. If you aren't confident about your computer knowledge, establish a relationship with a local supplier who can furnish you with recommendations and continued support after purchases are made.

There are computer consultants available who design systems based on your needs, help you get the best prices, provide tutoring and troubleshoot problems. Of course, you will be paying for their services in addition to the costs of hardware and software.

Once you know what you want, get supplier referrals from associates and friends. Call each one and explain your needs. Ask for price quotes, clarify what free bundled software comes with the system (some include word processing software, calendar programs and games), determine warranty information and ascertain service time frames. Discuss purchasing and leasing options. Obtain pricing on each component of your system and then ask for a package deal to include the entire system, training, maintenance agreement and support. Be sure to shop around in order to get the best price.

Should you decide on a PC or MAC clone, be sure the RAM chips are all made by the same manufacturer (otherwise you can have some very weird experiences) and that your vendor has been in business for at least five years. Buying a "home-made" clone can provide savings, but those savings erode into costly expenses if the vendor disappears. Unlike name brands such as IBM, Texas Instruments, Radio Shack, Apple or Compaq who stand behind their products, mom and pop computer builders may not be around when you need them and parts may become difficult to find.

Computer Features and Hardware Accessories

CD-ROM Drives: Many programs contain so much information that it's unwieldy to use floppy disks. Some programs (particularly those with a lot of graphics) are not available on floppy disk. CD-ROM drives are standard equipment on new computers. For older computers, you can mount a CD-ROM drive internally or work off the external parallel port (you can usually share the same port that is used for the printer). Avoid drives slower than 4X drives. (The nX refers to how much faster the data transfer rate is than the original CD player speed.)

Expansion Slots: Make sure you have enough slots to utilize all the features you want and then add at least one more.

Expansion Bays: Not everyone needs additional peripherals like a back-up drive or second hard disk—but if you do, make sure you have the bays available.

Fax/Modem: Put a fax/modem on your computer and you gain access to a vast amount of information and can easily (and inexpensively) connect with colleagues and clients worldwide. Different types of modems are available and choosing one depends on your need for speed. Don't settle for anything less than a 28.8Kbps model so you can surf the net with the best. Modems provide the physical means for electronically connecting to e-mail, the Internet and World Wide Web. You can choose from a variety of software programs for e-mail and Internet access.

A Fax/Modem provides you with fax capability to send and receive electronic documents. Someone with a fax machine can send a fax directly to your computer and you can send a fax from the computer to a fax machine or to another computer with a fax receiver.

Hard Drive: At the very least 500 MB and with today's programs, 1GB (gigabyte) is easy to fill up.

Main Memory: Don't go any lower than 16MB (megabyte) of RAM (random access memory). Be sure to check the requirements of your programs. At the time of this writing, 64 MB is becoming standard for programs and operating systems.

Microprocessor: The Intel 486 chip can still be useful for basic word processing and limited applications such as Quicken®. To save having to upgrade, it's suggested that you get the Pentium chip running at a clock rate of at least 75 megahertz (MHz); 100 MHz or more is preferable. For the Macintosh look for the PowerPC chip at the same clock-rate as the Intel chip.

Monitor Size: A 15-inch monitor is the standard for desktop computers. Graphics users prefer at least a 17-inch monitor. A larger monitor provides greater working space and vivid color—it's easier on your eyes and more fun to work with.

Monitor Image: Two things to look at are the dot pitch and refresh rate. The dot pitch is the distance between the centers of the colored dots that make up the screen.

Don't go above 0.28mm for sharp images. The refresh rate is how often the image on screen is drawn. The monitor's sharpness and speed is determined by the refresh rate. Look for 70Hz to 76 Hz (cycles per second) rate.

Physical Configuration: There are two basic types of enclosures—a box that sits on your desk (a "desktop") and a "tower" which stands vertically and usually is placed next to or under your work space with the monitor on the desk.

Sound: Macintosh always comes with built-in sound and now it's in stereo. Although it's becoming more standard for higher-end PCs to come with built-in sound capability, you may need to purchase the function separately. Look for 16-bit stereo sound.

Video Capability: The PCI (Peripheral Components Interconnect) local bus is standard on the Macintosh and new PCs. The amount of VRAM (video memory) determines the display resolution and color depth. One MB of VRAM is minimal for basic applications. If you work with graphics, consider at least two MBs.

Top 10 Reasons to Buy a Computer

1. Keep up with the Information Age.
2. Communicate with friends, family, colleagues and the online public.
3. Access information and research.
4. Manage your business.
5. Maintain client files.
6. Bill insurance electronically.
7. Create documents with desktop publishing.
8. Archive data.
9. Educate yourself.
10. Entertainment.

Top 5 Reasons to Wait

1. Cost of purchase and upkeep.
2. Time required to learn how to use it.
3. Misuse.
4. Lack of privacy.
5. Obsolescence.

Portable (Notebook) Computers ~

Portable computers have the same capacity and features as desktop computers, but give you the convenience of bringing them with you. A notebook (also commonly referred to as a laptop) computer can be used as your primary computer, a presentation tool (with multimedia programs) or a secondary computer while traveling.

Features to Consider

Additional Batteries: You need an additional battery if you plan to use your portable on a plane or in an area with no electrical outlet. The following are battery types in order of longevity: lithium ion, nickel-metal hydride and nickel-cadmium.

Battery Life: Your battery will usually last two to four hours with constant access to the hard drive. However, most portables come with software that helps manage power use to maximize battery life (generally doubling the minimum time).

Pointing Device: Your choices include trackballs, trackpads or keyboard buttons called trackpoints. The trackpad is the most popular (utilizing your finger as the means to get around the screen). Next are trackpoints and then the trackball. The standard mouse is awkward on the lap.

Power Supply: While most portables come with external AC adapters, some have built-in power supplies which means all you need is a power cord and an AC outlet.

Weight: You are looking at carrying around about six pounds plus the weight of an adapter, a cord, batteries, carrying case, disks and whatever else fits in your case. There are sub-notebooks available that weight around four pounds plus paraphernalia.

Once technology is out of the jar, you can't put it back in.
— Ervin L. Glaspy

Personal Digital Assistants (PDAs) ⚬

For many business people, notebook computers are unwieldy. PDAs are compact (hand-held) and travel easily. These units allow you to do limited computing and electronic communication. You can connect them to your computer and/or electronic notebook and transfer information. Most of these nifty devices come with rather small keypads but are equipped with electronic pens. These lightweight assistants can help you schedule meetings while on the run, take notes during meetings, track expenses, write letters while hanging in the air, make airline reservations, check your e-mail and do market research on the Net. There are many models on the market; the most popular ones are the Sharp Zaurus, the PalmPilot and Zion PSION. While they are high tech and really cute, they aren't as user-friendly as or as diverse in use as a portable computer.

Printers ⚬

The two most widely used printers are laser and inkjet printers. Inkjet printers spray tiny droplets of ink into patterns on a page. Inkjet printers are primarily used for color and can be purchased for under $300. If you mainly use your printer for black-and-white printing (e.g., correspondence and basic marketing materials) consider the laser printer. Laser printers use a laser to electrostatically imprint information on a page (this eliminates the smudging problems often encountered with inkjet printers). They are faster, quieter and provide the clearest print. Color laser printers are becoming more popular, although the cost is usually prohibitive for most businesses—with the exception of the graphics industry. At Sohnen-Moe Associates, Inc. we have several laser printers and one color inkjet printer (for producing announcements and overhead transparencies).

Features to Consider

Energy Use: Laser printers consume more electricity than most office equipment (except for copiers). Look for features such as a sleep mode to conserve energy.

Fonts: Laser and inkjet printers usually come with a variety of fonts. You can add more by downloading them from your computer.

Memory: If you are using only text, 2MB of RAM may be enough. Venturing into graphics or large files require at least 4MB.

Page Description Language (PDL): This is the built-in software that allows a page to print. The two most common languages are PostScript and Hewlett-Packard's Printer Control Language (PCL). Make sure to get the latest versions. PostScript is better for complex text and graphics combinations, but is usually an optional feature (which means more money).

Paper Capacity: Trays generally hold 50, 100, 250 or 500 sheets of 8.5 x 11 paper. Some printers have multiple paper trays in addition to a manual feed slot. Legal-size (8.5 x 14) and 11 x 17 trays are optional (although not all printers can accommodate these larger trays).

Resolution: 300 dots per inch (dpi) really doesn't make it any longer. 600 dpi in both laser and inkjet are affordable and provide far better graphic and text quality.

Speed: Usually four pages per minute is adequate, but can seem inordinately slow when you are printing large or complex documents. Many printers allow for added memory, which enhances speed.

Toner: You usually get 3,000 sheets of printed paper from a cartridge of toner. Of course it depends on the type of printing you do and how much dark area you use.

Weight and size: This can be important depending upon the amount of space you have in your office setting. Remember, you need to account for the paper feeder and how far it extends from the printer and whether it's in the back or front.

Software ⁓

Software programs can reduce the drudge work of financial record keeping, updating client files (computerize your records with a database to track and update information available at your fingertips), and correspondence (easy editing of letters and the ability to use "form" letters to save time). You don't necessarily need sophisticated database programs, WordPerfect® and Microsoft Word® may provide all the features

Before you purchase software or hardware, call the manufacturer's toll-free help line. How they handle your call (e.g., if you can't get through, are put on hold for what seems like an eternity or they don't promptly return messages) will help you determine whether you want to deal with them.

Client Management and Insurance Billing Software

Business Touch™
29 N Charlotte St
Lombard, IL 60148
708-691-8141
BizTouch@aol.com

Easy Billing™
524 Don Gaspar
Santa Fe, NM 87501
800-618-6136; 505-982-5321
easybilling@nets.com
www.nets.com/easybilling

you need. By using simple clip art you can create your own fliers, brochures and various mailings. These programs can also be a boon to marketing with the ability to print address labels with a push of a button or do mail merges for sending out groups of letters.

The software available today is astounding: word processing; accounting; list management; Personal Information Managers (PIMs) which includes calendars, schedulers, address books; 3-D interactive anatomy; desktop publishing; and just about anything else you might imagine.

What is exciting about computer technology is you can decide on what you need and create the system (software and hardware) that will serve you the best.

Features Software Can Provide

Accessing Information: Utilize database programs to provide accurate analysis of any part of your business by setting up fields for the information, compiling them into reports and printing them out—all in a matter of minutes. For example, you can choose a single client or group of clients to contact with information (all based on certain criteria you select, such as locale or profession), analyze how often certain modalities are being requested and can evaluate the effectiveness of your advertising (by setting fields to tell you which resources referred clients).

Record keeping and Financial Analysis: Simplify your bookkeeping efforts and reduce the amount of time spent in record keeping. This type of software allows you to print checks from your computer (thus eliminating multiple entries because it automatically puts the information in all the appropriate places). You can examine expenses by category and do financial projections. Preparing taxes becomes a matter of a simple command stroke and *voilà*! everything you or your accountant needs is in a printed report.

Personal Information Managers (PIMs): Computer calendars and address books help you manage your time and can automatically remind you about appointments, birthdays and follow-up calls....

Client Management: These programs range in features from keeping client charts, preparing insurance billing forms, analyzing information, invoicing and sending follow-up correspondence.

Marketing Strategies: Once you establish your marketing strategy, the computer can become your best line of assistance in implementing your plan. With the ability to set criteria, select appropriate clients and do functions such as mail merge and labeling, you can get yourself out to your target market quickly.

Desktop Publishing: Many programs are available to assist in the design of business cards, brochures, fliers, announcements and newsletters. Some word processing software programs include basic desktop publishing, but most people purchase a separate program. The price (and commensurate features) range from less than $50 to nearly $1,000. Most of these programs come with templates so all you have to do is type in the text. Several paper companies design products to work with these templates.

The Internet

The Internet is the focal point for the "information superhighway," providing electronic data access and exchange. The Internet is most popularly used for electronic mail (e-mail). What a blast to confer with colleagues around the world and keep up with the cutting edge in your field! There's an indescribable feeling when you open your e-mail and there's something for you from the Ukraine, Barcelona or Zimbabwe.

If you are interested in other features, such as research, you also need to connect to the World Wide Web (www). You access the Web through a web browser, such as Netscape® Navigator or Microsoft Internet Explorer.®

The SBA Small Business Classroom ofers Internet business classes. Go to www.sba.gov and click on "SBA Classroom."

See Chapter Nine, pages 332-333
for ideas on how health care providers utilize the Web to promote their practices.

• Insurance Reimbursement •

Accepting insurance can be an incredible boon to your business. Oftentimes it can be the determining factor in whether or not a potential client chooses you as their health care provider. Unfortunately, if you are not recognized by the insurance companies as a "primary" health giver, this process can be cumbersome. Insurance companies are more inclined to honor insurance claims if you work with a medical doctor or an osteopathic physician (and sometimes a chiropractic physician) and the doctor does the billing. The three types of major insurance claims are: third party (general medical health), workers' compensation and personal injury.

Let's look at the insurance industry itself. From a consumer's point of view, most of us think about health insurance as a way to ensure that our health care costs will be covered in case of a serious illness or accident and as a means to assist in the payment for our well-being (to prevent major illness). What we tend to forget is that insurance companies are just that—companies. And as such, one of their major priorities is to make a profit. Very few insurance companies hold altruistic beliefs as their main purpose for being in business; we must always remember that when contemplating the role of the insurance industry.

Currently insurance reimbursement is rather hit-or-miss, particularly with third-party claims. A lot seems to depend upon the mood of the claims adjustor. A company might honor a claim one time and refuse payment on the next submission. Each company has different general rules and regulations regarding coverage and payment. Keep in mind that each insurance company writes many different types of policies and each of those policies has its own guidelines. You may have conflicting experiences from the same carrier due to a difference in the terms of the policies. For example, you may have gotten prompt payment one time and then the next time been refused payment for the same exact service—the distinction being that it was with two different clients and thus two separate policies. It can be very confusing! Even if you are considered a primary health provider, it's recommended that you also verify each policy's specific requirements and allowances. You can't always predict if the company will authorize payments, the total amount they will cover or the number of sessions they will allow. Unfortunately, verifying the coverage of a specific policy doesn't guarantee payment. I know of an instance in which a massage therapist obtained verbal pre-approval for massage treatment (complete with an approval code number) for one of her clients, only to have the claim later rejected.

Workers' compensation supplies a significant amount of the money that goes toward health care. To receive direct payment under workers' compensation, you need to have a health care provider's number. If you are a primary caregiver, you can use your identification number in most states, while others require a separate number. If you are not the primary caregiver, you usually can still receive a code number, but you must also get a prescriptive referral from the primary caregiver for each case. You need to consult with the proper agency to get accurate information for obtaining your number and learn the required procedures for filling out the paperwork. There

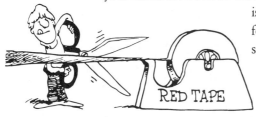

isn't a national bureau, so you have to contact the agency for your specific state. To find the agency, look under the state government section in the phone book for a category titled either "State Compensation Fund," "Industrial Workers' Insurance" or "Workers' Compensation Board." If you still are unable to locate the appropriate agency, call the general information number.

Personal injury claims are handled differently than most other types of insurance cases. Customarily, you submit the bill directly to the claims adjuster or the attorney. In most instances, they cover everything. Again, if you are not the attending physician, you need a prescription from one. One of the drawbacks to working with personal injury clients is that you usually don't receive payment for your services until the case is resolved (which sometimes takes years).

It's advisable to check with the insurance carrier for each client. You may need to call the local representative to get the name and number of the person with whom to talk at the main office. Getting pre-approval for services can be very helpful in receiving payment. **Always** note the name of the person you are talking with and (if possible) get a code for approved service. Obtaining written insurance verification provides you with the most protection.

See Appendix A,
pages 397-408
for insurance-related forms.

So many practitioners are pinning a lot of hopes on the insurance industry. Look what it has done in general to enhance the medical profession in terms of recognition and financial compensation. The most recent example of this benefit is evidenced in the chiropractic field. We've all heard people say how much the other health care providers' credibility will increase as more and more insurance companies cover their services. Perhaps so, but at what cost? Until recently, I was convinced of the enormous benefit that nationwide insurance reimbursement could be to the allied health care profession. If these services become acceptable billable modalities under all third-party insurance coverage, then it makes this field a much more viable career path because more money will be available to cover these services. And truthfully, we know that many people will only utilize health care services that are covered by insurance. Unfortunately, the costs are also very high. First of all, there's the tremendous amount of paperwork involved: Filling out appropriate records, keeping Subjective Objective Assessment Plan (SOAP) charts, and filing the proper claim forms. And then there's standardization of fees. But the area that concerns me the most has to do with the potential regulations and regimentation regarding the actual treatment.

Insurance companies are already actively dictating to the health care community the types of treatments they can perform. Since the insurance companies are paying for these procedures, they are imposing strict guidelines as to what is considered acceptable care and under what conditions. Even if they agree to cover additional services, what type will they cover? As insurance reimbursement becomes more common, the insurance industry will most likely impose more stringent guidelines. You may find yourself becoming more of a technician than a health care provider.

For instance, in British Columbia, massage is covered under its Medical Services Plan. Patients are able to see registered massage therapists (with a physician's referral) for up to 12 visits. Unless patients are exempt from paying the user fee, there is $10 co-payment per visit. The good side to this is that it makes massage available to anyone. Also, the demand for RMTs is very high. Yet all is not rosy. About 50 percent of the massage therapists have "opted-out" of the system, not wanting to conform to "performing" 20-minute treatments. Those therapists decided that having an essentially guaranteed income was not enough; they wanted the freedom to practice their own techniques.

As you can see, guaranteed insurance reimbursement is not necessarily great—it isn't the powerful panacea that many hope for in terms of providing additional sources of income. As we progress in this arena, we must strive to keep the integrity and diversity of our work intact. I think it's possible to have the whole spectrum of allied health care covered by insurance and be able to provide varied techniques. To accomplish this, we must make a concerted effort to educate the primary care providers and the members of the insurance industry about the different therapies and their specific benefits.

Choosing whether to accept insurance reimbursement clients (or even developing associations with primary care providers in order to gain referrals) is a major decision. The potential advantages are higher fees and an increased client load. The disadvantages include masses of paperwork, possible regimentation, the potential of not receiving compensation for your work and the time lag between provided service and remittance.

You can spend a lot of time in verifying policies and filling out paperwork. That is why many practitioners don't accept insurance claims. They require the client to pay them directly for the services, and then the client must submit a voucher to his own insurance company (or attorney) for reimbursement.

In the best of all possible worlds practitioners would be fairly and promptly reimbursed for delivering a competent service of proven effectiveness. Until (and even after) we reach that stage, you must weigh the tradeoffs inherent in tangling with the insurance bureaucracy, realizing that as your business grows, you may change your mind.

The following insurance reimbursement information is excerpted from *The Insurance Reimbursement Manual* by Christine Rosche, M.P.H. For individual and group consultations, contact Bodytherapy Business Institute at 1-800-888-1516.

Overview for Non-Primary Care Providers ⟞

The complementary health care field has grown to become more recognized as an insurance-eligible member of mainstream health care. Many insurance carriers, including recognized managed care companies such as HealthNet and Oxford Health Plans, are seeking qualified practitioners to join their pool of preferred providers. Medical doctors, chiropractors, physical therapists and many other primary care providers are referring more patients to complementary practitioners than ever before. As alternative health care centers open around the country, there is a growing need for qualified practitioners to join the staffs.

Consider these recent developments:
- In 1996, Washington became the first state to legally require all insurance companies to pay for alternative therapies, including massage therapy. Other states have similar legislation pending and a growing number of insurance carriers are including alternative therapies in their benefit plans.

- Many physicians, chiropractors, osteopaths and other providers want to see changes in laws and professional standards that support complementary health care therapies. They also support using case studies and articles which communicate the benefits of the specific services to insurance companies.

- Studies continue to show that consumers use touch therapy and other alternative services regularly and want insurance coverage for them. For example, in the *New England Journal of Medicine* (January 28, 1993) 34 percent of respondents in a survey reported using at least one unconventional therapy in the past year. In 1990, Americans made an estimated 425 million visits to providers of unconventional therapy and spent $13.7 billion. About 75 percent of these payments were "out-of-pocket," or not covered by insurance. This number exceeds the number of visits to all U.S. primary care physicians (388 million) and suggests a long-term shift in how patients choose their medical services and providers.

- The Touch Research Institute of Miami, Florida, has published numerous significant research findings on the clinical benefits of massage.

- The new Office of Alternative Medicine at the National Institutes of Health continues to fund ongoing research in complementary medicine.

- Television, radio, magazine and newspaper coverage calls attention to this "health care revolution." Traditional (allopathic) medicine and alternative/complementary therapies are blending and cooperating to offer more integrated treatment.

- *Life Magazine* (September 1996) ran a health care article with the headline, "Surgery or Acupuncture? Antibiotics or Herbs? Both are Better." The subhead underneath read, "More and more M.D.s are mixing ancient science and new science to treat everything from the common cold to heart disease." The August 1997 issue of *Life Magazine's* cover article featured "The Magic of Touch: Massage's Healing Powers Make it Serious Medicine."

The Medical Model ～～

To solve the insurance reimbursement puzzle you need to understand a few basic facts about medicine as it's practiced in the Western world and the insurance system that has grown up around it. In the West (meaning all those societies that trace their cultural and scientific origins from Greece and Rome), doctors have traditionally practiced what is called allopathic medicine based on the Western medical model. Common symptoms are classified into disease entities and scientific conclusions, which are based on verifiable observations. The Western doctor cures disease by treating the patient, who tends to passively receive it. Also, in the West health has been defined as the absence of disease or physical symptoms.

By contrast, Eastern medicine is based on what might be called the growth or balance model. The Oriental health practitioner studies life force or vital energy. She considers subjective sources of data, takes a broader view of the individual that includes his energetic and spiritual dimensions, and defines health as a range of states along a continuum of internal and environmental balance. This approach seeks to understand and consider all possible factors affecting a person's health and well-being. The Eastern practitioner (and her increasing number of Western students) sees the client as an active, contributing partner in the health treatment plan.

The Insurance Industry ～～

The insurance industry's operations can be quite complicated, but the idea behind it is simple. Insurance pools together the money of a large number of people in order to have a fund to reimburse the few individuals who experience a loss. Regardless of the kind of risk it protects against (e.g., fire, theft, accident, disease) an insurance company makes a profit by taking in more money in premiums than it pays out in claims. (A "claim" is a formal request by the insured to receive money to pay for his "loss.") The insurance company also makes money by investing its surplus funds in various profit-making ventures.

Given the above, it's understandable that insurance companies are concerned about the cost of health care. More people making more claims for more money reduces insurance company profits unless premiums are raised or people make fewer claims for less money. Faced with health care costs rising even faster than the rate of general inflation, insurance companies have worked to both raise premiums and reduce the number and size of medical insurance claims.

In deciding what is a valid claim under a medical insurance policy, the insurance industry has structured itself to fit the Western medical model of disease. As a practical consequence, insurance companies pay only for the treatment of disorders or diseases diagnosed by a health care professional who is licensed to practice in his or her state. The amount of reimbursement for such services varies with each insurance company, but the client must have a diagnosed disorder or recognized medical condition in order to be eligible for reimbursement.

Although insurance companies increasingly recognize the role of prevention and early detection of disease in holding down health care costs, the health insurance system is still based on reimbursement for treatment of a diagnosed disorder or disease. Only some consumer-oriented insurance companies reimburse for preventive services and check-ups. Usually, services which aim only to enhance well-being or prolong life without correcting or relieving a diagnosed disease or disorder are not eligible for coverage. In short, insurance pays to relieve sickness but not to enhance wellness.

Fortunately, more doctors and health care providers are willing to consider the Eastern view of health and disease, and to take a whole person approach to health care. They understand the need to see health as a process of internal and external balance. For example, lifestyle factors such as stress and tension are becoming recognized as important contributors to one's overall health profile. What this means for practitioners whose discipline is based on the Eastern model is that health care centers are being formed which recognize the importance of adding the services of complementary health care providers to traditional Western medical treatment. For example, a clinic may include several medical doctors working with acupuncturists, psychologists, chiropractors and touch therapists. Also, traditional doctors and clinics frequently refer their patients for various adjunctive services which have proven helpful.

Therefore, until insurance companies reimburse routinely for the services of alternative health care practitioners, the only way you can get paid by insurance companies is to establish a legally-acceptable, medically effective relationship with a licensed primary care provider who will refer clients to you as part of a supervised treatment program.

Once a licensed primary care provider establishes you as an effective adjunct to regular prescribed treatments, then many insurance companies will pay for your services.

Licensing Regulations ~~

The word "license" may be used in at least two different ways that often lead to confusion for health care practitioners, especially those just getting started. You must understand the difference between 1) a license to provide health care; and 2) a business license from your city to practice your profession.

A licensed provider of health care is a professional who has passed licensing examinations by his state professional board (such as the Board of Medical Quality Assurance in California, the State Medical Board in Ohio and the Florida Board of Massage Therapy) after completing degree and educational requirements. For example, licensed primary care providers include medical doctors, chiropractors, osteopaths, registered physical therapists, psychiatrists and clinical social workers.

A business license is simply legal permission from a city or county to sell a product or perform a service for money at a certain location.

To summarize, in a licensed state you may work independently with a client who has been referred to you by a doctor who supervises your work. (Be sure to confirm your eligibility for reimbursement when you verify coverage with the insurance company.) Many insurance companies may recognize you as a practitioner, since you have met the state requirements for your professional license, and you are considered to be an adjunctive therapist.

In an unlicensed state, the insurance company requires the practitioner to work directly under the license and supervision of the primary health care provider who is referring the patient. For major medical and Workers' Compensation insurance claims the doctor must be on the premises at least 50 percent of your work week. For personal injury claims such as car accidents you may bill from your own office with a doctor's referral letter.

"Responsible and Necessary" is the phrase used by insurance companies to validate a treatment modality.

See Chapter Eight, pages 231-233 for ideas on how to keep accurate client files.

Basic Steps for Submitting Claims ⌇

1. The requirements for reimbursement include a prescription from a referring doctor which indicates the name of the therapy, the number of visits per week and the diagnosis for which it's prescribed (e.g., soft-tissue therapy, two times per week for three weeks for cervical strain and sprain).

2. Verify Coverage: confirm with the company that the client has insurance, what it covers and that you are eligible for reimbursement (see Figure 6.1). A key part of getting insurance reimbursement and getting paid promptly is to develop an effective business relationship with a claims adjuster. Be sure to ask for the adjuster's name and number when you first verify coverage and address any letters or bills directly to that adjuster.

3. The claim is either submitted manually (paper forms are filled in by hand and sent in the mail to the insurance company) or by computer (forms are printed out on your computer system and submitted in the mail). In some cases claims may be filed by a service bureau (an independent firm uses raw information you provide to prepare and submit claims under contract) or via electronic billing (claims are submitted by your office as raw data files sent over computer networks).

Figure 6.1

MARLIN THERAPEUTICS
JULIA HARSHBARGER, L.M.T.-N.M.T.

Specializing in
Neuromuscular Therapy
and
Injury Rehabilitation

Certified Neuromuscular
Specialist
License # MA000095221
Provider # K526

Authorization Confirmation

Date: _4-20-2001_

Time of Call: _1:35 p.m._

Insurance Adjuster: _Steve Jones_

Phone No.: _(206) 555-9721_

Insurance Company: _Be-Well Insurance_

Address: _123 Grant Avenue_

City: _Seattle_   State: _WA_   Zip: _98000_

Dear _Mr. Jones_,

I am writing this letter to confirm the verbal authorization of benefits given to me on
_4-20-2001_ at _1:35 p.m._ .   Please verify the following:

Percentage of coverage _70%_ for _10_ sessions of massage therapy by
Tracy Smith , licensed massage therapist.

Please sign below and mail or fax to 206-555-5556.

Steve Jones
(Signature of Adjuster)

Thank you.

690 Seaside Way, Suite 210 • Mariner Business Park • Seattle, WA 98000
206-555-5555 • Fax # 206-555-5556

4. The procedures for filing an insurance claim varies with the payment policy of your office and the payment arrangement with the client. For example, if your policy is that cash payments are due at the time of the client's visit, the client would pay at each visit and then receive a superbill (pre-printed billing form from the health care provider that contains all the information needed by the insurance company including the diagnostic and procedure codes, the dates of service and amount paid as well as provider, patient and insurance information). The client submits this form to his insurance company for reimbursement.

   If your office accepts Assignment of Benefits and is prepared to bill the insurance company for clients, the clients present your office (on or before the first visit) all the necessary information and paperwork (including claim forms from their insurance companies).

   Your office fills out all the required paperwork including dates of service, procedure and diagnostic codes, amount billed and insurance/patient information required. Your office collects a percentage of the total amount of the balance due from the patient at each visit (usually 20 percent or the amount of the co-payment). The office then receives the payment from the insurance company directly, usually in four to six weeks. In this case the office is also responsible for collecting from the patient any outstanding balance after the insurance company has paid.

5. The office keeps an insurance log of all claims sent out and payments received as well as accounting records of paid claims.

Diagnostic and Procedure Codes ∞

Diagnostic and procedure codes are a critical piece of the insurance puzzle. All insurance carriers require diagnostic and procedure codes to process insurance claims. These numbers, which are used by doctors and licensed health care providers, identify the diagnosis of a medical condition and the specific procedure done, as well as the length of treatment time.

The Physicians' Current Procedural Terminology (CPT) manual defines the services you provide. For example, Number 97124 in the CPT book refers to massage therapy lasting 15 minutes.

The diagnostic codes for licensed health care providers are listed in an ICD-9-CM (*International Classification of Diseases-Ninth Revision-Clinical Modification*) code book. These codes are used by physicians when diagnosing and prescribing therapies for their patients.

All health care providers, whether certified by a professional board or licensed in their state must be aware of the laws and guidelines in their state for using the diagnostic and procedure codes. To diagnose, you must be a licensed health care provider such as a medical doctor, acupuncturist, licensed clinical psychologist or chiropractor.

Lists of Codes

The Insurance Reimbursement Manual
by Christine Rosche
Bodytherapy Business Institute

The Medical Code Manual for Massage Practitioners
by E. Denning and D. Hecht
Therapy Associates

To use the procedure codes you must be licensed by your state professional board or work directly under the supervision of a licensed health care provider. Be sure to check with your state professional board for detailed requirements for your profession.

The absence or misuse of medical codes cause many claims to be rejected. The American Medical Association publishes a CPT book annually and the ICD book is frequently published by the U.S. Department of Health and Human Services. Both books are available at medical school libraries and medical school bookstores. You can also order them directly. Many companies produce booklets that list the common codes used for specific professions. Check your professional journals or contact your professional associations to find vendors.

Troubleshooting Delinquent Claims ⌁

Before you learn why reimbursement gets delayed or refused and what to do about it, you must be sure insurance companies and their claims representatives understand the medical value of your services. It's imperative that this groundwork be in place for you to receive reimbursement.

Many insurance carriers do not know that your services offer clinical, therapeutic benefits in conjunction with a doctor's treatment plan. Instead, they see your services as offering only relaxation or cosmetic benefits. Perceiving complementary health care professions in this way, they think paying such claims would waste money on something of no medical value.

They often deny claims by saying they do not pay for preventive or wellness services. They also reject claims because they require your services be performed by a registered physical therapist or medical doctor. They may disallow claims in states where practitioners in your field are not licensed, since lack of licensure means to them "not a medical professional."

The root of refusal problems is widespread ignorance of the scope and value of complementary health care services. While Europe and Asia have traditionally seen the value of complementary health care services and include them in their modern health care and hospital systems for medical rehabilitation, U.S. insurance companies and physicians don't recognize the clinical value as an adjunctive treatment.

Research showing effectiveness and cost-saving implications of these services should appeal to those trying to limit health care costs. But more outcome studies are needed, and the results must reach those who can make decisions in your favor.

Therefore, you can help both yourself and your profession by educating insurers and their claims representatives to the efficacy and cost-effectiveness of your services. For example, you can pave the way for reimbursement by sending insurance carriers a well-written, professional letter describing your services along with copies of doctors' testimonial letters and reputable outcome studies demonstrating the significant clinical benefits of your type of services. Further, you may even consider giving a 15-

20-minute free demonstration on a claims representative. This can be a highly effective way to show the value of your services.

You should also point out the hours of education and training you receive to practice your professions. For example, touch therapists have an average of 300-1,000 hours of training in soft-tissue therapy. This contrasts with physical therapists, who usually receive only 15-30 hours training in massage therapy (yet they can bill for soft-tissue treatments).

Further, explain to claims representatives that you are uniquely qualified to perform these services, and your fees are significantly lower than a medical doctor's for the same services. The sooner you establish these facts with insurance company executives, the sooner you will begin to receive reimbursement. For example, a massage therapist spends 45-60 minutes with a patient and charges only $65, while a physician may charge at least $200 for a service not commonly part of his practice. In brief, the massage therapist can write that massage therapy has specific clinical therapeutic value, she specializes in it, she has far more training in it than any other profession and charges two-thirds less than physicians.

Finding the Solution to Reimbursement Problems

When you have difficulty getting paid by an insurance company (claims are delayed, reduced or rejected) the solution can be found in one of four places:

1. Your Office: Correct errors in your paperwork and office procedures.

2. The Doctor's Office: Have them give timely, accurate and complete information on patient, diagnosis and procedure.

3. The Insurance Company: Insist it meet its payment obligations (time and amount) under the patient's policy and state laws.

4. Your State Insurance Commissioner: Ask for an investigation of reimbursement problems.

If a claim is not paid within a reasonable amount of time (four to 10 weeks depending on the insurance company and the type of claim) the doctor's office or the practitioner may send an inquiry letter to the insurance company (also called an insurance tracer). The purpose of the tracer is to determine the status of a claim to find out why something is missing. Along with your tracer, include a copy of your detailed progress notes and any other documentation to support the medical necessity of your services.

If a claim is not paid within 30 days, the provider can also re-bill both the insurance company and the patient. Be sure your re-bill includes language to the insurance company stating that if unpaid within 30 days you will file a written complaint with the state insurance commissioner. It also helps to call the claims representative within a week to say, "I want to verify you have received a re-bill for this unpaid claim." When you re-bill the patient, remind them that they are responsible for any amounts unpaid by their insurance.

When a claim is denied, notify the patient by mail or telephone as soon as possible to keep them informed. Always retain the correspondence from the insurance company so you can retrieve it quickly for patient inquiries.

When a claim is denied or inadequately paid, the recourse is to appeal (which is a request for more payment) by asking for a written review. Usually appeals carry time limits, so it's important for you to read and understand the Explanation of Benefits form.

If you establish an ongoing rapport with a claims representative, you can significantly shorten these kinds of delays. You can also speed up your collection times by establishing regular office procedures and claims management techniques (e.g., insurance claims register, tickler file.) These support systems enable you to follow up quickly and correctly. They can even allow you to recover payment after a claim has been denied in whole or in part.

By following the above suggestions and staying in touch with the claims representatives, you can get paid promptly and in full.

Claims Provisions

Many details on what's covered and who may be reimbursed are spelled out in the detailed language of the client's policy. To make the insurance reimbursement system work for you in building your practice, you must understand and follow these crucial details. Remember, an insurance policy is nothing more than a contract between a company and a person or group. Essentially, the insurance company agrees to pay money, IF you and the patient meet specific requirements.

Time, or when things must occur, is a key requirement in all policies. For example, individual health insurance policies require the company to pay benefits promptly after they receive a claim. However, how quickly they must pay varies from one company to another.

In addition, the person making the claim must notify the insurance company of a loss within a certain time period, or the insurer may deny benefits. If the insured disagrees with the company on the amount it paid for the claim, he can begin a lawsuit only within three years after submitting the claim.

Another common provision says an insured cannot bring legal action against the insurance company until 60 days after submitting a claim. If a payment problem develops and the insurance company ignores, denies or is too slow to pay a claim, you or the insured may ask the state insurance commissioner to intervene on your behalf. The insurance commissioner does not have the power to force a company to pay a claim, but his authority does include the following:

1. Hold a hearing to determine whether licensed insurers, brokers and agents have complied with state laws.

2. Review a policy's provisions to determine if the insurer's denial of the claim has violated its obligations under the insurance contract.

3. Advise the patient whether the company has violated the law. (This may pave the way for the client to sue the insurance company.)

Electronic Billing 〜

The tools of the information/technology revolution can add real power and efficiency to your billing once you understand and use them. Electronic billing for insurance reimbursement also speeds up your business growth.

Electronic billing (a form of electronic data interchange), dates from the late 1960s. In simplest terms, two computers talk back and forth by wires inside a building, outside telephone lines or by radio waves.

An electronic claim is one you submit to the insurance carrier using no paper. Instead the claim is in digital form (1s and 0s) and sent directly (computer to computer) on a magnetic medium (such as a tape or diskette) or as a digital fax.

Professionals of every kind have adopted these tools because they remove hassles and save money (often a lot of money) at every step of billing and collection. Sometimes the savings are direct and immediate (less than a penny to send a claim form hundreds of miles over a telephone line or by satellite in seconds versus 32 cents in U.S. postage in one-four days). Occasionally the savings are slower but much larger. For example, electronic claims are nearly 100 percent accurate, which means you don't have to spend money for staff time (or your own time) to tediously follow up on what are usually clerical errors.

The best reason for learning to use electronic billing is accurate claims get processed and paid much faster. For your income growth, that means much less waiting while "the check is in the mail." Because of what's called "the time value of money," a check you receive in two weeks is worth more to your business than one you wait three months to receive. Thus, whatever anxiety or hesitation you may have about the electronic revolution, your ability to collect insurance claims promptly more than compensates for your time and effort in learning how to use these new tools.

Fortunately, putting the technology at your service doesn't mean you have to understand electronics and the workings of a computer any more than driving a car means you have to understand electronic fuel injection or compression ratios. To drive a car, you learn the rules of the road, get a driver's license and a car owner's manual. To use electronic billing, you obtain (or get the use of) the right kind of computer, the right computer program and some brief training in how to use it for record keeping, billing and follow up. Or, you hire someone to do it for you.

To standardize the process (and save more money), in 1981 eleven major insurance companies formed the National Electronic Information Corporation (NEIC). This industry group provides a national network and clearinghouse to electronically receive, process, edit, sort and transmit claims to insurers for payment in two weeks or less. By comparison, claims submitted the traditional way by first class mail are usually paid within four to six weeks.

The NEIC system benefits physicians and health care providers by letting them use one version of software to communicate with a variety of insurers. (Imagine the headache of having to learn and use 11 different electronic billing programs.) You can submit claims directly to NEIC for routing to your client's insurance company.

You can also do your billing through a network of independent software companies, clearinghouses and billing centers. A clearinghouse, also called a "third-party administrator" (or TPA), receives claims (you don't have to submit them one at a time, but can batch them together), separates them and sends each to the correct insurance payer. All this information is sent as fast as electricity flows and requires little or no intervention by error-prone, human operators.

Nearly 90 percent of all insurance companies use electronic claims submission to drastically lower their costs in staff salaries and office space. Electronic claims require no signing or stamping, searching for an insurance carrier's address, postage or trips to the post office, or filing and storing of paper forms. Also, electronic records leave an audit trail, which means you can track when and where the data went, when it was received, by whom and who may have altered it.

Electronic Billing Benefits
- Better cash flow
- More time for patient education
- More time for collection efforts
- Lower labor costs
- Much higher accuracy rates
- Fewer disputes of the "We never received the claim, please resubmit it" variety, because proof of receipt is generated at the insurer's end.
- Faster problem resolution. The office is notified of rejected claims faster, allowing quicker follow-up with corrected data.

How to Make Electronic Billing Work for You

To begin using electronic billing, contact your major insurers for a list of vendors approved to handle electronic claims processing. The carriers know which systems meet their criteria and work with their special electronic billing requirements. If you cannot link your system with the insurance carrier, use a clearinghouse, which forwards a batch of claims to insurers. For your benefit this means that you can send every claim electronically rather than having to fall back on the payer system for some of them.

Clearinghouses charge a flat fee per claim or a percentage of the dollar volume. In addition to electronic billing, computer programs can provide similar help with your internal billing. If you properly choose, install and use it, a computerized office billing system will save you enormous amounts of time. Plus your records will be easily and quickly accessible in one place. Some systems even offer formats for patient notes, bookkeeping and follow-up progress reports.

Managed Care ⚍

An exciting new trend in health care in general, and insurance in particular, is the growing acceptance of so-called "alternative therapies." As acupuncture, chiropractic, counseling and touch therapies continue to prove their effectiveness and cost-saving value, insurers under managed care are more open to including these professions in their organizations.

Why should you care about being on a list of providers? Depending on the state where you practice, it can increase by 10 or 20 times the number of people who can see you with insurance coverage, IF you are willing to accept a 20 percent discount below your regular fees.

What are HMOs and PPOs?

A health maintenance organization (HMO) is a prepaid group practice sponsored and operated by an insurance company, clinic or hospital/medical plan. "Prepaid" means the health care provider agrees to treat all the covered illnesses of everyone in the group for a year at a fixed total price.

Like any business, if the provider spends less than it takes in, it shows a surplus or profit. If it spends more to deliver its services (expenses) than it takes in (revenues), it runs a deficit or a loss. Insurance companies have supported creating HMOs because this form of organization forces the providers to maintain their profits or minimize their losses by holding down their expenses. Providers reduce their expenses by delivering fewer services and/or less expensive services.

A preferred provider organization (PPO) contracts with a group of "preferred" providers to deliver care to members. Unlike HMO members, PPO members are free to choose any physician or hospital for services, but they receive more benefits (or pay less of the cost themselves "out of pocket") if they choose a preferred provider. A PPO plan usually requires filing claims and paying deductibles and co-payments. HMOs largely eliminate this paperwork.

Good News for Complementary Health Care Providers

As of September 1996, several managed care companies have added acupuncture, chiropractic, massage and other complementary therapies as covered services. Many more are considering adding them to their pool of providers. For example, Steve Gorman of Alternative Health Insurance Services, Inc. (AHIS) of Thousand Oaks, CA, (800-966-8467), says his company is developing a network of holistic, complementary health care providers, including touch therapists on behalf of a number of insurance companies. Similar to a conventional PPO, the network (AHIS) contracts with providers who offer reduced fees to network subscribers (clients who buy their insurance plan) in return for exposure to many new patients. Because the requirements for providers are still being formed and vary from company to company, you should call them directly to get the latest information as it applies to your specific situation.

Another example is WellTouch Corporation of Dallas, Texas, which is enrolling and certifying 7,500 professional massage and touch therapists nationwide. WellTouch is also negotiating managed care contracts with some of America's largest corporations, including IBM, Ford Motor Company, Xerox, General Dynamics, Blue Cross and Blue Shield. These contracts will enable nearly six million people to receive treatment from contracting massage therapists. WellTouch is an affiliate of the Wellness Corporation, which sees massage therapy as a core component in the future of health and preventive medicine.

WellTouch imposes stringent credentialing and educational requirements on therapists applying for membership and insists providers offer clients the highest professional standards. Massage/touch therapists must also agree to accept 20-30 percent lower fees, depending on the region of the country. This fee arrangement is similar to that followed by doctors, pharmacies, dentists, chiropractors and eye care professionals. For more information, call WellTouch at 1-800-WELLTOUCH.

Another new HMO worth investigating is Oxford Health Plans Inc., a highly profitable HMO in the Northeast. Oxford has a strong marketing reputation and has the most extensive program to date, covering many complementary therapies including acupuncture, chiropractic and massage/touch therapy for wellness care and prevention as well as illness care for a diagnosed disease or injury.

As with other HMOs, Oxford prefers therapists who are licensed by their state or are nationally certified, have at least two years experience and are graduates of schools with the highest educational standards in the field. Also, they require continuing education hours each year. For more information on becoming a provider, write to: Kerry MacKenzie, Oxford Health Plans, 800 Connecticut, Norwalk, CT 06854.

Think of how much fuller your appointment schedule will become as larger numbers of clients can receive reimbursement for your services. Becoming a preferred provider or joining an HMO is a practice-building opportunity to consider, IF you are willing to accept lower fees in exchange for many more clients becoming available to you.

The driving motive behind insurance companies accepting alternative practitioners is what else? Money. A study of one 15-month period (January 1995 through March 1996) looked at the percentage of premiums collected by the Alliance for Alternatives in Health Care it paid out to members. For every dollar collected in premiums, it paid out only 59 cents in claims. The remaining 41 cents it kept to pay expenses and return profits to its owners. This "59 percent claims ratio" is better than average for the insurance industry and tends to encourage other companies to follow along.

Insurance companies make their profits by paying out less in claims than they collect in premiums. They profit when they pay less as well as when they delay payment even for a month. Why? The answer lies in a concept called "the time value of money." To banks, large companies, governments or anyone with large amounts of money, a dollar today is worth more than a dollar in the future. As individuals, we usually don't notice this because the amounts involved are small. The company owes you $225. What difference does it make if you wait one month or two?

But imagine the insurance company owing $225 to 1,000 practitioners spread out over your state. That $225,000 it holds for a month can be "put to work" earning interest or helping to pay for some other profit-making aspect of its business, especially since the insurance company does not owe you interest on unpaid or delayed claims, even when it causes the delay.

On the other hand, and for your long-term benefit, companies have a strong incentive to pay for therapies that reduce their higher-cost claims. For back pain, for example, an effective therapeutic massage, biofeedback and exercise program may cost 1/50 the price of prescription drugs and back surgery.

Insurance companies are also more open to covering increasingly popular "alternative therapies" because they see financial loss to themselves if they don't catch up with consumer demand. As many as one in three Americans now use some type of non-traditional treatment, according to a landmark 1993 survey published by Harvard Medical School. And the spending on non-physician, non-prescription treatments is huge: $14 billion compared to $1 trillion on conventional health care.

The point for your profession is that when insurance executives see consumers turning toward alternatives not covered by insurance, they see the threat of losing policy holders who opt out of their coverage and pay for these services themselves. The companies want to prevent losing the potential revenue and profits by including these services in their coverage.

"Consumers are already voting with their out-of-pocket expenditures that these services work," says Alan Kittner, a consultant who helps HMOs set up alternative providers. Not only do favorable profit figures show that insurance companies can benefit significantly when they include alternative/complementary therapies, studies also show that when alternative therapies are available, members use fewer health care services and make fewer claims. As more companies use alternative therapies and realize lower overall health care costs, more managed care companies will want qualified therapists to join their provider pools.

• Hiring Help •

This information can also help if you desire to work for someone else.

As your business builds, you will most likely reach a point where you have more work than you can handle by yourself, find yourself in a position of not possessing the skills or expertise needed, decide you don't want to do certain tasks that must be done, determine that it's more cost effective to have someone else do the job, or simply want to take an extended vacation. This is the time to consider outside help; either as employees or independent contractors.

Many of the duties involved in running a business need not be done by just you. Expanding your practice by bringing in other practitioners or office personnel can free you to focus on what you do best. This relates to honoring yourself and valuing your time; often we do everything ourselves instead of delegating tasks. Usually this isn't the wisest use of our time. For example, let's say you charge $50 an hour for your services and it takes you three hours per week to clean your office. Most cleaning services charge between $15-$20 per hour. If you were to hire a service rather than do the cleaning yourself, you could spend those three hours working with clients. It would cost you approximately one hour's worth of service ($50). This leaves you with two extra hours in which to make a profit of $100.

Refer to Chapter Three, pages 41-43 for more information on risk taking.

I realize this isn't as simple as it sounds. Often it means taking a risk because you might not get those extra appointments booked. Consider, though, that the more you focus on income producing activities, the more profitable your practice becomes.

Office management is also a major area to contemplate in hiring others. Administrative tasks such as scheduling and confirming appointments, keeping client files, doing follow-ups, typing, organizing and purchasing supplies can usually be done efficiently and cost-effectively by someone other than yourself.

Financial matters such as bookkeeping, tax preparation, payroll and filing insurance claims can easily be assigned to another person/firm. Many of the operational duties in your practice can be handled by janitorial and laundry services.

Some health care providers hire a marketing consultant to coordinate their promotions and advertising, organize special events, oversee the graphic design and printing of promotional materials, and schedule speaking engagements.

The most common manner in which practitioners enlist additional help is by including other health care providers in their business. This usually occurs when a practice has grown to the point where there is a client overflow or the owner wants to expand the scope of modalities and services offered to current clients.

Many sources exist for getting assistance with your business. You can hire independent contractors, consultants or employees. You may even be able to find someone as an intern or apprentice. You can contract with a company that provides specific business services (e.g., secretarial, answering service, laundry, bookkeeping, janitorial). Or you may hire a "temporary employee" through an employment agency or even an employee leasing company—then you won't have to worry about all the paperwork because those agencies are responsible for withholding taxes, paying appropriate fees such as workers' compensation and filing all the governmental forms. Another option is to form associations with other business owners to share tasks and expenses.

Deciding whether to hire an employee or subcontract for the services you need can be a difficult decision. You may want to incorporate a variety of people and service providers in your business support team. Most companies would prefer to hire independent contractors, consultants or service firms than employees.

With employees, in addition to the responsibility of having enough money for their paychecks, you need to do the following: match their FICA (Social Security and Medicare) deductions; pay FUTA (Federal Unemployment Taxes) which is calculated at a percentage of the employee's first $7,000 of wages annually; pay state unemployment taxes; provide workers' compensation; withhold state and federal taxes; deposit withheld taxes (the requirement varies from weekly to monthly to quarterly, depending on the amount); file regular returns; send W-2 forms to employees annually; and in most instances offer fringe benefits such as health insurance, paid vacations, sick leave and retirement plans.

Two of the employment forms you need are SS-4, Application for Employer Identification Number and Form W-4, Employee's Withholding Allowance Certificate. Check with your state employment department for requirements, fees and forms. In addition to a Federal Employer's Identification Number (EIN) you need a state EIN. All employees must also fill out Form I-9, Employment Eligibility Verification (from the U.S. Department of Justice, Immigration and Naturalization Service).

You do not have to withhold income tax or social security tax from independent contractors. But if you pay an independent contractor $600 or more during the year in the course of your trade or business, you must file a form 1099-MISC at the end of the year. That form is optional if you've contracted with a service company.

When you hire an employee, your status changes from simply being a practitioner to also being a manager. It takes considerable time and excellent communication skills to be a good boss. You have to train your staff so they understand the type of work you do and can explain it to potential clients. You need to organize your business to make certain there's enough work to be done, hold staff meetings, give employees regular feedback and be willing to delegate.

In most instances it's much easier and less risky to terminate a contract than to fire an employee. Also, your liability is reduced in terms of malpractice if you have hired an independent contractor, who is required to carry her own insurance.

The potential pitfalls of working with non-employees include paying a higher price for their services and not having control over their work in terms of timeliness and quality.

Contact the IRS
Request Publication 15, Circular E—Employer's Tax Guide, which contains detailed information on federal regulations.

State and federal law requires all employers to report each new hired employee to the State Directory of New Hires.

See Chapter Seven, pages 177-190
for detailed tax information.

I may seem to be making a strong case for not hiring employees. Au contráire! Many practitioners and clinic owners claim they could not be where they are without employees—particularly clerical support staff. It can be extremely helpful and comforting to know that someone is going to be at your office every day taking care of business. A strong bond tends to develop between employees and the business owner, particularly in a small business. The peace of mind and sense of stability this creates is invaluable. You also receive the other benefits as previously mentioned when you are able to focus in on your high priority activities. If you decide to hire an employee but are concerned about the regulations and paperwork, you can pay a bank, accountant or payroll service to do it for you.

The IRS guidelines for determining employment status are fairly clear when it comes to clerical staff: in most instances an office-person is an employee. A gray area exists in hiring other health care providers. In researching numerous spas, clinics and group practices, I discovered many of them walk a very thin legal line. A significant number of the so-called independent contractors they have working for them would most likely be classified as employees under the IRS guidelines. Just calling someone an independent contractor doesn't make it so.

Independent Contractor Status ⟿

See pages 144-151
for sample contracts.

As an employer, you take a considerable risk by deeming a worker an independent contractor. If the IRS determines that your independent contractors are (or were) indeed employees, you may be required to pay fines (of up to 100 percent of the tax) in addition to the back income taxes and social security taxes. This can easily add up to a sizable amount. In the eyes of the IRS, it makes no difference if you signed an agreement that states you are contracting with an independent contractor—although a written agreement is advisable.

To assist your understanding of this vital topic, I am providing the following information (adapted with permission) from IRS Publication 937, Business Reporting:

Under common-law rules, anyone who performs services subject to the will and control of an employer, as to both **what** must be done and **how** it must be done, is an employee. It doesn't matter that the employer allows the employee discretion and freedom of action, so long as the employer has the **legal right** to control both the method and result of the services.

Two usual characteristics of an employer-employee relationship are that the employer has the right to discharge the employee and the employer supplies the employee with tools and a place to work. (Now don't assume that you can get around this by having your "employee" provide his own specific supplies. "Tools" is a broad term that can include the equipment required in running a practice such as telephones and copiers.)

If you have an employer-employee relationship, it makes no difference how it's described. It doesn't matter if the employee is called an employee, associate, partner or independent contractor. It also doesn't matter how the payments are measured, made or what they are called. Nor does it matter whether the individual is employed full-time or part-time.

The IRS has developed the following list of 20 factors that they use to determine the status of employee or independent contractor. The degree of importance of each factor varies according to the profession and the conditions in which the services are performed. The most important factor is control. If the business owner has the right to control how and when a person works, then that person is most likely to be considered an employee.

An Individual Is Likely to Be Considered an Employee If S/he:

1. Is required to comply with company instructions about when, where and how to work.
2. Has been trained by the company to perform services in a particular manner.
3. Has her services integrated into the company's operations because the services are critical to the success of the business.
4. Must render services personally.
5. Utilizes assistants provided by the company.
6. Has an ongoing, continuing relationship with the company.
7. Has set work hours established by the employer.
8. Is required to work the equivalent of full time.
9. Works on the company's designated premises.
10. Must perform services in the order or sequence determined by the employer.
11. Must submit regular progress reports.
12. Is paid in regular intervals such as by the hour, week or month.
13. Is reimbursed for all business and travel expenses.
14. Uses tools and materials furnished by the employer.
15. Has no significant investment in the facilities that are used.
16. Has no risk of loss.
17. Works for only one person or company.
18. Does not offer services to the general public.
19. Can be discharged by the company.
20. Can terminate the relationship without incurring liability.

You can still qualify an individual as an independent contractor even if some of these factors are present in your working relationship. The key elements to differentiating between employee status and independent contractor status in the health care industry involve the following: who regulates the type of work done and how it's performed; where and when the sessions occur; who determines the fee structure; who receives the money from the clients; who provides the equipment and supplies; who pays for client-related expenses; and who generates the clientele.

You can minimize the risks of your independent contractors being reclassified as employees by taking the following steps: make certain independent contractors have

In general, it's wise to consider an individual as an employee until you can prove otherwise.

multiple sources of income; sign "independent contractor" contracts which clearly state the requirements of all parties while making it clear the contractors are able to pursue other clients; require contractors to provide their own tables, linens, products, music and other supplies; allow contractors to set their own schedules (no more than 20 hours per week); have clients pay contractors directly; request copies of the contractors' tax returns; and require contractors to provide their own insurance and workers' compensation coverage. Complying to these suggestions still doesn't guarantee independent contractor status. If in doubt, you can have the IRS determine whether a worker is an employee by filing Form SS-8.

If you decide to hire other health care providers as independent contractors, be sure to create a thorough contract. Hire a lawyer to review the contract. The several hundred dollars it may cost you in attorney fees is minimal compared to the potential fees and penalties the IRS are wont to impose.

The Anatomy of a Contract

Legal forms and agreements are an integral part of any business relationship, yet all too often people avoid written contracts. Whether you are interested in a one-time only interaction or a long-term affiliation, it's wise to delineate in writing your roles

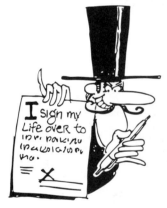

and expectations. Clear written agreements serve several purposes: they help avoid problems, provide a pre-determined method for resolving conflicts and keep you focused on your goals.

This information can be applied to any type of contract (massage therapy examples are used to clarify the specific points). It's my hope to provide you with guidelines sufficient to make informed choices and protect yourself legally. I've heard so many horror stories about people terminating relationships, filing lawsuits and of the IRS seizing funds. Most often this was due to simple misunderstandings or lack of knowledge. A little prevention in the form of a clear contract would have averted most of these problems.

Your contracts should reflect the specific nature of your business and eliminate confusion about expectations of all parties involved. As an employer, you have the opportunity to create a fair and equitable contract. When someone asks you to sign an employment agreement or an independent contractor agreement, the document is most likely geared to protect the hiring company. I recommend that you be prepared with your own contract—or at the very least a list of questions and concerns. Keep in mind that contracts are negotiable.

Probably the major reason most people don't have a good contract is the lack of models. The standard employment and independent contractor agreement forms (available at office supply stores) just don't quite fit well for health care providers. Their scope is extremely limited due to the enormous potential liability involved in publishing a more complete, specific contract.

The following checklist covers the major elements to include in your contracts. Sometimes this information may be provided in separate documents, although it's best to have it in one contract that's signed by all parties. Ideally, you would come to the negotiating process with a sample of your own contract and the checklist, review the hiring company's contract, and create a specific contract that is mutually agreeable to both of you. If the hiring company insists on only using their contract, make sure you have responses (preferably in writing) to all the items in the checklist (see figure 6.2, Contract Checklist).

I realize this checklist is quite substantial, albeit most of these issues can be addressed in a one- to two-page document. This can even be done in an informal letter, sans legalese. You may be tempted not to use it for presumably simple transactions, particularly if it's just a "one-time" deed. Yet it's usually those seemingly negligible events that you live to regret! Invest the time in clarifying what is truly important to you in a business relationship. Even if you are currently involved in a business relationship and don't have a contract, you can always design one now. Each situation is unique and one contract will not suit all situations, although once you have the basics done, you will find it much simpler to alter any contract.

The Complete Legal Guide For Your Small Business
by Paul Adams
John Wiley & Sons

The Legal Guide for Starting & Running A Small Business
by Fred S. Steingold
Nolo Press

Figure 6.2

Contract Checklist

1. Names and addresses of all parties involved.

2. A short description and mission statement of the hiring company.

3. A statement summarizing the desired role of the contracted party. This section describes the focus of the work performed (e.g., to provide relaxation treatments, therapeutic massage or stress reduction); the type of massage modalities used (such as Swedish, acupressure or sports massage) and the typical duration of session (15, 50, 60 minutes).

4. A classification of the business relationship. Many business relationships are possible in this field. Some of the most common titles are that of a salaried employee, a commissioned employee, an independent contractor, a lessee or a licensee. You need to know exactly what your status is and the ramifications of same. Your legal and financial obligations vary according to your status and the specific agreements in your contract.

    A misunderstanding of the nature of your business relationship can affect you in many other ways than drawing the notice of the IRS. For example: you decide to purchase a new car. On the loan application under employer, you put ABC Health Club (you have been doing massage there for two years). The loan processor calls the club and is told that you are not an employee. The loan company thinks you lied on the application and denies you the loan. How could this have happened? Well, when you started working at the club, you signed an Independent Contractor's Agreement and, as such, you are not listed anywhere as an employee. Regardless of the legalities of whether or not you are an independent contractor or an employee, you have misrepresented yourself to the loan company and thus inadvertently besmirched your credit rating.

5. A detailed description of what each party promises to provide. Compile a list of the equipment and supplies required and who is responsible for providing and maintaining them. Be sure to include linens, oils, lotions, table, chair, music and sound system. Also delineate any marketing and management services (e.g., appointment booking, insurance billing, client files and fee collection).

6. A timetable of when the work is to be performed. Clarify the hours you will work (primary shifts, back-up shifts, on-call), when you must be on the location and when to check-in for appointments.

7. Location of where work is to be performed. Specify the sites(s) where you will be providing your services. Will you be working at the hiring party's location (e.g., a special therapy room at a hotel, spa or clinic)? Will it be necessary for you to go to different client's locations such as a hotel room, office or home? Will the work location vary from day to day (particularly common when doing massage at corporations and conventions)? Or will you be required to be available for a combination of the above?

8. The duration of the contract. Contracts may be for a single specific event, a series of events (e.g., all the bike races for a particular team for the next six months), or ongoing until either party decides to terminate the contract.

9. Payment method and schedule. Common methods of payment include a straight commission, per client rate, hourly wage, salary or a combination of the above. Payment schedules range from daily, weekly, twice a month, monthly, at the end of the contract or even whenever the insurance company feels like remitting payment.

10. Fringe benefits. Items to consider are health insurance coverage, facilities privileges, sick time, paid vacation and discounts on products and services.

11. Opportunities for increases in financial remuneration. Determine the parameters for direct increase in compensation for your services (such as an annual cost-of-living increase or a percentage increase after working on a specified number of clients). Oftentimes you are not limited to income solely from primary services. You may be able to bill for adjunct services, sell your own products or receive a commission on selling products that the hiring company carries.

12. Insurance coverage provided. One of the major concerns you need to address is insurance coverage. Find out if the hiring company provides workers' compensation, premise liability insurance, fire and theft insurance and medical health insurance. If you are an independent contractor, I strongly recommend you also obtain general liability insurance. It covers negligence toward clients, employees and the general public while you are on their premises. General liability insurance is wise to have anyway—particularly if you do any on-site work or even public demonstrations. Unfortunately, none of these policies cover *you*, so be sure your medical health and personal disability insurance provides adequate protection.

13. Insurance coverage required. Most companies require practitioners to provide their own malpractice/professional liability insurance. Malpractice insurance is usually limited to protecting you against claims due to loss incurred by your clients as a result of negligence or failure on your part to perform at a professional skill level.

14. Guarantees. Usually the practitioner guarantees his/her own work and doesn't charge a fee if a client is dissatisfied.

15. Financial obligations of the contracted party. This is usually included when the contract involves subcontracting and is mainly to protect the hiring party in case you do not perform your services adequately. For example, let's say a convention coordinator contracts a local company to provide 10 massage therapists for their convention. The local company hires you as a subcontractor but for some reason you don't show up. The convention coordinator could require compensation from the local hiring party and then the local hiring party would pass that on to you.

16. Conditions for termination of the agreement. Some conditions to consider are violation of the hiring company's policies and procedures, poor or non-work performance, mismanagement of funds and untimely payment of fees due.

17. Guidelines for transfer of the contract. The ability to transfer your contract to another person/company is always desired, although it won't work in all cases. Since health care is such personal work, the hiring party may be reluctant to have a different practitioner provide the service. You will most likely be able to include a transfer clause if you are truly an independent contractor. For example, let's say you were hired by a company to provide their staff with on-site massage for eight hours per week. After a while you decide that it isn't in your best interest to do this anymore (perhaps you've moved or the other aspects of your practice are requiring all of your time). Since you were the one responsible for getting the contract (marketing, negotiating the original contract and providing the services for a time) you could easily charge a fee to another therapist for the privilege of taking over the contract.

18. Who retains custody of the client. Many health care providers work in other practitioners' offices, health clubs, salons, spas and clinics in the hopes of building up their private clientele. Problems can arise if the expectations and boundaries aren't clear. Consider the following example: You provide massage services for a health club. Several of your clients decide they would prefer to receive their sessions at home. Your ability to ethically take them on as private clients depends upon your agreement with the club. The club owner might not care whatsoever, particularly if she mainly views your services as an added value for membership. But an upset might arise if the health club regards you as a significant revenue-producing adjunct.

    Another common occurrence is changing locations. For whatever reason, you may no longer want to work at the hiring party's location. You will avoid a lot of hurt feelings (and possibly a lawsuit) if you've clearly defined how you'll deal with the allocation of clients.

19. Arbitration. This clause usually states that if an irreconcilable problem arises, the parties will take the matter before a mutually agreed upon mediator.

20. Who is responsible for legal fees if a breach of contract occurs. Most often contracts state that the party who breaches the contract is responsible for the other party's legal costs.

21. The location and contact to send communications regarding the contract.

22. Signature lines and date the contract is signed.

Sample Employment Contracts ~~

These sample contracts are for illustrative purposes only to show the differences between independent contractors and employees and not intended for use as legal documents. Most employers do not create written employment agreements for support staff (although it isn't a bad idea). Please confer with an attorney before finalizing any legal agreements (to specify financial arrangements and to ensure the document meets IRS guidelines).

Figure 6.3

Massage Therapy Independent Contractor Agreement

This agreement, dated July 4, 2001, is by and between Holistic Health Clinic ("Clinic"), with principal office located at 1776 Independence Way, Washington, D.C. and Frank Benjamin ("Contractor"), with principal office located at 1912 Thomas Jefferson Blvd., Washington, D.C.

Status as Independent Contractor
Contractor is an independent contractor and not an employee of the Clinic. As an independent contractor, Clinic and Contractor agree to the following:

a. Contractor has control of the means, manner and method by which services are provided.
b. Contractor furnishes all necessary supplies and materials used in the performance of services (e.g., oils, lotions, linens and music).
c. Contractor has the right to perform services for others during the term of this Agreement. Contractor shall not solicit or provide services to Clinic's clients for private practice during the term of this Agreement or for one year after termination. Upon termination of Agreement, Contractor and Clinic shall discuss which clients, under what conditions and with what compensation Contractor may maintain continuity of service. All client records shall remain the property of the Clinic unless otherwise agreed.
d. Contractor shall indemnify and hold Clinic harmless from any loss or liability arising from services provided under this agreement.
e. Contractor is responsible for maintaining appropriate certification and licensure (including all costs thereof).

Services to Be Provided by Contractor
Contractor agrees to provide massage therapy services within the scope of licensure. Contractor agrees to dress in a style consistent with the Clinic's image. Contractor shall maintain client records in a mutually agreed manner.

Services to Be Provided by Clinic
Clinic shall provide the following: a safe, clean environment; a room furnished with a hydraulic table, chair, stool, settee, hydrotherapy equipment and storage area; receptionist services; appointment scheduling according to Contractor's stipulated hours; insurance billing; and marketing.

Other Provisions
All Contractor's marketing materials which include any information about Clinic must be approved in advance.

Fees, Terms of Payment and Fringe Benefits

Contractor shall set the amount of fees for services provided to clients. Clinic shall retain 30 percent of all fees collected on behalf of contractor to cover operating expenses, room rental, equipment usage and marketing (see Other Provisions). In cases of deferred client payment, Clinic shall reimburse Contractor within 30 days of receipt. Contractor acknowledges that Contractor is not eligible to receive any employee benefits.

Local, State and Federal Taxes

Contractor is responsible for paying and filing all applicable local, state and federal withholding, social security and Medicare taxes.

Workers' Compensation and Unemployment Insurance

Clinic is not responsible for payment of Workers' Compensation and Unemployment Insurance. If Clinic is a corporation, Contractor must provide Clinic with a certificate of Workers' Compensation Insurance prior to performing services.

Insurance

During the term of this agreement, Contractor shall maintain a malpractice insurance policy of at least $2,000,000 aggregate annual and $1,000,000 per incident.

Term of Agreement

Either party may terminate this agreement, given reasonable cause, as provided below, or by giving 30 days written notice to the other party of the intention to terminate this Agreement:

a. Material violation of the provisions of this Agreement.
b. Action by either party exposing the other to liability for property damage or personal injury.
c. Violation of ethical standards as defined by local, state and/or national associations and governing bodies.
d. Loss of licensure for services provided.
e. Contractor engages in any pattern or course of conduct on a continuing basis which adversely affects Contractor's ability to perform services.
f. Contractor engages in any pattern or course of conduct on a continuing basis which adversely affects Clinic's or Clinic's associates' ability to perform services.
g. It is agreed that any unresolved disputes will be settled by arbitration, including costs thereof.

This constitutes the entire agreement between Contractor and Clinic and supersedes any and all prior written or verbal agreements. Should any part of this agreement be deemed unenforceable, the remainder of the agreement continues in effect. This agreement is governed by the laws of the District of Columbia.

Signatures

Contractor: _Frank Benjamin_   Date: _July 4, 2001_

Clinic: _Marshall Taylor_   Date: _July 4, 2001_

Witness: _Joy Cronkite_   Date: _July 4, 2001_

Figure 6.4

Massage Therapy Employment Agreement

This agreement, dated July 4, 2001, is by and between Holistic Health Clinic ("Employer"), with principal offices located at 1776 Independence Way, Washington, D.C. and Frank Benjamin ("Employee").

Services to Be Provided by Employee

Employee agrees to provide massage therapy services within the scope of licensure. Employee is responsible for maintaining appropriate certification and licensure (including all costs thereof). Employee agrees to dress in a style consistent with the Employer's image, including uniforms. Employee shall maintain client records in the manner prescribed by employer.

When Employee isn't engaged in treatments, Employee shall assist with other office duties as directed, including but not limited to:

a. Assisting other practitioners with clients.
b. Performing clerical duties.
c. Cleaning and organizing the clinic.

Services to Be Provided by Employer

Employer shall provide the following: a safe, clean environment; a room furnished with a chair, stool, hydraulic table, settee, hydrotherapy equipment and storage area; receptionist services; appointment scheduling; insurance billing; marketing; and all necessary supplies and materials used in the performance of services (e.g., oils, lotions, linens and music).

Other Provisions

a. Employee has the right to perform services for others during the term of this Agreement, however such services are not to be performed on Employer's premises.
b. Employee shall not solicit or provide services to Employer's clients for private practice while employed or for six months after termination of employment, except as noted in "c."
c. Upon termination of employment Employer and Employee shall discuss which clients, under what conditions and with what compensation Employee may maintain continuity of service.
d. All client records shall remain the property of the Employer.
e. All Employee's non-clinic marketing materials which include any information about Employer must be approved in advance.

Fees, Terms of Payment and Fringe Benefits

Employee shall be compensated at the base rate of $10 per hour, with an additional $5 per half hour massage and $10 per hour massage, not to exceed 30 hours per week. Employee shall be paid biweekly. Employee shall receive payment on all services performed regardless of the collection time. Employee is eligible to participate in any of the following fringe benefits: health insurance, vacation time and employee pension plan (see policy manual).

Local, State and Federal Taxes

Employer is responsible for paying all required local, state and federal withholding, social security and Medicare taxes.

Workers' Compensation and Unemployment Insurance

Employer will provide Workers' Compensation and Unemployment Insurance.

Insurance

During the term of this agreement, Employee shall maintain a malpractice insurance policy of at least $2,000,000 aggregate annual and $1,000,000 per incident. Employer shall maintain insurance coverage for liability, fire and theft.

Term of Agreement

Either party may terminate this agreement, given reasonable cause, as provided below, or by giving 30 days written notice to the other party of the intention to terminate this Agreement:

a. Material violation of the provisions of this Agreement.

b. Action by either party exposing the other to liability for property damage or personal injury.

c. Violation of ethical standards as defined by local, state and/or national associations and governing bodies.

d. Loss of licensure for services provided.

e. Employee fails to maintain the standard of service deemed appropriate by Employer.

f. Employee engages in any pattern or course of conduct on a continuing basis which adversely affects Employee's ability to perform services.

g. Employee engages in any pattern or course of conduct on a continuing basis which adversely affects Employer's or other employees' ability to perform services.

h. It is agreed that any unresolved disputes will be settled by arbitration, including costs thereof.

This constitutes the entire agreement between Employee and Employer and supersedes any and all prior written or verbal agreements. Should any part of this agreement be deemed unenforceable, the remainder of the agreement continues in effect. This agreement is governed by the laws of the District of Columbia.

Signatures

Employee: _Frank Benjamin_____ Date: _July 4, 2001_

Employer: _Marshall Taylor_____ Date: _July 4, 2001_

Witness: _Joy Cronkite_____ Date: _July 4, 2001_

Figure 6.5

Independent Contractor Agreement

THIS AGREEMENT, made this 10th day of September, 2001, by and between TYRONE POWERHANDS (hereinafter called Licensed Massage Therapist or L.M.T.) and NATURE'S GENTLE HANDS, INC. (hereinafter called NGH), an Oregon corporation.

I
TERM

The term of this Agreement shall be for a period of one (1) year, commencing on the 1st day of October, 2001, and terminating on the 30th day of September, 2002, with a provision for a thirty (30) day written Notice of Termination of Contract due to dissatisfaction by either party.

II
NATURE OF RELATIONSHIP

The parties acknowledge and agree that the Licensed Massage Therapist is an independent contractor and is not an employee or agent of NGH for any purpose. NGH expects the Licensed Massage Therapist to perform without any additional training, direction, supervision or control on its part, except that NGH retains the right to specify from time to time the results to be achieved. NGH also retains the right to confirm that the expected standards are met and results achieved (as stipulated in the attached addendum). NGH will notify the Licensed Massage Therapist of any deviation from expected standards or results and direct the correction of such deviation(s).

NGH charges, on a sliding fee scale from $12.50 to $37.50, for space and table rental, fees for laundry, utilities and professional services based on individual L.M.T. usage. NGH will submit an invoice for services and costs on the last day of each month. The L.M.T. agrees to pay NGH on the 1st day of the month following the date of the invoice for the above services and rental costs. NGH will collect fees on behalf of the L.M.T. and distribute such fees at two week intervals with the first payment due October 15, 2001.

III
DUTIES

NGH shall provide to the Licensed Massage Therapist, the non-exclusive use of a designated area within NGH from which the Licensed Massage Therapist may administer services. The Licensed Massage Therapist's use of this room shall be limited solely for the purpose of administering massage treatments. The performance of services shall be available to the general public and not be limited in any way. The L.M.T. has a choice of time blocks, in which the treatment rooms and table are available. During these time blocks, the L.M.T. is not required to be on the premises between clients. (However, if the L.M.T. stays on the premises, walk-in clients may be obtained.) NGH will provide trays for the L.M.T.'s personal use to store oils and other personal supplies on the premises. NGH policy on out-calls is that referral service will be provided. A referral fee of $10 for the first visit and $5 for each visit over the next six months will be charged. The L.M.T. sets fees for outcalls.

The Licensed Massage Therapist shall obtain and maintain any and all required professional licenses and permits, and shall be solely responsible for the reporting and payment of all applicable federal, state or local income, sales and service taxes, licensing and permitting fees, and any other tax or assessment levied by governmental authorities relating to the performance of the Licensed Massage Therapist's duties under this agreement. NGH requires a copy of the L.M.T.'s license, business card, and liability insurance carrier to be kept on the premises.

The Licensed Massage Therapist shall keep the Treatment Rooms in good order and in a clean, sanitary condition.

NGH will have no liability for any services rendered by the Licensed Massage Therapist.

IV
ASSIGNMENT

The Licensed Massage Therapist may assign its rights and obligations to any person or entity, without restriction. Such assignee shall be placed in the stead of the assignor wherever mentioned in this Agreement, as of the date of such assignment. NGH expects 24-hour notice if the L.M.T. or assignee are not able to cover assigned time blocks. The L.M.T. and assignee are responsible for finding replacements. As a courtesy a phone tree of other therapists will be provided.

V
INSURANCE

The Licensed Massage Therapist is required to carry comprehensive general liability insurance with combined limits of one million dollars ($1,000,000.00) during the term of this Agreement, and will deliver a certificate of coverage for the term of this Agreement, with such insurance being deemed primary as to NGH, whether or not NGH has other insurance coverage. L.M.T. will provide NGH with thirty days written notice prior to cancellation of said coverage.

VI
REPRESENTATIONS

The Licensed Massage Therapist warrants and represents the following:
1. That L.M.T. is currently licensed by the Oregon Board of Massage and shall keep such license active and current during the term of this Agreement.
2. That L.M.T. will satisfactorily perform the services stipulated by this Agreement and shall provide services at all times in a lawful and professional manner, consistent with the high standards of NGH.

The parties hereby acknowledge and agree that notwithstanding anything contained in the Agreement to the contrary, in the event of a breach by the Licensed Massage Therapist in the performance of this Agreement, including, without limitation, a breach of any of the above warranties or representations, NGH may, in its sole discretion, immediately terminate this Agreement by giving notice to the Licensed Massage Therapist as provided for in Article XI below.

VII
INDEMNIFICATION

The Licensed Massage Therapist exonerates, protects, defends, indemnifies and saves harmless against and from any and all claims by or on behalf of any person, firm or corporation arising out of this Agreement, the relationship of the parties or the actions of the Licensed Massage Therapist or L.M.T.'s employees or agents and against and from all liability in connection with any and all costs and expenses reasonably incurred with respect to any such claim or any action or proceeding brought against NGH hereon, including without limitation, attorney's fees and costs (including attorney's fees and costs of any appeals).

VIII
REPAIRS

The Licensed Massage Therapist is responsible for any repairs or replacements made necessary by the act, neglect, fault, misfeasance or malfeasance of or by the Licensed Massage Therapist.

IX
SIGNS

The Licensed Massage Therapist shall not place any sign, other advertising material or other thing of any kind anywhere on the exterior or in the interior of the NGH building at without first obtaining the prior written approval from NGH. Such approval may be withheld for any reason whatsoever, including, without limitation, aesthetic reasons. In the event that NGH approves signage, advertising material or other things, the Licensed Massage Therapist shall maintain such item in good condition and repair at all times and shall promptly remove the same at the end of the term of this Agreement, if requested to do so by NGH within thirty (30) days from the end of the term of this Agreement.

X
CONDITION

The Licensed Massage Therapist acknowledges and agrees that the L.M.T.'s use of the Treatment Rooms shall be non-exclusive and that the L.M.T. has inspected the same in its present state and accepts it in "as is, where is" condition and shall vacate it at the end of the term of this Agreement in the same condition as received. Repair of normal wear and tear and damage caused by others or additions to the Treatment Rooms may not be made without first obtaining the prior written approval of NGH. Such approval may be withheld for any reason whatsoever, including without limitation, aesthetic reasons.

XI
NOTICES

All notices required by this Agreement shall be in writing and be delivered via United States Certified Mail, Return Receipt Requested, addressed to the party to whom such notices are directed. Either party may change its address for notices hereunder by giving notice to the other party in the same manner as provided herein.

XII
GOVERNING LAW

This Agreement shall be governed by and construed in accordance with the laws of the State of Oregon.

XIII
COMPLIANCE WITH LAWS AND ORDINANCES

The Licensed Massage Therapist agrees to comply with all laws, ordinances, rules and regulations applicable, from time to time, with respect to this Agreement and the operations stipulated herein.

XIV
ENTIRE AGREEMENT

The Licensed Massage Therapist acknowledges that NGH has not made any statement, promise or agreement, or taken upon itself any engagement whatsoever, verbally or in writing, in conflict with the terms of this Agreement, or which in any way modifies, varies, alters, enlarges or invalidates any of its provisions. This Agreement sets forth the entire understanding between the parties and shall not be changed, modified or amended, except by an instrument in writing signed by the party against whom the enforcement of any such change, modification or amendment is sought. The covenants and agreements herein contained shall bind, and the benefit and advantage hereof shall inure to, the respective heirs, legal representatives, successors and assigns of the parties. Whenever used the singular number shall include the plural and the plural shall include the singular and use of any gender shall include all genders. The headings set forth in this Agreement are for ease of reference only and shall not be interpreted to modify or limit the provisions hereof.

IN WITNESS WHEREOF, the parties hereto have caused this Agreement to be executed by their duly authorized officers, the day and year first above written.

Licensed Massage Therapist

_Tyrone Powerhands_____   Date: _September 10, 2001_
Tyrone Powerhands

Nature's Gentle Hands, Inc.

_Terry Terrific_____   Date: _September 10, 2001_
By: Terry Terrific
Its: President

Clerical Support Staff ⚉

Your clerical support staff is one of the quintessential operational assets of any small business. They are often the first encounter a potential client has with your business. In those first few minutes (as well as in the continuing relationship with established clients), your support staff establishes the persona of your business, its image and philosophy. Therefore, hiring the right type of person with the proper skills for your particular job requirements and client service is critical.

The first step is to identify what type of support you need. What are the job duties? Are you looking for a receptionist, secretary, bookkeeper, administrative assistant or operations manager? Each type of position has differing job duties and responsibilities. Some common office tasks are typing, filing, answering the phones, taking messages, producing monthly reports, filing insurance claims, analyzing data, marketing, maintaining databases, managing inventory and proofreading. To screen your candidates, interview effectively and hire intelligently, the position must be specified clearly and succinctly. Determine whether the position is part or full time; what hours you require; and the wage rate according to the demands of the position and the skill level required.

Motivate employees, train them, care about them, and make winners of them. At Marriott we know that if we treat our employees correctly, they'll treat the customers right. And if the customers are treated right, they'll come back.

— Bill Marriott Jr.

Once you have established the position's duties, responsibilities and the personality you need to project the persona of your business, design your interview questions to elicit the most information about your candidates and whether they will fit into the mold you have established for the job. Consider the following (true) story: A manager had gone through five secretaries in one year. She finally admitted that obviously something was amiss, otherwise, why would five different secretaries quit within a one-year period? The manager established that she needed to know what would make an individual person quit. Hence, in the interview, one of the questions she asked was simply, "What would make you quit a job?" She also got feedback from her previous employees and established a certain "personality" that she knew was needed in order to work together effectively and harmoniously.

Therefore, by identifying your position well and designing your interview effectively you enable yourself to choose the best possible support staff. Not just for yourself and your business persona, but for those you serve.

Managing Your Staff ⚉

As a manager or owner you are responsible for literally "supporting" all the members of your team, including your support staff. Simply establishing positions and hiring the appropriate people isn't the end, it's the beginning of a working "relationship." One of the most important concepts to grasp is that you are working "with" someone. This establishes a sense of teamwork and camaraderie. Remember, you will be working with your staff at least eight hours a day, five days a week. Quality intercommunication is essential. If issues arise regarding job performance, they need to be handled diplomatically and quickly.

Be certain to listen to all the team members as they are the ones who deal with daily tasks and generally have some very creative, imaginative and efficient methods of conducting their work. Never underestimate your staff. They may have some surprising abilities that when allowed to come forth will be assets to your business. They may not all have college degrees and the support staff may not be versed in the intricacies of your profession, but don't insult their intelligence.

It's also important to allow individual autonomy and not be over-controlling (micro-management). Give your staff the authority to make decisions. Make certain they understand your policies and know when they can determine the proper action and when they must first confer with you. It's okay to oversee your staff and review their actions, but don't monitor their every move. Identify barriers to effective teamwork and eliminate them.

One of the reasons people stop learning is that they become less and less willing to risk failure.
— John W. Gardner

Institute annual performance reviews which not only evaluate job performance, but also establish goals and objectives for the coming year. Review the position duties and responsibilities and make adjustments according to the changing needs of your office operations. Make this performance review a two-way communication. Ask your staff to clarify:

1. Their perception of their duties and responsibilities.
2. What contributions have they made to the position other than the mechanics of the job?
3. What goals and objectives do they have for the coming year?
4. What additional seminars, lectures or outside activities would they like to participate in relative to their position and enhanced job knowledge and performance?

Answer these questions from your own perspective and then sit down together to review them. This allows each of you to jointly assess the previous year, while lessening the opportunity for misunderstanding and poor communication about each of your expectations and needs. Included in this performance evaluation should be an objective review of performance (e.g., Quality of Work, Quantity of Work, Communication, Timeliness).

A well-designed performance evaluation is an excellent management tool promoting effective, clear communication and establishing a sense of teamwork. This helps form a satisfying working relationship.

Don't wait until the end of the coming year to informally discuss progress and concerns. Conduct informal reviews quarterly, if not monthly. This provides an occasion for you to affirm exceptional performance, correct minor difficulties before they become major problems and initiate changes in operational needs in a timely manner. It also allows your staff the opportunity to discuss those matters of concern they may have in their working relationship with you or your clients.

In addition to reviews, you need to hold staff meetings. These should be at least once per month and preferably once per week. These meetings serve to build camaraderie as well as provide a forum to discuss problems, learn new skills, brainstorm ideas and set goals. It also keeps each other informed about what is being done and fosters better understanding when people are aware of each other's projects and deadlines.

Unfortunately, in any business, you find the "Jobs That Nobody Wants To Do." These tasks are either boring, unpleasant or difficult to accomplish. It isn't uncommon for resentments to arise around these noxious tasks. As a manager you need to find a way to balance these duties among your staff. This can be difficult when you only have one employee or if you are the only person in your business. If you're lucky, you will find someone who loves to do those tasks that everyone else hates. Alas, these people are rare. So, the next best option is to hold a staff meeting and brainstorm ideas for dealing with these tasks. Conducting brainstorming sessions and including your staff in some of the decision-making processes will make them feel as though they are part of a team—and when people feel that they are working as a team, they are less apt to feel resentful over having to do those "awful" assignments.

One of the outcomes of a brainstorming session might be a change in the company's operations and procedures. Sometimes a slight alteration in the execution of a task can alleviate the dread associated with it. Frequently, tasks can be simplified or even eliminated. Changes don't occur very often because people rarely take the time to evaluate policies, procedures and goals. Another outcome of the brainstorming session may be that the staff decides to rotate these unpleasant tasks. Whatever the results of this session are, it's imperative that you follow through and monitor the progress.

See Chapter Three, pages 43-44 for more information on motivation.

People are motivated most by recognition, appreciation and participation. Each person on your team requires a different type of encouragement. Get input from your staff and develop incentive programs.

The net result in the proper management of your team is the optimum in working harmony, efficiency in working capacity, the building of good working relations with your staff, establishing goodwill with your clients and a bottom line that shows black.

• Private Practice Issues •

Running a one-person practice is very different than working in association with other health care providers, being part of a clinic, or providing treatments at a spa or salon. You still have to perform the basic practice management activities, though in a different manner for each arrangement. Also you may need to incorporate additional activities.

At some point in their careers, most health care providers work alone, either out of a private office, home or out-call. A private practice provides freedom, flexibility (e.g., you choose the attire, clients, environment, music, lighting, ambiance, creativity, modalities, fees and scheduling) and you can essentially do anything you want as long as it's legal, ethical and moral. In addition to the general practice management activities mentioned in this chapter, the sole practitioner must contend with other issues as follows.

Autonomy ~

Along with the freedom of being on your own is the potential for loneliness and isolation. You are the one responsible for making certain everything is done, which often means YOU get to do it all—until you can afford to hire an assistant.

Tips

- Establish a support system of colleagues and advisors to assist you in creating a healthy, profitable private practice.
- Trade tasks with colleagues (e.g., you balance her checkbook and she helps you develop your marketing plan).
- Join at least one networking group.
- Attend conferences and expositions.
- Hire someone to do tasks so that you can focus on providing quality health care services. In other words: Do The Math. If you pay someone $10 an hour for 10 hours a week ($100) and that frees you up to do 8 more sessions at $50 each ($400), you'll net $300, plus you won't have to do those tasks you abhor.

Safety ~

Safety should always be a concern for any business owner, but even more for the person in private practice. You don't always know who the clients are the first time they come to your office or the neighborhood you'll be entering if you do out-calls or on-site services.

Tips

- Ideally, only work hours when someone else is in the building (or your home).
- Lock your treatment room door so uninvited people can't wander in.
- If you are the only person in your office, call a friend (while the client is nearby) and tell him that you will call him after your session. This precaution also works well when you are on an out-call.
- When working at night, make sure the area is well-lit.
- Keep your car in good condition and adequately fueled.

Finances ∾

When you are the only source of revenue in your business, you may not have the cash flow to purchase items when you want them. Oft times you need to delay financial expenditures such as expensive equipment (e.g., an office copier, computer or hydraulic table).

Tips

- Create a reserve account specifically for purchasing high-ticket items.
- Prepare (and update) a cash-flow forecast.
- Barter.
- Lease equipment.

Benefits ∾

The only "employment benefits" you receive are the ones you pay for yourself (which kind of defeats the whole concept of "perks"). As a sole practitioner there are no true paid vacations, holidays or sick days.

Tips

- Set up a savings account for "paid" days off.
- Purchase appropriate health and disability insurance.
- Verify that your auto insurance covers lost income if you are in an accident (this isn't standard).

• Group Practice Issues •

Group practices can be formed as an association or partnership. (In most instances, health care providers prefer to form associations rather than partnerships). The benefits of a group practice include: the potential for more interaction with others—easing the sense of isolation; the synergy that gets created when there's two or more people; offering a wider variety of services and thus attracting a larger market; working off each other's strengths; increased safety; having backup (someone to work on your clients as well as another source of income to cover costs) if you are ill or want to take a vacation; reduced overhead; projects a higher professional image; easy access to peer support; increased buying power (better discounts on quantity supplies and inventory for resale); and it's usually more fun and rewarding to share your space with others.

See Chapter Five, pages 74-79 for information on legal structures.

Unfortunately, too many people develop these alliances without creating a proper structure. The following scenario demonstrates how easy it is to set yourself up for problems when working in a group practice.

Group Practice Scenario

A massage therapist (Steve) decides to share an already established office with another therapist (Terry). The office is situated in a prime location and Steve has been feeling rather isolated in his practice. He has known Terry for several years and respects her work. Steve asks Terry to create an association agreement, but Terry refuses and acts offended (this should have immediately sent Steve running in the opposite direction). Steve decides to proceed anyway. After all, they are both caring, responsible adults, and he feels confident they could work out any problems. Things go fairly well for several years. Terry starts getting involved in accounts that take her outside of the office, so she brings in another massage therapist (Stacy) to work with clients in her treatment room. This is done without consulting Steve. Now there are three people sharing the total space, yet Steve is still paying half of the expenses. Resentment brews. Then Steve discovers something that sends him over the edge: Several times clients had called to book sessions with him when he wasn't in the office. Stacy talked with the clients and instead of trying to figure out another time when they could schedule with Steve, she booked the appointments for herself. He is unable to resolve these issues and no guidelines had been set for how to deal with unresolved conflicts. So, Steve gives notice. He wants to leave as soon as possible but agrees to stay for several months. Meanwhile, things go from bad to worse. He feels uncomfortable in his own office. He realizes that communication is difficult, so when the time nears for him to leave, he submits a written 30-days notice. The next day, Steve goes to work only to discover that the locks to the office had been changed. Ultimately, the situation gets resolved, but not without unnecessary grief and anger, not to mention the intervention of an attorney.

The Partnership Book by D. Clifford and R. Warner Nolo Press This book is filled with excellent information and sample forms for developing partnership agreements that can also be adapted for association agreements.

You can avoid these pitfalls and garner the benefits of working with others by observing the following practice management considerations.

Self-Assessment ᨠ

The first phase in choosing an associate or partner is clarifying your reasons for wanting to share your business (or space) with another person. For instance, are you doing this because you want to or is it mainly stemming from financial desperation? It's vital that you assess your temperament to determine if it's appropriate for you to have another person involved in your business. Think about how you want to share your space and how much control you need to exert: if you are uncomfortable when things aren't done in a specific manner, it may become difficult for you to share an office, let alone be in partnership. If you decide to go ahead with the idea, you need to be clear about the desired relationship between yourself and your potential associate/partner. Do you want this person to play an active role in your business or would you rather just have someone to share ideas and expenses?

Memories fade. You can avert problems by referring to a partnership document.

Tips

- Clarify your reasons for considering a group practice.
- Make a list of the characteristics of your "ideal associate/partner." Then highlight those qualities that are absolutely essential.

Interviews ᨠ

After you have clarified your reasons for wanting an associate/partner and have envisioned his/her qualities, it's time to conduct interviews. Your closest friends or colleagues may not be the wisest choices. Invest the time required to do this well; after all, this is someone you may be seeing day in and day out. Share with each other your dreams, goals and concerns. Some of the questions to consider are: How long do you intend to stay in this location? What kind of work schedule do you prefer to keep? What type of atmosphere do you want to have? Who do you want as clients? Do you ultimately want additional associates or employees? Do you plan on incorporating other services or products?

Look for the commonalities and possible areas of conflict. Do your businesses complement each other? Are your fee structures similar? Also, get to know each other's communication style and see if your personalities are compatible. Everyone has their own personality and way of doing things and these styles don't always mesh well in a business setting. For example, if you prefer a methodical approach to business and your partner tends to work best under pressure or in chaos—you may be in for a tempestuous association.

Tips

- Identify your strengths and limitations.
- Write job descriptions for yourself and potential associates/partners.
- Pick people not just because they're friends, but because as a group you're more powerful than as single entities.

Roles, Goals and Expectations ~~~

If you have decided that indeed you would like to become associates or partners, the next step is to delineate—**in writing**—your roles and expectations. List all of the things that are important to each of you in running your business.

In addition to writing your shared vision, goals, roles and expectations, I strongly encourage you to create a dissolution (or buy-out) agreement. Who knows what the future holds? People's goals change or major life-altering circumstances may occur. Make sure that all parties have a realistic means to ethically and amicably part ways. If you decide to become partners (and not just associates), I highly recommend you design a full business plan before the partnership is official. In the process of developing your business plan you will be compelled to evaluate your strengths and weaknesses, clarify your financial arrangements, delineate your roles, determine legal responsibilities and refine your business vision. Also, memories aren't always accurate; you can avoid many misunderstandings by referring to a written agreement.

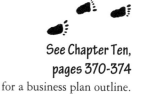

See Chapter Ten, pages 370-374 for a business plan outline.

Tips

- Clarify roles and expectations. Delineate them IN WRITING! Make sure that you share a vision on where you want to go with your business and the image you wish to portray.
- Create a written association agreement which includes dissolution terms.
- Include a section in your association agreement on procedures for handling problems (conflict resolution).
- Develop a business plan as well as written office policies and procedures.
- Adopt a Code of Ethics.

Legal Status ~~~

Most group practices are associations and not partnerships: that is, the practitioners get together to share resources and expenses, keeping separate business identities. A partnership is two or more people contributing assets to a jointly-owned business and sharing in the profits or losses (although not necessarily equally). To be considered a partnership you do not need to use the term "partner" or have a written partnership agreement. The operative phrase is "jointly owned." In many states if you're *perceived* to be a partnership, you could be held liable for something your associate does. Legalese aside, your reputation could be on the line if anyone else within your group does something unprofessional.

Tips

- Create an association or partnership agreement.
- Clearly post an announcement that states each person in the office has his/her own separate business.
- Purchase appropriate insurance.

Image ～

It's important to decide the image you wish to portray. Nothing is quite as frustrating as sharing space with others who don't hold a similar vision or standards.

Tips

- Include a section on image in your association/partnership agreement. Cover items such as the way clients are greeted, practitioners' attire, physical layout of the office, beverages you make available, music and noise level.
- Coordinate office furniture so it doesn't appear hodge-podge.
- Develop telephone scripts for consistency.
- Decide ahead of time what your budget and goals are for office embellishments (e.g., flowers and holiday decorations).
- Make certain the types of therapy offered aren't in conflict. For example, a massage therapist who works with elderly clients and does a lot of quiet guided meditations would not coexist well with a counselor who does Primal Scream Therapy (which can get very noisy).

Product Sales ～

Product sales are a great diversification method and the profits can be used to defray overhead expenses. The three biggest problems are choosing the product lines, determining who is responsible for overseeing sales, and calculating who gets what profit (particularly when a client sees more than one practitioner in the group setting). Note: if your business is a partnership, then the funds can be commingled.

Tips

- As a group, create an action plan for product sales, including goals and a budget.
- Associates Option One: Even though you may place orders as one entity, each practitioner is responsible for paying for their share of the inventory and collecting revenues from sales.
- Associates Option Two: Assign one person to oversee product sales, from stocking inventory to processing sales through her account. Allow her to keep a percentage of the profits to cover time in managing product sales. Apply the rest of the profits to lower shared overhead expenses (e.g., rent, linen service, telephone and marketing).

Marketing ~

Many marketing activities and expenses can be shared even when group practices are associations and not partnerships. Actually, this is one of the strongest benefits to being in a group practice. The combined energy, expertise and financial resources can provide diversity and afford you the opportunity to experiment with avenues that were previously unaffordable or infeasible.

Tips

- Determine what percentage of marketing is to be done jointly.
- Develop a marketing plan with goals, target dates and a budget.
- Before placing long-term advertising (e.g., a Yellow Pages ad), create a payment agreement to cover the possibility of an associate leaving.

Finances ~

Financial obligations can be a major source of entanglement in an association. Usually one person is required to assume responsibility for each major account (e.g., rent, utilities and telephone). If you commingle too many funds then you are in essence creating a partnership.

Tips

- If at all possible, have everyone's name included on the lease.
- Clarify the group's shared budget and do financial projections (be cautious when jointly making major purchases unless you are indeed partners).
- Draw up contracts outlining each person's financial obligations.
- Determine how profits are to be split.

Interaction Levels ~

Some people get involved in a group practice merely to share expenses while others desire more contact and camaraderie. Although communications and time spent together will vary, it's important to clarify your desired levels of interaction. It takes time, energy and concern to maintain decent relationships.

Tips

- Clarify the purpose, level and types of desired interactions.
- Hold regular "office" meetings.
- Determine the types of preferred peer support and schedule meetings.
- Establish a schedule for doing office tasks and marketing.

Office Logistics ～

Logistics mainly encompasses the day-to-day activities in running the business, such as preparing the office for clients, stocking supplies, cleaning and coordinating repairs. Most people in group practices develop a task list and share those activities.

Tips

- Clearly define the levels of cleanliness required. Every person has their own standards of quality, so it's vital to establish agreed-upon parameters.
- Set up a cleaning schedule.
- Coordinate schedules to cover hours of operation.
- Create objective consequences for when a person doesn't fulfill her obligations.

Booking Clients ～

In most group practices each individual is responsible for booking his own clients. This gets fuzzy when clients come in from shared marketing activities (particularly a Yellow Pages ad). You can avoid many misunderstandings and resentment by creating a new client booking policy.

Tips

- Make a list of all the practitioners and then place a check next to each one's name every time she gets a new client. In general, it's best to match the first caller with the first practitioner on the list and then proceed down the list. This isn't always possible when a client wants an appointment at a certain time (or desires a specific service) and the only person available is the one who received the last referral. But if you review the list, whoever answers the phone knows that practitioner B gets first choice of the next new client.
- Develop a telephone script.
- Keep everyone's appointment schedule next to the main telephone.

• Clinic Issues •

A growing trend for health care providers is working in clinic environments. This provides many potential benefits such as: increased opportunity to interact with other health professionals and do case management; the possibility of walking into a full practice with little marketing; being able to provide a larger scope of services for your clients' well-being; starting out with a ready-made professional image; being part of an office with clear and established boundaries; reduced paperwork (there's usually a secretary, nurse or assistant who manages the office); the ability to focus on hands-on work; access to better and more varied equipment and supplies; excellent built-in referral base; and it's usually easier to get insurance reimbursement if you are not already a recognized primary care provider.

The old cliche is true: "An ounce of prevention is worth a pound of cure."

The major concerns are: working with other's visions, policies and procedures; the possibility of needing to alter your style and scope of practice; and the controversy of being hired as an independent contractor versus employee.

I realize that some of the following suggestions require a major time investment on your part. However, the time expended is well worth the savings in effort, disappointment and potential legal problems in solving conflicts. It's best if you can cover as many of the tips as possible prior to signing a working contract. If you are unable to complete all the activities prior to employment, prioritize them and achieve them as soon as possible.

Image ⤳

Be sure the clinic attracts the kind of clients with whom you want to work, provides opportunities for you to use your favorite modalities, and allows you to work at a pace and style in which you're comfortable. Keep in mind that the environment may be more sterile than you prefer and require regimented policies and procedures. If your style is holistic, then you probably won't be happy in an allopathic setting. Many clinics approach dress formally (e.g., uniforms or lab coats) while others are more casual and allow you to choose your apparel. Some have stringent hygiene policies such as long hair pulled back and in a bun, no facial hair and no perfume. It's important that the personalities, styles and philosophies of the various health professionals blend—otherwise, conflict can arise over working conditions and what's best for the client/patient.

Tips

Before agreeing to work at the clinic, do the following:
- Sit in the waiting room at various times on different days to see who shows up and experience the ambiance (e.g., furniture, music, scents, comfort and friendliness of staff).
- Discuss the types of clients who are seen in the clinic (target markets, conditions addressed and health philosophies).

- Examine the appointment book to see how often your type of service is being (or could be) utilized and to determine the treatment time allotted.
- Meet with each staff member and practitioner to determine if styles mesh. Create scenarios and discuss how to handle the situations. (Let them dominate the conversation.)
- Review the clinic's mission statement and policies.
- Obtain copies of all promotional materials.

After joining the clinic:
- Discuss ideas for changes at staff meetings.

Interaction Levels ～

One of the prime advantages to working in a clinic environment is the opportunity to do case management. You can better serve your clients when they have access to a variety of health care providers under one roof who actively work together for the optimum well-being of clients. For this to succeed, what's required is communication, time, cooperation and shared values.

Tips

Before agreeing to work at the clinic, do the following:
- Make sure that you hold a similar philosophy toward well-being as the clinic members, (i.e., are your approaches compatible and are they committed to the same level of customer service as you are).
- Agree on the definition of case management and what it entails, including the degree of interaction between the providers.
- Make sure that you're educated in the proper terminology to readily communicate with the other health professionals in their language regarding patient care.

After joining the clinic:
- Set weekly meetings to discuss case management goals.
- Review the next week's client/patient load prior to the weekly meetings. Update your treatment plans and be prepared to discuss them.
- Present your treatment plans concisely and with supporting data to gain cooperation.
- Be willing to compromise for the client's best interest, setting aside ego.
- Allow time daily to consult with each other on last-minute issues or walk-in clients.

Client Contact ～

Most practitioners discover that they need to alter their treatments in a clinic setting. The time you spend with clients and the actual work you do may be determined by the lead primary care provider. You could be told what to do, how to do it, when to do it and the time allowed. You may even experience a sense of detachment from the client because someone else usually handles the greeting, scheduling, payment, paperwork and at times the follow-up (on the positive side, this may provide you with more hands-on time with your clients). Clients benefit by your being in a clinic because it provides access to managed care as well as state-of-the-art equipment (that you otherwise might not be able to afford). Also, your schedule may be more standardized given that few clinics are open late evenings or Sundays.

Tips

Before agreeing to work at the clinic, do the following:
- Visit the clinic as a "new patient." Experience how everything is handled. This will give you good insight into the clinic even though you might get treated a bit more carefully (since they know who you are).
- Covert operations: send a friend as a "new patient" and debrief afterward.
- Give the referring providers a mini-session and then a full treatment so they can experience the difference.
- Discuss your vision with the other providers. Allow everyone to share their preferred treatment styles and create treatment guidelines.
- Establish an agreement that allows you to develop and maintain your own client base and utilize the clinic's facilities.

After joining the clinic:
- Make sure the front office staff are aware of your time requirements for working with clients.
- Take the time to do a short post-session interview with each client. Utilize this information for enhancing your further work with the client and making any alterations in service, environment or operational procedures.
- Review all client files monthly and do appropriate follow-up.
- Educate the staff and providers on the benefits and scope of your services.
- Review the specific client's file just prior to the actual session.
- Given that someone else may be using your space, make sure your room is clean and stocked with necessary supplies before your client arrives.

Finances ～

Clinic finances tend to be complex, especially considering the necessity for providing fairness in shared expenses, clients and revenues from product sales. If you are dealing with insurance reimbursement, you may not receive payment for months after you've done the work. You also may ultimately be responsible for generating your own clientele if the other practitioners aren't consistent in their referrals.

It's vital to create clear agreements to avoid entanglements and misunderstandings. For instance, a conflict of interest might arise if you're only working there part time and you have clients of your own whom you don't want to come into the office because of the percentage you'd have to give up. This can escalate to an ethical dilemma.

Clinic Scenario

You work at a clinic four days a week and maintain a small home-based practice. A clinic client (Tensio Muscalia) has received his total insurance-covered massages for the current year. He is still in need of further treatment. Your rates at the clinic are substantially higher than your home-based practice. Tensio has somehow discovered this and has requested private sessions. What do you do?

If you had previously set up guidelines, this issue could be avoided or at least resolved with minimum conflict.

The other major source of financial concern is employment status. Oftentimes, practitioners are "hired" as independent contractors, yet as defined by the Internal Revenue Service they are usually deemed employees.

Tips

Before agreeing to work at the clinic, do the following:
- Clarify your employment status. Determine which category best suits your needs and fits with IRS guidelines.
- Your financial arrangements are determined by which category of employment is chosen. For instance, an employee isn't responsible for clinic expenses nor shares in revenues whereas an independent contractor would be expected to pick up certain expenses and receive a percentage of revenue. This would affect the amount you charge and the bottom line of what you receive per client session.
- In the case of independent contractors, profits generated from product sales could be applied to lowering the overall expenses.
- Define parameters for working with clients outside of the clinic.
- Establish an agreement that allows you to develop and maintain your own client base and utilize the clinic's facilities.
- Determine client status and any fees or percentages incurred in the event you leave.
- Consult with a business coach, attorney or financial advisor before signing on at the clinic.

After joining the clinic:
- Do cash flow forecasting to budget (particularly if you will be receiving deferred payments).
- Be proactive in financial matters regarding the clinic.

Logistics ∿

Logistics entails the day-to-day clinic operations. You need to know what the expectations are of you when you're not directly working with clients (e.g., paperwork, janitorial chores, clerical duties, assisting the other practitioners, providing treatments for staff and marketing). Whether you get paid for these activities depends upon your employment status.

Tips

Before agreeing to work at the clinic, do the following:
- Determine your boundaries and what activities you will consent to doing.

After joining the clinic:
- Establish guidelines for non-hands-on activities.
- Clarify the performance parameters for each given task.
- Prioritize logistic activities.

• Spa and Salon Issues •

Spas and salons are expanding their scope from simply furnishing beauty services to offering health care services. It's commonplace to find health care providers (e.g., touch therapists, acupuncturists, estheticians, energy workers and nutritionists) in both of these settings.

Spas and upscale salons provide a luxurious atmosphere. Working at this type of location can be quite nice. The equipment tends to be first rate and products are of high quality. Staff is available to do the scheduling, place confirmation calls and handle financial transactions. Plus, there is a team environment.

Working in these settings also requires conforming to a set image and structuring your treatments to align with the company's schedule. Many practitioners hire on at a spa or salon part-time to augment their private practices. This can be boring, frustrating and financially disadvantageous unless you work where the schedule is fairly full or you receive a base pay when no clients book sessions.

Image ∿

Spas range in image from holistic wellness centers to posh pampering resorts. Salons range from crowded bustling turnstiles to lush elegant day spas. The requirements in terms of attire, interactions and skills vary with the environment. Some spas advocate practitioners expand their skills so they can perform other services when not doing their primary service (e.g., hydrotherapy, wraps and paraffin treatments).

Treatment rooms in spas are likely to be roomier and more well-appointed than in salons. Often salon treatment rooms are very close to other activities, lack temperature control units in the rooms and are not well-insulated from sounds and odors.

Before hiring on at a spa or salon, determine if it attracts the type of clients you want to work with and allows you to work at a comfortable pace and style. Consider the people who frequent these establishments, the kinds of services they require and the manner in which they expect to be treated.

Tips

- Make sure your personality matches the setting (e.g., customer-service-oriented to the max, perky, happy, warm, nurturing yet detached, in-the-moment ability to appreciate the person and session, flexible, willing to do grunt work).
- Clarify expectations.
- Find out if uniforms are required. If so, ascertain if the company furnishes them (and how many) or if you must purchase them. If they furnish them, do they also launder and press them?
- Make sure that if there are no separate room temperature controls, you have a portable heater and fan in the room.
- Meet with the health care practitioners, staff and other service providers to determine if styles and personalities mesh.
- Review the company's mission statement and promotional materials.
- Attempt to share a room with someone whose cleanliness and taste is compatible with yours.
- If you work in a salon, see if you can arrange it so that the treatment room isn't adjacent to drying or chemical stations.

Interaction Levels ⚞

Spas and salons offer you the opportunity to contact a wide variety of people, both colleagues, associates and clients (versus the isolation of working at home or in an office alone). The camaraderie and team environment can be very appealing and stimulating. The down side is contending with workplace politics and gossip (which can be rampant in salons).

Tips

- Practice conscious detachment.
- Be cautious in all communication.
- Keep a positive attitude and encourage others to do the same.

Finances ∼

Salons and spas usually have distinct financial arrangements. Salons customarily rent rooms to practitioners. Salons rarely have more than three health care providers (usually touch therapists and estheticians) on site whereas spas often have 20-50 active practitioners. Some spas hire practitioners as employees and others as independent contractors (the independent contractor status is being challenged nationwide by the IRS because these establishments tend to treat practitioners like employees, yet classify them as independent contractors to reduce paperwork and cost). Compensation varies greatly between spas: some pay on commission, others offer a combination of base salary with a commission. The average wage is in the mid $20 per hour range (this is for hours when the practitioner is actually giving treatments).

If the spa isn't well-known with a high guest count, there might not be a lot of work available for the practitioners—meaning your shift would not be filled. When slots go unfilled, the therapists may not be required to do any other type of work, which means they are also not paid for the time. For example, one spa in Arizona only pays practitioners for the actual client treatments. While the practitioners are not required to do other work or stay on the premises, they must be able to return on a half-hour's notice if paged during their scheduled shift.

Spas often base salaries and preferential scheduling on seniority. This tremendously impacts your finances, particularly if residing in a location where the numbers of clients hinges upon the season.

Working in these settings does avail certain perquisites. You can receive discounts on services and products. If you work at a spa, you may be able to use the facilities and get free or low-cost meals. When hired as an employee, the benefits can include health insurance, paid vacations, paid sick days, pension plans, profit sharing and reimbursement for continuing education.

Tips

- Get seniority.
- Develop a small private practice as well (in your home or part-time office space rental).
- Clarify your employment status.
- Create clear financial contracts.

Client Contact ∼

Clients are usually happy and upbeat—they go to spas and salons to look better and feel better. They may desire long-term benefits, yet rarely expect major therapeutic work; although in salons there's an air of expectation that it's also therapy central (as people are used to confiding in their hairdressers).

You may need to alter your style, modalities and length of your sessions. Most spas maintain fairly rigid schedules, but salons are usually a bit more flexible. You don't get to choose your clients, whereas you have greater control with a private practice. Salons and spas tend to provide a safe environment. You don't have to worry about sexual impropriety from clients—it rarely happens, and if it does, assistance is nearby.

Spa work provides minimal opportunity to mark progress or make lasting connections because clients rarely return regularly. You end up with less emotional investment in clients' issues than when you work with someone consistently. Given the nature of spas, practitioners usually do a variety of treatments; this is less taxing on the body, reduces the likelihood of repetitive stress syndrome and keeps work interesting.

Tips

- Keep client files. (Spas: Indicate which clients are locals.)
- Develop an intake form that can be completed quickly or even done during the first few minutes of the treatment.
- Maintain clear boundaries.
- Review locals' files monthly and do appropriate follow-up.

Marketing ~~~

In a spa, you technically don't have to do the marketing or scheduling of clients, but there is no guarantee that your work hours will be filled. Most practitioners discover (to their dismay) that they need to market their services when working in a salon. For instance, massage and other health treatments are of primary concern to spa visitors whereas massage is one of the least utilized services in salons. Sometimes salons downplay massage so much that it isn't even listed on the services board. Rarely do you find massage prominently displayed in salon marketing materials.

The majority of spa guests are from out of town; salons mainly draw local residents and yield repeat business. Working in a salon provides potential for easy marketing because of the sheer volume of traffic. People visiting a salon have the mindset of looking better and it's a short transition to wanting to feel better. Salons offer clients a one-stop shop for health **and** beauty care.

Salons provide you with a built-in clientele of people who *need* your services—the other employees!

Tips

- The best way to ensure referrals is make sure that everyone who works at the salon experiences your services.
- Confirm new clients yourself.
- Have good signage.
- Whenever you have empty slots, connect with clients who are waiting in the lobby. If you are a massage therapist, offer to give free five-minute sessions. If you are an esthetician, you can give product demonstrations.
- Offer referral incentives.

- Put your marketing materials in the lobby.
- Hold educational meetings for your co-workers. Explain the benefits of your work, give demonstrations and show them tips for self-care.
- Discuss marketing ideas with management.

Logistics ～

Logistics entails day-to-day business activities. The major areas of concern are the physical space, products, supplies and what you do with your time when not working on clients.

In salons, you usually have to share the treatment room with other practitioners. In spas, the room you work in constantly changes (musical-chairs-syndrome). It becomes a challenge to focus when the room isn't yours—lacks your personality and the layout may not be what you prefer. Additionally, the rooms may not be adequately sized or insulated and the equipment may vary from room to room.

Most spas provide you with all equipment and supplies (e.g., linens, oils and music). Unless the salon offers a variety of health care services, you may need to supply everything yourself (particularly linens).

The expectations surrounding what you do when not working with a client depend upon the company philosophy and your employment status. Some facilities expect practitioners to assist wherever they're needed—from greeting clients to cleaning. Oddly enough, these expectations can be present even when you aren't getting paid for non-client interactions.

Tips

- Review policy and procedure manuals.
- Clarify ambiguous policies.
- Determine who prepares the room for a session.
- Arrange to have a room that gets assigned to you whenever possible.
- Set explicit duties and responsibilities.

Booking Clients ～

Most receptionists are not very proactive when it comes to marketing health care services. This is understandable (to a point) given the vast number of available services. The other problems inherent in having someone other than you do the scheduling are that the receptionists might not know enough about your treatments to answer questions and inspire clients to try your services, they may be less than enthusiastic about you and your work, or worse—play favorites.

Scheduling is another concern. You may not have the autonomy to decide what clients you work with and the types of sessions you do. Some companies expect you to work a complete shift without a break. For instance, you may find yourself booked for four deep tissue sessions in a row with no time in between to recuperate. Although the schedule can be flexible, most facilities are open on weekends. Spas tend to stay open on holidays and have extended hours. Last-minute cancellations are common in salons.

Tips

- Be at peace with periodic "breaks" and have personal activities ready to do (e.g., books to read, correspondence, workout and meditation).
- Have clear procedures for booking sessions.
- If you work in a salon, have your business cards and brochures on display at the reception desk.
- Have the receptionist send your brochure to new clients.
- Set clear cancellation policies.
- Develop a script for receptionists.
- Call all the people who inquired about your services. Don't rely on the receptionists to secure new clients.

• Job Interviews •

It's wise to learn interviewing skills—even if you are or plan to be self-employed. Much of the basics in being adept at interviewing center on having excellent communication skills. You must be confident, and most important of all, you must be prepared.

Successful Interviewing Skills

- Be well-poised, centered and relaxed.
- Maintain good eye contact.
- Listen to what is really being said.
- Dress appropriately and be on time.
- Use positive wording and take control of the interview.
- Avoid telephone interviews.
- Ask specific questions and don't give vague answers.
- Look for closing signals.
- Avoid discussing salary and benefits in the first interview.
- Be prepared. Have necessary documentation available.
- Bring an appointment book and a classy pen.

After you have honed your interviewing skills, you must learn how to get an interview.

- Create a list of potential employers. Get their addresses, phone numbers and the names and titles of the people who have hiring authority.

- Network. Network. Network. Talk to people, let them know you're available. Ask for leads. Remember, quite often it's who you know that gets you the job.

- Set up initial contact on the phone. You must be well-organized, know your purpose and goals for this call. The primary goal, of course, is to get an interview.

- If you don't get an interview from this initial contact, send a resumé with a cover letter or just send a letter.

- If you have not gotten a response within five days of the potential employer having received your letter, call them.

- In some cases, endurance pays off. If you keep yourself so visible that an employer is fully aware that you really want to work for her company, you may get the job out of sheer persistence.

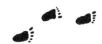

Refer to Chapter Nine, pages 314-319 for more specifics on networking.

Before your personal interview, prepare yourself. Research the company; know how long it's been in business, the number of employees and the services it offers. Be ready with answers that the employer is likely to ask. Role-play the potential interview with a friend. Get feedback. Make any changes necessary so that you can have an excellent interview.

Resumés

The purpose of a resumé is to get you a job interview. Rarely is anyone hired solely on the basis of a resumé. Indeed, most employers use resumés for the initial screening of job applicants. A resumé that inspires a potential employer to interview you is one that conveys your talents and clearly demonstrates your ability to produce results that align with the particular company's goals. This is why it's so important to research your potential employers. Make certain you know to whom you are writing: learn about the company's history, its mission, needs and problems; determine the ways in which your skills can contribute to the company's success; and finally, ascertain the name and title of the person in charge of hiring (which isn't always the personnel administrator).

Your cover letter is an integral part of your resumé packet. This is where you establish rapport. Keep your tone friendly and use terminology that's appropriate to your field. Open your letter with something you find interesting about the company. Inform them how you can be of direct benefit to the company. Close your letter by requesting an interview.

In the health care field, your resumé may be very different from the traditional ones, where the focus is demonstrating results, and that may be difficult for you to do. It's important to think of your resumé not in terms of a biography, but as a prospectus for your future.

The two major types of resumés are chronological and functional. The chronological resumé is used when you want to emphasize a good work history that is directly related to your desired job. The functional resumé is used when you want to emphasize your talents, abilities and potential—not your work history. In most instances health care providers use more of a functional resumé or sometimes even just a targeted personal letter.

Targeted Personal Letter

A targeted personal letter is appropriate when you have a specific job in mind. It's particularly valuable when you want to focus on your abilities—regardless of whether or not you've had much experience or training. You must determine the type of job you want and specify it up front with a title (e.g., Spa Coordinator, Massage Therapist, Staff Counselor, Speech Therapist), and possibly include a short description if the title doesn't fully convey the job description.

As with a cover letter, the first thing to do is develop rapport. Then discuss your desired job position and give a concise, dynamic summary of your experience, capabilities and achievements that directly relate to the targeted job. You may want to include specific work history and education, but keep the focus on what you have to offer. Close the letter by suggesting a time to get together. Type this on letterhead stationery and keep the length to one page.

The closest most people come to perfection is when they fill out a job application.
— Don L. Griffith

Chronological Resumé Format

Heading

Name, address and phone. Centered at top of the page.

Work Experience

Start with your present or most recent job. It isn't necessary to give the month and day, just the year. List your employer, job title and a brief description of your duties. Emphasize your major accomplishments and abilities. You don't have to list each position change within a company.

Education

Include year graduated, name of school, degree(s), certification(s) and any awards or honors. If your education is within the past few years, it should be the first thing listed after the heading, otherwise put it at the bottom.

Personal

This is optional. Only include information you feel is valuable toward getting you the job.

Functional Resumé Format

Heading

Name, address and phone. Centered at top of the page.

Function

List your strongest abilities or accomplishments in four or five separate paragraphs—put them in order of relevance to desired job. Have a major headline for each paragraph (e.g., Sports Psychology or Staff Management)

Work Experience

(Optional.) List a brief summary at the bottom of the page. Include dates, employers and titles.

Education

Put at bottom unless it was within three years.

Personal

Again, this is optional.

A resumé is a useful tool for promotion, even when you are a business owner. If nothing else, the process of developing your resumé clarifies your strengths and reinforces your self-esteem. Before you prepare a resumé, I recommend that you read a book on resumés. It may give you many useful ideas and insights, and can suggest attractive and appropriate layout styles.

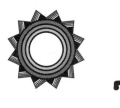

7

Financial Management

• Bookkeeping •

Bookkeeping is often viewed as an evil chore or an arcane art to deaden the psyche. Since most people will do almost anything to avoid chores, many practitioners do not keep accurate records, if they keep records at all. Thus, they tend to miss numerous legitimate tax deductions. Keeping records is a habit that must be developed. It's highly recommended that prior to setting up your books you consult with a bookkeeper or an accountant and most definitely confer with an advisor when it's time to file tax returns. The manner in which you keep your records can be simple and straightforward despite complex tax laws that seem to change every other week.

Maintaining accurate records is vital for any small business. Bookkeeping entails more than keeping a ledger for tax purposes. The information you glean from your records assists you in running a smooth profitable business. It's difficult to make prudent decisions without all of the facts. The checkbook alone doesn't always give an accurate account of the business' financial standing. Many business owners make the mistake of believing they are generating a profit because they have plenty of funds in their checking account, while unpaid bills accumulate and upcoming expenses are forgotten. For instance, it's mid-month, all of your monthly expenses are paid and you have $5,000 in your checking account. Your first impulse is to buy that expensive entertainment center you've been dreaming about for months. You look at your cash flow projections and notice that you have several major business expenses in two months and you haven't put aside money to cover those expenses. Instead of purchasing the entertainment unit you put $500 in a special savings account (for the future purchase of the unit) and leave the balance in your account to cover imminent business expenses. Had you not checked your cash flow projections, you could have found yourself in dire financial straits.

Many people find themselves in a precarious financial position come tax time because they haven't set aside money for taxes. I advocate opening an interest-bearing business savings/money market account and regularly depositing money in that account. My accountant made a brilliant suggestion: every time you pay yourself, deposit 30 percent of the money into your savings account. For example, you want to pay yourself $1,000: write one check to yourself for $700 that you deposit into your personal checking account and another check for $300 that you immediately deposit into your business savings account.

Your bookkeeping can be quite simple if you operate a small sole proprietorship with no employees. All you really need is a bank account and a ledger system with income and expenditure sheets. It's not necessary to spend a fortune on a bookkeeping system. Sometimes simple columnar sheets from an office supply store will suffice (or use sample ledger sheets from Appendix A). The records required and the complexity involved escalates with added business dimensions such as employees, product sales, partnerships and corporations.

The rule of thumb regarding record keeping is: keep all receipts. Also, write down expenses when receipts are unavailable. Keep all receipts in one place and post them on either a weekly or monthly basis to ease the paperwork burden at income tax time.

Some people use hand-posted ledgers for all their bookkeeping activities. I highly recommend using a computer as much as possible. Several inexpensive, user-friendly accounting programs are available for both PCs and Macs. These software programs can print your checks and post the information in the appropriate places. The software usually includes a tutorial that walks you through setting up your accounts—it poses questions and your responses enable the computer to determine how to organize your files. It's so much easier to know where you stand and to plan the future because the information is right there. You simply go to the "Reports" icon where it lists all the major standard reports. All you have to do is highlight the dates (e.g., "Last Month" or "Current Fiscal Year to Date") and in a matter of seconds, a report is prepared—one that could easily take hours by hand. You can also examine expenses by category such as creating a report of all your automobile expenses for the year. The reports can combine information from all of your accounts (e.g., checking, credit cards and petty cash). Let's say that XYZ Supplies sends you a notice for an outstanding invoice. You're fairly sure you paid for it, but you don't remember the payment method. If you only kept manual files, it could take you 20 minutes (or more) to sort through all the various ledger sheets and receipts. With a computerized accounting package, it takes moments.

Prosperity is the fruit of labor. It begins with saving money.
— Abraham Lincoln

The Institute of Certified Financial Planners
800-282-7526
www.icfp.org

Int'l Assn for Financial Planning
(free consumer information)
800-945-4237
www.iafp.org

National Assn of Personal Financial Advisors
888-333-6659
www.napfa.org

This is not an accounting book. The material in this chapter is provided to assist you in developing your bookkeeping system and inform you about basic IRS tax regulations. It has been streamlined as much as possible.

Small-Time Operator
by Bernard Kamoroff, CPA
Bell Springs Publishing

Minding Her Own Business
by Jan Zobel, EA
EastHill Press

Creating a Separate Identity ⌐

Creating a separate identity is important for personal and financial reasons. Many sole proprietors are extremely lax about setting business boundaries (corporations have regulations that require financial divisions between the business and the business owners). One of the best ways to set boundaries is to keep business and personal finances separate. Open a business bank account—this can be a "personal" account with your name (e.g., Mary Jones, D.C.), although I recommend establishing yourself as a business with a "business" account.

Deposit all income (checks and cash) into the business checking account. If you accept credit cards, the monies collected should be directly transferred to the business checking account.

Pay your business bills by check. This provides better documentation than cash. If you also use credit cards for purchases, note the charges on a ledger sheet and pay the monthly statement with a business check. Avoid paying for business expenses with cash or personal checks. If you find yourself in a store with only a personal check, don't worry. Just make sure that when you return to the office, you post the expense under Petty Cash and make a note of which checking account was used and the check number. Then write a check to "petty cash" for the same amount to cash.

Basic Do's and Don'ts ⌐

Don't:
1. Throw away any business-related receipt.
2. Pay bills until they are due—unless you receive a discount for early payment.

Do:
1. Have a separate business checking account.
2. Keep records for at least seven years.
   A. Receipts
   B. Bank statements
   C. Copies of tax returns
   D. Ledger sheets
      • Income Received: Record all pertinent information on checks received: client's name, check number, amount, date and type of income.
      • Check, Cash and Credit Card Disbursements
      • Accounts Receivable (when clients don't pay in full and make payments)
      • Summaries
      • Profit & Loss Statements
      • Balance Sheets
3. Keep lists of inventory, equipment and furniture.

4. Maintain client files.
5. Make cash flow projections.
6. Keep automobile mileage logs.
7. Maintain daily records.
   A. Keep an appointment book/diary.
   B. List all incidental cash expenses (e.g., mineral water while waiting for a client...it adds up) in a daily diary and then record on a cash disbursement ledger sheet (or petty cash fund sheet).
   C. Keep activity tracking sheets.
8. Prepare monthly bank reconciliations.

Figure 7.1

Accounting Definitions	
Assets	The total resources (current, fixed or other) of the sole practitioner or business—tangible and intangible. Assets may include cash in the bank, invemtory, goodwill, accounts receivable and equipment.
Liabilities	Current and long-term debts of the practitioner or business. Liabilities may include accounts payable, long-term debts, (e.g., a car loan), payroll taxes and credit card balances.
Accounts Receivable	The amounts owed to you by another person or business.
Accounts Payable	The amounts you owe another person or business.
Capital	Essentially it's the net worth of a business—the difference between the assets and the liabilities.
Capital Account	The total money invested by the owner.
Journal	A book of original entry for recording complete information on all transactions (e.g., Monthly Receipts/Income Journal and Monthly Expense Disbursements Journal).
Ledger	Summary sheets—final entry.
Credits	Entries made on the "right side" of an account. Credits reduce Asset and Expense Accounts, and increase Liability, Capital and Income Accounts.
Debits	Entries made on the "left side" of an account. Debits increase Asset and Expense Accounts, and reduce Liability, Capital and Income Accounts.
Drawing Account	Sole proprietors may withdraw cash for personal use. It's similar to a salary except you don't take out withholding taxes (instead you pay self-employment taxes). Withdrawals can reduce owner's equity.
Petty Cash Fund	Cash on hand to pay for incidental expenses. Put a voucher in the petty cash drawer and record each transaction. Do not put cash received from a client into the petty cash fund. When the fund is low, write a check (and cash it) to bring the fund back to the desired level (most likely between $20 and $100). Be sure to transfer the transactions to your Petty Cash and/or Disbursements Journals.

Business Income 〰

Business income includes all monies received: cash, checks, credit cards and barter. Record income at least twice a week; daily is preferred.

Credit Cards

Many pros and cons exist in offering your clients the option of paying with a credit card. Traditionally, health service businesses haven't taken credit cards, but a lot can be said for making it easy for your clients to pay you. I do recommend taking credit cards if you sell products (e.g. vitamins, herbs, books and tapes) or offer classes. The advantages are that transactions are easy for your clients, people from out-of-state can buy gift certificates and it might make it more appealing for your clients to buy a series of sessions and to make large product purchases. People are willing to spend more if they can pay on credit—plus there's the impulse buy factor.

The disadvantages are that the set-up fees can range from $25 to $250, the charges range from 1.79 percent to seven percent of the gross sales (plus with some systems, you have to pay 15 to 35 cents each time you call in a charge), there is usually a delay (up to seven days) in getting access to the money, and the client has up to six months to refute a charge. If you operate a home business, you may find it difficult to get a merchant account. Call several banks and ask them about their policies and rates on setting up a merchant credit account. Also check the phone book under "credit cards" for other companies that issue merchant numbers and credit card plates.

In the past, the costs and the hassles of taking credit cards haven't been worth it; but today we live in a society that relies heavily on plastic.

Gift Certificates

Gift certificates infuse income into your practice and provide an easy way for clients to share your services with their family, friends and colleagues. I view gift certificates as a tool to increase your client base, so it's in your best interest that they get redeemed. In one of my workshops, a massage therapist shared the following method for successfully integrating gift certificate sales: Whenever he sells a gift certificate, he posts who bought the certificate and the name and phone number of the intended recipient (if this is unknown at the time the certificate is bought, he checks back with the purchaser in a month or so). His gift certificates include a six-month expiration date (see Figure 7.2). One month prior to the expiration, he calls the recipient to give notice that a session needs to be booked before the certificate expires. After six months elapse without redemption and he is unable to contact the recipient or the recipient doesn't schedule an appointment, he contacts the original purchaser and tells her that the gift certificate reverts to her use. He sells a lot of gift certificates and has a redemption rate in the high 90th percent! His clients feel comfortable about purchasing gift certificates from him because they don't have to worry about the certificates (and their money) going to waste.

See page 186 for a Sample Weekly Income Ledger Sheet.

Card Service International
800-675-6573

The universe operates through dynamic exchange...giving and receiving are different aspects of the flow of energy in the universe. In our willingness to give that which we seek, we keep the abundance of the universe circulating in our lives.
— Deepak Chopra

I recommend that you put at least half of all gift certificate revenue into a savings account and transfer the funds into your checking account when the certificate is redeemed. Otherwise, if you sell a lot of gift certificates, you could find yourself in the position of working for an extended period of time without receiving "new" income.

Figure 7.2

Sample Gift Certificate Register									
Date Sold	Exp. Date	Purchased by	Phone #	Issued To	Phone #	Services	Products	$ Amount	Date Redeemed

Business Deductions ∼

Business owners are entitled to numerous deductions. Most of these expenses (except for those such as draw) are recognized as full deductions on Schedule C—although some of these allowances have strict guidelines and ceilings.

A legitimate expense according to the IRS must meet the following guidelines: it must be incurred in connection with your business; be ordinary (similar expense to others in your profession); and be necessary.

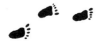

Refer to page 185 for a list of Common Business Expenses.

Here is a partial list of fully deductible expenses: office supplies (e.g., appointment books, stationery, tissues, pens, postage and thank-you notes); marketing; telephone; bank fees; legal and professional services; business insurance; interest on business debt; office rent; sales tax collected; utilities; inventory cost of goods; and business books and trade publications. Office furniture, computers or other equipment may be written off up to a cap of $18,500 per year, or else they need to be depreciated. Educational expenses can only be deducted if they relate to improving your current line of work. You cannot deduct education expenses for starting a new career. For instance, if you are a physical therapist or a chiropractor and you want to expand your practice by offering massage, it would most likely be deductible. But if you are an artist and want to sculpt muscles instead of clay—it would not be deductible.

Expenses most often questioned during an audit are connected with home business use, travel, entertainment and transportation. These are also areas that rarely receive full expense deductions.

Business Use of Home

You can deduct expenses that are related to using a part of the home regularly and exclusively as either a principal place of business or as a place to meet clients. The percentage of business use of a home is determined by dividing the square feet of the business space by the total square feet of the home. If the space was used for less than a full year, you must prorate expenses for the number of months used for the business.

One hundred percent of the cost of decorating, furnishing, repairs and maintenance of the business-use space is deductible or depreciable. The business percentage of permanent improvements that benefit the entire home (e.g., new roof or temperature control unit) are depreciable.

Deductions for the business use of a home may not be used to create a business loss or increase a net loss from a business. Deductions in excess of that limit may be carried forward to later years (subject to the income limits in those years). Also, if you deduct office space in your home, you may be subject to a capital gains tax upon the sale of your house. Certain time parameters are involved, so consult with an accountant and plan appropriate strategies.

To claim a home office expense, you must file Form 8829 (Expenses for Business Use of Your Home) with your Schedule C.

Travel and Entertainment

It's essential to keep accurate records to substantiate all travel and entertainment expenses. In regards to gifts for clients, you are allowed to declare $25 per client per year. The deduction for business-related meals and entertainment is limited to a maximum of 50 percent (the IRS frowns upon lavish meals that include magnums of Dom Perignon). If you have to travel any distance for business, the transportation and lodging costs are usually wholly deductible (although an unusual number of trips to exotic locales might spark an audit).

The records you keep must be supported by adequate evidence such as receipts, canceled checks and credit card statements. Keep a journal that denotes (for each expense) a description of the expense; the amount spent; date, time and place; business purpose; names and business relationship of person(s) entertained or gifted; and any other pertinent information.

Transportation

The customary and necessary expenses incurred on operating and maintaining a vehicle for business purposes are deductible according to the actual percentage of business use.

The two methods for computing allowable expenses are the actual expenses (at the business-use percentage) or the total business mileage (using the IRS determined allowance). You must use actual costs if you use more than one vehicle in your business.

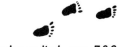

See Appendix A, page 386 for a Mileage Form.

The best evidence to support a transportation deduction is a logbook/journal that shows the date, business purpose, destination and mileage of all business travel.

Assets Owned Prior to Business Establishment

A common question asked by new business owners is, "Can I deduct the expenses of the equipment and books I bought while I was a student?" If you are a sole proprietor, anything that was your personal property and is now being used solely for your business can be declared as owner's equity (e.g., inventory, merchandise and supplies such as oils) or as a fixed asset (e.g., massage table, office furniture, stereo equipment); which then gets depreciated as of the date you place it in service in your business. The basis used for depreciation is the lower of the actual cost or the fair market value of the item when placed into service, not the original cost.

Pro Bono Work

Many people wonder if they can legally take a deduction for their *pro bono* work. Alas, no. This work doesn't "cost" you money. What it costs is your time. Even though we know time is money, the IRS doesn't view it in those terms. So, choose wisely to whom you give your *pro bono* work, be it for an individual, organization or event. Most people do *pro bono* work to help a needy individual, support a specific cause or group, or to further establish themselves in the community. The services you give to charity should be considered an act of goodwill, motivated by compassion.

Depreciation

Depreciation is a tax term that describes the loss in value of an asset over time. An asset is a tangible commodity that will last for more than one year (e.g., a computer or a building). When you purchase more than $20,000 worth of assets in any given year, the IRS requires the cost to be deducted over years (since the asset's life is greater than one year).

The amount of depreciation allowed depends on the category of the asset and its value. Depreciation rules change almost every year and can be quite complicated to calculate. This is a prime example of why you need an accountant.

Figure 7.3

```
┌──────────────────────────────────────────────────────────────────────┐
│                                                                        │
│  Common Estimated Business Expenses                                    │
│                                                                        │
│  Initial Expenses:                            Estimated Cost:          │
```

Common Estimated Business Expenses

Initial Expenses: Estimated Cost:

Opening Business Checking Account	$ 500.00
Telephone Installation	$ 200.00
Approximately $100 deposit per line,	
$80 connection fee, plus wiring charges	
Equipment	$?
First & Last Month's Rent & Security Deposit	$ 1,000.00
Business Cards	$ 100.00
Stationery & Envelopes	$ 150.00
Brochure	$ 250.00
Logo	$ 250.00
Advertising Package	$ 1,000.00
Ads in local papers, magazines, radio	
Decorations	$ 150.00
Office Supplies	$ 300.00
Furniture, Music System, Tapes, Clothes	$?

Annual Expenses:

Property Insurance	$ 175.00
Auto Insurance	$ 800.00
Business License	$ 100.00
Liability Insurance	$ 250.00
Professional Society Membership	$ 300.00
Legal & Accounting Fees	$ 400.00

Average Monthly Expenses:

Rent	$ 400.00
Utilities	$ 50.00
Telephone	$ 75.00
Bank fees	$ 10.00
Supplies	$ 50.00
Networking Club Dues	$ 40.00
Education (seminars, books, journals)	$ 50.00
Medical Insurance	$ 200.00
Auto (payments, gas, repairs)	$ 300.00
Promotion	$ 200.00
Postage	$ 25.00
Entertainment	$ 50.00
Repair & Maintenance (also cleaning service)	$ 70.00
Travel Expenses	$ 30.00
Yellow Pages (approximately $8 per line)	$ 24.00
Inventory	$ 150.00
Business Loan Payments	$?
Personal Draw/Salary	$?

Figure 7.4

Sample Weekly Income Ledger Sheet

Month _____ Day _____ Year _____ Page _____

Date	Client Name	Amt Paid	Ck #	Services	Products	Type	Location	Company	Notes
4/2	Perry Winkle	20	911	20	0	O	Outcall Office	ABC Corp	
4/2	Astria Ames	20	123	20	0	O	Outcall Office	ABC Corp	
4/2	Sandy Lott	35	709	25	10	O	Outcall Office	ABC Corp	
4/2	Maureen Dock	25	312	25	0	O	Outcall Office	ABC Corp	
4/2	Brad Jones	35	1947	25	10	O	Outcall Office	ABC Corp	
4/2	Amy Allen	40	417	40	0	N	Office	Humane Society	
4/2	Bill Peters	0	Prepay	0	0	O	Outcall Home	Attorney	Prepaid Services
4/3	Warren Piece	45	Cash	45	0	N	Office	Evans & Assoc	
4/3	Shirley Ujest	0	Prepay	0	0	N	Office	T&J Accounting	Gift Certificate
4/3	Weldon Rod	75	Cash	40	35	O	Office	Artist	
4/3	Les Moore	50	Promo	50	0	N	Office	Stars R Us	Knows many people
4/3	Helena Montana	50	653	50	0	N	Office	Thornton Co.	
4/4	Gail Windser	90	712	50	40	O	Outcall Home	Mattson Corp.	Prepaid Services
4/4	Hope Esperanza	0	Prepay	0	0	O	Outcall Home	N/A	
4/4	Holly Fields	80	211	40	40	N	Office	N/A	
4/5	Morris Katz	45	506	45	0	O	Office	School District	
4/5	Grover Funk	45	614	35	10	O	Office	TMJ Corp.	
4/5	Butch Smalls	50	430	50	0	O	Office	Allied Assoc.	
4/5	Truly Scrumptious	60	Cash	40	20	O	Office	Carpenter	
4/5	Harry Beardsley	50	Barter	50	0	N	Office	N/A	Barter for bookcase
4/6	Sam Iyams	0	Prepay	0	0	O	Outcall Home		Prepaid Services
4/6	Somer Days	100	347	40	60	N	Office	Model	Referred by Moore
4/6	Clyde Dales	155	940	155	0	O	Office	Burns & Assoc	Series of 5
4/6	Penny Cash	45	Cash	45	0	O	Office		
4/6	Sylvia Goldsmith	65	810	45	20	N	Office	Data Tech	
4/6	May Springman	40	Cash	40	0	O	Office	M&M Inc.	

Total Income: $1,220   Service Income: $975   Product Income: $245   # Sessions: 26   New Clients: 9   Ongoing: 17

Figure 7.5

Sample Monthly Disbursement Ledger Sheet

Month _____ Day _____ Year _____ Page _____

Date	Description	Amt Pd	Ck #	Rent Util	Maint Phone	Suppl Postage	Promo Fees	Travel Auto	Furn Equip	License Dues	Educ Ins	Books Inv	Bank Fees Ent.	Misc. Draw
4/2	ABA	250	140							D 250				
4/2	Jones Cleaning	27	141		M 27									
4/2	Paul 'd Auto	17.30	142					A 17.30						
4/2	Sunset Bld	350	143	R 350										
4/3	Gas To Go	9	Cash					A 9						
4/4	RJ Office	6.21	144			S 6.21								
4/4	Pace Printer	29.50	145				P 29.50							
4/4	Last Cafe	12.70	Cash										E 12.70	
4/10	The Garden	18.40	146										E 18.40	
4/12	Phone Co.	65.90	147		T 65.90									
4/12	Success 1st	20	148							D 20				
4/17	Career Sem	50	149								E 50			
4/17	Draw	800	150											D 800
4/18	Discount Sup	8.14	Cash			S 8.14								
4/19	Western Bank	8.20											B 8.20	
4/20	Ace Ins.	200	151								I 200			
4/21	USPS	25	152			P 25								
4/25	Earth Time	60	153				P 60							
4/25	AAA Util	50	154	U 50										
4/26	Discount Sup	20	155			S 20								
	Total	2027.35		400.00	92.90	59.35	89.50	26.30	0.00	270.00	250.00		39.30	800.00

Please note that not all expenses are 100% deductible. Please consult current tax laws.

Figure 7.6

Sample Cash Flow Projections Sheet

	May	June	July	Totals
Beginning Cash	1,850	2,740	440	1,850
Plus Monthly Income From:				
Fees	2,800	1,800	3,200	7,800
Sales	0	0	0	0
Loans	0	0	0	0
Other	0	0	0	0
Total Cash and Income	4,650	4,540	3,640	9,650
Expenses:				
Rent	400	400	400	1,200
Utilities	50	55	50	155
Telephone	75	75	75	225
Bank Fees	10	10	10	30
Supplies	75	10	65	150
Stationery & Business Cards	0	150	0	150
Insurance	0	650	0	650
Dues	75	0	325	400
Education	25	200	0	225
Auto	300	700	300	1,300
Advertising & Promotion	100	150	250	500
Postage	25	0	40	65
Entertainment	40	30	60	130
Repair & Maintenance	80	50	80	210
Travel	0	70	0	70
Business Loan Payments	0	0	0	0
Licenses & Permits	0	0	75	75
Salary/Draw	500	1,000	500	2,000
Staff Salaries	0	0	0	0
Taxes	0	0	600	600
Professional Fees	35	50	25	110
Decorations	20	0	0	20
Furniture & Fixtures	50	0	0	50
Equipment	0	0	425	425
Inventory	50	500	0	550
Other Expenses	0	0	0	0
Total Expenses	1,910	4,100	3,280	9290
Ending Cash (+ or -)	2,740	440	360	360

• Federal Taxes •

The topic of taxation has become enshrouded in an aura of mystique. Many people believe that cutting taxes means hiring high-priced experts to find "loopholes" in the law (an option only for rich people). The law is the same for everyone, and tax-cutting strategies are available to all.

No one is required to pay more tax than the law demands. Some of the more common tax-cutting strategies are:

* **Splitting income** among several family members (age 14 and older) or between legal entities in order to get more of the income taxed at lower brackets.
* **Shifting income** from one year to another in order to have it fall where it will be taxed at lower rates.
* **Shifting deductions** from one year to another in order to place them where the tax benefit will be greater.
* **Deferring tax liability** through certain investments and pension plan contributions.
* **Structuring your business** to obtain a tax deduction for some expenses paid for things that you enjoy (e.g., travel).
* **Investing your money** to produce income that is exempt from either (or both) federal and state income tax.

The information provided here is a general overview. Tax laws change regularly so keep apprised of current regulations. IRS Publication 334 (Tax Guide for Small Business) is published annually and contains tax information for sole proprietors, partnerships and corporations.

I highly recommend you consult with an accountant regarding tax matters. Unless your financial affairs are extremely simple, chances are that you will overlook deductions and credits to which you are entitled. A professional tax preparer knows what to look for and what's available to reduce your tax bill. While it's important for you to be familiar with the general workings of tax planning and the tax law—leave the technical details to your accountant.

Think of this in terms of your own practice. The general public might be able to handle their well-being on their own, but they come to you because you are supposed to have a higher degree of knowledge, experience, objectivity and techniques than they possess. If you expect people to use your services, it behooves you to also utilize appropriate allied professionals.

Tax Reporting

The following information concerns federal tax reporting. Check the IRS guidelines to ascertain filing dates for tax returns. Generally, state tax returns are due the same as federal returns. Some states follow the same tax law as the IRS and others don't. Check with your state taxing agency to verify requirements.

Sole Proprietors

A sole proprietorship is not an independent entity from its owner, so the business does not file a separate tax return. Income or loss is reported on the owner's personal tax return. If you are a sole proprietor you must file:

- Schedule SE: Self-Employment Tax
- Schedule C: Profit or Loss From Business (Sole Proprietorship)
- Form 1040:   U.S. Individual Income Tax Return
- Form 1040 ES: Estimated Tax For Individuals (quarterly— if you will owe taxes)

Generally, you must pay estimated tax if you expect to owe (after subtracting your withholding and credits) at least $500 in tax for the current year, and you expect your withholding and credits to be less than:

1. 90 percent of the tax to be shown on current year tax return; or
2. 100 percent of the tax shown on the previous year tax return (given the return covered all 12 months).

The exception to this is if your previous year tax return showed a refund or the tax balance due was less than $500. Plan ahead: If your income level requires you to pay taxes (even if you can avoid making prepayments to the IRS this year), set up a "savings" account for that money.

Partnerships and LLCs

Partnerships and LLCs are taxed similarly to sole proprietors. A partnership doesn't pay taxes. Income or loss is reported on the individual partner's tax returns. The partnership must file the following (plus include a copy with their personal tax returns):
- Form 1065:   U.S. Partnership Return of Income
- Form 1065 K-1: Partner's Share of Income, Credits, Deductions, etc.

Corporations

Corporate annual returns are due by the 15th day of the third month after the close of the corporation's fiscal tax year. Corporations must file the following:
- Form 1120:   U.S. Corporation Income Tax Return (or short form version, 1120A)
- Form 8109:   Federal Tax Deposit Coupon (quarterly estimated tax payment)

Employer's Forms

As an employer, you are required to file the following:
- Form 941:   Employer's Quarterly Federal Tax Return
- Form W-2:   Wage and Tax Statement
- Form W-3:   Transmittal of Wage and Tax Statements
- Form 940:   Employer's Annual Federal Unemployment Tax Return (FUTA)
- Form 1099:   Miscellaneous Income (any business that pays more than $600 to a self-employed person must report that payment to the IRS and the sub-contractor)
- Form 1096: Annual Summary and Transmittal of U.S. Information Returns

Record Keeping ～

IRS regulations require taxpayers to keep records and receipts for as long as they may be applicable to the enforcement of tax law. For income and expenses, this is usually the later of three years from the date the return was filed or two years after the tax was paid.

Records related to the basis (cost) of property should be kept indefinitely (e.g., papers related to the purchase of real estate and equipment). Copies of tax returns should be kept for at least 10 years.

If you are documenting your work and keeping accurate accounts, tax preparation becomes a natural extension of your bookkeeping activities.

• Work Smarter with Barter •

Barter is the exchange of goods and services. This cashless transaction method is not confined to primitive societies. It's the preferred method of managing finances for some, while others use barter only occasionally to control their cash flow. Bartering is not a casual activity. According to the International Reciprocal Trade Association (the governing body in the barter industry), approximately 300,000 companies (mainly small businesses) transacted more than $8 billion in sales in 1995, with a projected growth rate of 15 percent annually. It's estimated that more than one third of all world trade is done through barter.

Technological advances in electronics (e.g., computers, fax machines, modems and e-mail) have expanded barter from a face-to-face interaction to a global transaction. This enables the small business owner the opportunity to participate in an arena that previously was dominated by large corporations.

Barter affords you a simple, legal method to conserve cash outlays. If you can trade for something you need, then you can use your cash for other purposes. I've traded for office supplies, printing, advertising and cleaning. You may need your office rewired, your taxes prepared, flowers delivered or your back adjusted. Bartering is also an excellent method for expanding your client base. Many people who've never received the services of a complementary health care provider might be more open to scheduling an appointment if they didn't need to pay in cash. I know I have made several training contracts with companies that probably would not have hired me or anyone else if it meant dipping into their cash reserves. Even though I didn't receive cash, the trade was useful and those clients have referred cash-paying clients to me.

Direct Barter ～

Many health care providers already barter on a direct basis. They identify services and products they need and then approach appropriate business owners with a trade proposal. Quite often, too, a client will be the one to initiate a barter transaction. These direct trades work best if the items or services are of equal value. You can use gift certificates for trades and get gift certificates or vouchers from the person with whom you are trading. For instance, if you are bartering chiropractic services with a printer, have the printer give you a voucher for the amount you normally charge for an office visit. Then when you are ready to do a printing job, you can redeem your vouchers. Here's another example: Let's say a restaurant owner wants to trade you meals for acupuncture treatments. You charge $45 per visit. One method is to have the restauranteur provide you with a $45 voucher for each treatment. Another idea is to transact a trade for a set amount, such as 10 acupuncture certificates for $450 worth of restaurant vouchers (in varying denominations). The beauty of the latter idea is that the certificates and vouchers can be redeemed by anyone. If you don't want to eat $450 worth of food at that restaurant, you can give the vouchers as gifts or use them for trading with someone else. Your client can do the same with the acupuncture certificates you give, which can ultimately bring you additional cash-paying clients.

Two major problems with direct barter arise from inequitable trades and trading for things you don't really need. The following scenario demonstrates the first concern: *You want to have someone clean your office. You don't really have the cash to pay for that service, so you consider approaching someone to barter. Although you may find an office cleaner, it probably won't work for long. The person is likely to become resentful when five hours of labor (at $10 per hour) equal one hour of your services.*

The second problem relates to setting good boundaries. It can be so tempting to accept a barter offer from a potential client, particularly if you feel that the only way the person will utilize your services is if you agree to trade. If this occurs, remind yourself that your time is valuable. If the trade is not for something you want or that you can give to another, then you will essentially be giving away your session if you agree to trade. Both of these problems can be eliminated by membership in a barter network.

Developing your own direct barter network takes some thought and a bit of research. Start by listing all the goods and services you need in your business. Then make a second list of the items you would like for personal use. Make a third list of friends, colleagues and clients and the services and goods they offer. Then compare all three lists. You may match a lot of your needs with people you already know. Build your network by telling people that you are interested in bartering—let them know your needs and what you can offer in return.

While I do some direct bartering, most of my bartering is done through Business Exchange International (BXI). Join a barter exchange if you plan to incorporate more than the occasional barter into your practice. Contact the National Association of Trade Exchanges or the International Reciprocal Trade Association for listings of barter organizations in your city.

Business Exchange
Int'l (BXI)
333 N Glenoaks Blvd #400
Burbank, CA 91502
818-563-4966

Int'l Trade Exchange (ITEX)
10300 SW Greenburg Rd,
Suite 370
Portland, OR 97223
503-244-4673
800-213-5496

National Assn of Trade
Exchanges (NATE)
27801 Euclid Ave #610
Euclid, OH 44132
216-732-7171
www.nate.org

Int'l Reciprocal Trade Assn
(IRTA)
6305 Hawaii Ct
Alexandria, VA 22312
703-916-9020

Barter Exchanges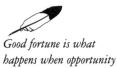

More than 600 barter networks exist in the United States. BXI and the International Trade Exchange (ITEX) are the two largest trade organizations. BXI has 28,000[+] members and ITEX has 16,000[+] members.

Essentially barter organizations work by members selling their goods and services to other members in exchange for trade dollars which are valued at the equivalent of cash dollars. With each transaction trade dollars are debited from the buyer's account and credited to the seller's account. The seller can then spend these trade dollars with other exchange members.

Good fortune is what happens when opportunity meets with preparation.
— Thomas Edison

You are given either a credit card or checkbook with which to make your transactions. A client getting a treatment from you either charges it and you call it in to the exchange office (a similar procedure to processing bank credit cards) or writes you a barter check which you deposit (just like a bank check). The organization charges 10-15 percent commission (in cash) on the value of the actual trade. Usually the commission is applied against the buyer's account, but some exchanges split the charge between buyer and seller.

Barter exchanges function like a bank. They handle transactions, debit and credit accounts, charge fees and send monthly statements. The exchanges will usually work with you in setting up your account. They may even offer a payment plan or extend a line of credit.

Most barter organizations act as a broker or agent. In addition to providing account management services, barter companies provide advertising and sales support to expand your clientele base. The main tool to accomplish this is the barter directory. Your company name and a brief description of your services get published in the barter exchange's directory. Many exchanges also send members weekly faxes with announcements, special offers and addresses of new members. Other methods which exchanges employ to help promote their members are: inserting fliers and brochures into directory mailings; profiling members in the directory; publishing members' articles in the directory; hosting fairs; and displaying members' products in the exchange office.

Most barter exchanges require an initialization fee of up to $600 and charge an annual fee ranging from $100 to $600 (usually a portion in cash and the rest in trade); some have a single lifetime fee of approximately $1,000. Another fixed cost is a monthly maintenance charge ranging from $5 to $35 (usually in trade dollars).

Bartering Tips

Successful barterers embrace the trade concept and utilize the barter system **before** resorting to cash. The downside to barter is that you aren't always able to get the items you want according to your desired specifications and/or time frame. You need to be creative, flexible and patient. Your broker can assist in getting your needs met.

Maintain good records so you don't allow your account balance to get too high (unless you are saving up for a large purchase). If you notice that you have accumulated too many trade dollars, you can always go on "standby." Here you notify the barter organization that you are temporarily not accepting new trades. The organization then notifies the other members. You tell the organization when you want to resume active trade status.

Treat barter as cash; after all, it's taxable income. The trade dollars you spend on business expenses are deductible; the personal expenditures are usually considered draw. The barter exchange organization reports each member's income to the IRS via the 1099-B form.

To keep control over the amount of trade revenue generated, you can issue a limited number of gift certificates or scrip to the barter organization. Members buy the certificates directly from the organization and your account gets credited. Although some people prefer this method to standby, it isn't the best technique for health care providers. You may lose potential clients because many won't want to be bothered going through extra steps before being able to schedule an appointment.

Don't pay more for an item through barter than you would pay in cash. Before making a purchase, check prices with other vendors. Most barter members are ethical, but some charge higher prices to trade customers than cash customers.

Take the time to build a strong relationship with your broker. Explain your anticipated purchases and when you'll need them. Also discuss ways to expand your clientele.

Don't accept bartering transactions that you can't fulfill. For example, a barter member wants you to provide ongoing chair massage to 50 employees. At first, this seems great but then you realize that this would take between 16-20 hours per week of your time. This would not allow you much time for cash clients. This transaction becomes more feasible if you know another therapist who could work with you.

Choosing an Exchange ~~~

Contact the National Association of Trade Exchanges and the International Reciprocal Trade Association for listings of trade exchanges in your area. Request information from the local exchanges and compare the services. Ask what the total membership is, the specific types of member businesses and the number of members on standby. Ask the exchange to send you a copy of its directory. Find out whether the organizations you are considering have members that offer items on your lists of business and personal needs. Talk with some of the members about their success with the particular exchange. Also do a random survey of service providers in the organization to ascertain whether their fees are within the average range. Check to see how many other people in your specific profession are members. If the total membership of a prospective exchange is under 200, and if five of the same type of practitioners are members, you may want to consider a different group (because there might not be a large enough potential client pool to be shared). Once you have done your research, compare the different exchanges in terms of contract requirements, fees, membership and support services.

Figure 7.7

Typical Barter Offerings

Most barter exchanges have members representing a wide spectrum of services and products. These are some common offerings:

Accountants	Dentists
Acupuncturists	Education
Advertising	Electricians
Alarm systems	Entertainment
Alterations	Estheticians
Answering services	Furniture
Appliance repair	Gifts
Architects	Graphic artists
Artists, artwork and supplies	Health clubs
Athletic trainers	Hotels
Attorneys	Massage therapists
Automotive: dealers, repair and services	Office supplies
Beauty salons	Painters
Bed & breakfast	Pets: boarding, care, grooming, supplies
Brokers	Photographers
Bulk mailing	Physicians
Business equipment: sales, services	Plumbers
Carpet sales and cleaning	Printers
Caterers	Psychotherapists
Child care	Real estate
Chiropractors	Restaurants
Cleaning service and products	Salons
Clothing	Spas
Computer: classes, consulting, sales, service	Travel
Construction	Typesetting
Consultants	Veterinarians
Cosmetologists	Window coverings

• Recession-Proof
Your Practice •

You are part of a very small percentage of the population: those people who are doing what they love (and making a difference) for a living. But how much of a living are you really making? A substantial number of health care providers are finding it difficult to earn enough money to adequately support their families. One of the biggest drawbacks to this profession is the finite number of hours you can work directly with clients. Depending on the type of work you do, you may only have the physical and emotional stamina to work directly with clients for 25-30 hours per week. Imagine that you see 25 clients per week, 50 weeks per year. At $50 per session, that's $62,500 per year. Not bad, except that figure is **before** expenses. Depending on your setup, you may clear less than $25,000 per year after deducting business expenses.

It is my contention that it's hazardous (physically, emotionally and financially) to rely on your hands-on work as the sole source of your livelihood—particularly if your work requires intensity. You can increase your income potential in several ways: reduce your overhead, increase your number of billable hours, hire support staff to free up your time, raise your rates or diversify your practice.

Diversification is the key to long-term financial success. The most common methods of diversification are to vary the scope of your practice by incorporating additional billable modalities, hiring other practitioners, teaching and selling products.

Product Sales ～

Of all the above diversification techniques, selling products has the potential for being the most lucrative. Some disciplines discourage (or even prohibit) their members from selling products. I can understand their concern: as a health care provider, a power differential exists between you and your clients. Clients assume that you are the authority and they may feel influenced to purchase products out of a need to please you or because they think you know everything. Even if you take great care not to exploit this power differential, it still exists. You must be careful not to manipulate or coerce your clients.

Ethical sales are based upon educating your clients on the benefits of certain products and then allowing them the opportunity to purchase them from you. Only sell products that you know are reliable, are suitable for use by your clients and are a natural extension of your business. For instance, if local statutes permit, it's totally appropriate for a massage therapist to sell health care products that are designed to assist in the relief of pain and promote well-being. Examples of these items are hot and cold packs, ice pillows, books, relaxation tools, support pillows and similar ergonomic devices, herbs, supplements, remedies, essences (such as aromatherapy), sports creams, self-health books and videos. A counselor might sell books, hypnosis tapes and batakas. A reflexologist might carry pain erasure balls, wallet-sized reflexology cards, specialty lotions, tea tree oil, aromatherapy oils, foot sprays, pumice stones, loofah pads, foot bath equipment/products and arch supports.

Selling products is not about hype or "hard-sell" tactics. The income you receive from the items your clients purchase is not going to make you rich, but it can be a decent source of supplemental (passive) income. The point is providing your clients with easy access to high-quality products that are going to help enrich their well-being.

Focus on products that fit into the type of work you do. The following examples demonstrate how to incorporate different products into your practice:

- Display your products and promotional literature in the waiting area. If you carry self-health videos, play them before and after sessions.
- At the start of a session have your client pick a "thought-for-the-day" card. Discuss how the card relates to issues that the client is experiencing and then work it into the session.
- Utilize products during the treatment: play a tape (just be sure that it doesn't zone YOU out); apply a hot or cold pack (be aware of contraindications—and while you're at it, tell your client about what they may be); give your client an appropriate formula such as Bach Flowers; or include aromatherapy applications.
- Print fliers that describe all the products you carry. Give these to your clients and mail them for special promotions.
- In the post-interview, recommend any reference materials, relaxation tools, support devices, books and supplements that are appropriate to the client's goals. Be certain to demonstrate any products and explain all procedures.

Don't carry too many different products—it can be too overwhelming for your clients.

As a health care provider, your clients depend on you to give them accurate information. You must know every one of your products well and be able to convey that information to your clients. Let's say your client really enjoyed the cervical hot pack you used during the session and wants to purchase one. You need to educate the client how to use the pack and under what circumstances not to use it.

Your clients will lose faith in you (and then no longer be your clients, not to mention the loss of goodwill) if you fail to adequately inform them about the appropriate use, benefits, limitations and possible side effects or contraindications of products sold.

Just carrying a product isn't going to sell it. Because people are more inclined to buy something they've experienced, remember to incorporate your products into your practice and take the time to educate your clients. Always keep in mind that the major focus of product sales is to enhance your clients' health and well-being.

Ultimately, selling products is like "selling" your services—simply share your enthusiasm about them. If you make your products visible, accessible, attractive and affordable, your clients will buy them when it's appropriate.

Nutritional Supplements

In the quest to diversify their practices, many practitioners are selling nutritional supplements. The major concern is that practitioners may be working beyond their scope of practice—unless they are a nutritionist or herbologist (or extremely well-versed in this subject).

The use of herbs and vitamins has expanded so much that a new industry term of "nutriceuticals" has been coined. And given that it sounds like medical-ese, you can be sure that the government has its eye on regulating it. I remember in the 1970s when the Food and Drug Administration (FDA) attempted to reclassify chamomile as a narcotic—it almost succeeded. Comfrey became a recent target and now herbs such as ephedra are under scrutiny. The FDA on more than one occasion has said that certain supplements are not safe, and what qualifies us to say they are (other than our innate distrust of bureaucracy)?

Recently legislation was pending to require these types of supplements to be prescribed by a physician. The bill didn't pass, but just the idea of it frightens me. I don't want anyone to take away my freedom to choose and purchase my supplements from wherever or whomever I desire. Unfortunately, the more that people haphazardly sell products without proper education, the more likely the government will intercede.

There is no security on the earth, only opportunity.
— General Douglas MacArthur

I have been in some health care providers' offices where the waiting room looks like a small health food store. I'm willing to wager that those practitioners know little about all the various products they carry. You might be thinking that store clerks don't know that information either, so what's the problem? Essentially, the problem is that you have a client/therapist relationship, which differs from a consumer/retailer relationship (see preceding section on the power differential).

But what happens when you've taken a product that changes your life (or someone you know has experienced profound change)? How can you **not** sell it? After all, your role is to support your clients in their overall wellness.

If you have a product(s) that you really believe in and want to make available to your clients, educate yourself on the product: the contents, suggested applications, possible adverse reactions and contraindications. Keep in mind that just because something works for you, doesn't mean it's beneficial to the next person. Also, "works" is a tricky word. Results aren't always proven or reliable. The possibility exists that the product could even be harmful to someone else. When discussing nutritional supplements with clients, you need to discuss the potential side effects (such as a healing crisis) in addition to explaining the benefits.

The more informed you are about the products you carry, the less risk is involved for yourself and your clients. If you are interested in herbs and vitamins, consider taking courses on the subject—or even pursue a degree in nutrition or herbology. Another option to help ensure that you are providing your clients with information and products that are in their best interest is to team up with a nutritionist or herbologist.

The U.S. market is flooded with nutritional supplements and the general public is looking for direction. As health care providers, your clients naturally rely upon you to provide them with information, products and services to enhance their well-being. When it comes to incorporating nutritional supplements into your practice, I recommend that you proceed cautiously.

Value-Added Service ～

Most health care providers have a rather extensive repertoire of techniques and services they use on a regular basis. Even though these modalities may usually be incorporated into treatments without additional charge to clients, you may want to consider expanding some of those services and charging a fee. For instance, instead of doing a three-minute energy balancing technique at the end of a treatment, you could do a full 20-minute energy balancing session.

Let's use massage therapy as an example. Other techniques that can be full sessions in and of themselves are: modalities such as reflexology, acupuncture and craniosacral therapy; crystal/stone therapy; sound treatments; chakra clearing and balancing; breathwork; stretching/exercise; biofeedback; and vibrational treatments. Many complementary services such as facials, pedicures, hypnotherapy and ear-coning can be performed after the massage or even at the same time by another practitioner.

Another arena to consider is the use of products or equipment that take very little of your time yet are of immense benefit to your clients. This includes hydrocollator packs, hot pads, ice packs, ginger fomentations, herbal compresses, paraffin treatments, aromatherapy, heated gloves and booties, as well as special equipment such as steam units, passive movement tables, anti-gravity machines, flotation tanks and "brain-gym" equipment. Again, some of these treatments can be part of your primary treatment or done before or after the session.

A terrific advantage to utilizing these products and equipment is your ability to be doing other things such as paperwork, phone calls or exercising while your client is receiving the treatment. They provide you with an innovative means to serve your clients' well-being and earn money without much of your hands-on time. Also, most of these items are a pure profit-generator after the original cost of the equipment is paid for. For instance, you can purchase a paraffin unit for $150. It would only take between 15-20 sessions to recoup your initial outlay for the cost of the unit plus the extra wax. A great side benefit is that you can utilize the equipment to take care of your own hands and feet. A steam canopy is another example of a tool which provides a profitable adjunct service to your practice. For less than $1,000 you can own a piece of equipment that virtually costs nothing to use and takes very little of your time. This is my idea of working smarter—not harder.

You have to gauge what is a billable modality and what isn't. For instance, some massage therapists charge extra for using aromatherapy oils or hot packs while others don't—they consider it a way of differentiating themselves from other therapists. The questions to ask yourself to determine whether to charge an additional fee for a

Champions keep playing until they get it right.
— Billie Jean King

service are: Does this cost me much in time or money? Are others charging for this service? Will my clients be able to easily perceive the benefits? Does this make MY job easier (e.g., a hot pack will loosen muscles so I don't have to put in as much effort/pressure to achieve the same results)? Will offering this service at no extra charge **increase** the number of referrals and enhance client retention? Is incorporating this service the most effective use of my time?

Package Example

Francine Feelgoode is a massage therapist who is trained in several energy balancing techniques and aromatherapy. In addition to her massage equipment Francine has a steam canopy, a paraffin unit and a set of heated gloves and booties. She offers several different packages to her clients:

- 1-hour Massage — $45
- 90-minute Massage — $65
- 20-minute Steam Treatment — $15
- 20-minute Aromatherapy Steam Treatment — $20
- 30-minute Energy Balancing Treatment — $25
- Hand and Foot Paraffin Treatment — $20
- Deluxe Session (1-hour Massage and Aroma-Steam) — $55
- Mini-Spa Session (90-minute Massage, Aroma-Steam and Paraffin) — $85
- Total Health Session (90-minute Massage, Aroma-Steam, Energy Balancing and Paraffin) — $100

As you can see the discounts increase with the number of services included in the package. The beauty of this customer service based marketing approach is the client receives a wide variety of services without costing the therapist much in time or product (the steam treatment is done without the therapist needing to be present and the paraffin treatment can be done during the massage). Using the Total Health Session as an example, the time required for Francine to be directly working with a client is approximately two hours. She is earning more than her standard hourly massage rate and the client receives an incredible treatment. This is what win-win is all about.

Offering adjunct services and treatments to your primary service is beneficial to both you and your clients. It increases your clients' awareness of the scope of available modalities and gives them the power to take more responsibility for their wellness by designing their ideal treatment sessions. Keep in mind that most people appreciate options as long as the list of choices isn't too overwhelming. It also helps you avoid burnout from doing one session after another, gives you a competitive edge and increases your income potential.

• Inventory Control •

Practitioners who sell products need to keep track of what has been ordered, how long it will take to receive merchandise and what is in stock. You don't want to run out of your best-selling item (particularly if it takes weeks to obtain more). Also it isn't wise to carry too much stock that has a relatively short shelf life—oils that can go rancid or magazines that are published monthly.

If you carry a limited selection of products, daily inventory can be checked visually and a written tally (often referred to as a physical inventory) taken at least twice per year. A more formal approach to inventory is recommended if you stock a wide variety of goods. Most accounting software packages include inventory record keeping. These programs keep track of inventory on hand and alert you when stock gets low. Even if you rely on computerized inventory control, it's wise to do a physical inventory at least twice each year; posting errors can occur and adjustments need to be made.

Forgetting to place an order can easily happen when you are busy with all the other aspects of running a practice. Charting inventory activities reduces the chances for errors and provides you with a quick at-a-glance overview.

Figure 7.8

Sample Inventory Record

Item: _____ Vendor: _____

Address: _____ Phone: _____

Date Ordered	Quantity Ordered	Date Received	Quantity Received	Posted on Computer	Quantity Sold	Balance	Date of Physical Inventory

Whenever you sell retail products, you must collect sales tax (unless you live in a state that doesn't have it). Contact your State Department of Revenue for a Transaction Privilege Tax License. Usually the first year you have this license, you make monthly reports. Then depending on your sales volume, you may only need to file quarterly or even annually.

• Selling a Practice •

Until recently, I was rather disenchanted with the possibilities of selling a practice. After all, because most practices are founded on the individual qualities of a particular practitioner, how could another health care provider successfully take over someone's practice? But I changed my attitude after interviewing a business broker who was extremely optimistic about the selling potential of health care practices. The purpose of this section is to walk you through the selling process, explain how to set a value on your practice and present you with techniques to set up your business so it can sell.

People have many reasons for selling their businesses. The standard ones are burnout, relocation, serious injury or permanent disability, the desire for a career change, death, boredom, disagreement with a business partner, lack of capital and retirement. Just because you want (or need) a change, selling isn't the only avenue. Many alternatives exist. You can cut back your hours, find partners, incorporate other practitioners, change the business structure, get help, give the business away, sell part of it, franchise or expand.

The topic of selling a business is fraught with misconceptions, the biggest one being that a buyer will come out of nowhere and make the seller wealthy. Another common fallacy is that selling a business is like selling a house. Everyone needs a place to live, but no one needs to buy a business. Also, unlike real estate, there are generally no accepted ways to set a selling price and you can't compare selling prices of other health care practices. The most frequent assumption is that buyers fully appreciate the years of sacrifice it took you to build your practice; in most instances they don't. Another major misconception is that the less information you give the buyer the better. Nothing could be further from the truth. Uncertainty is always discounted and buyers always pay less for less information. Also, legal ramifications can occur if you fail to disclose full information (also known as fraudulent inducement).

Most small business owners either sell or close their business within 20 years. I have no idea what the average is for the various types of health care practices. Through the mid 1990s, the only practitioners that seemed to sell their practices were primary care providers (mainly medical doctors and dentists). There still isn't much in the way of statistics on other practitioners.

See Chapter Five, pages 70-73 for related information on buying a practice.

With traditional businesses the majority of sellers hope a family member or employee/associate will buy their business, but in reality only 25 percent of businesses are sold to a family member and 10 percent are sold to an employee. Over half of the buyers are found through brokers.

Most businesses are bought by individuals. Employees usually don't have the money and competitors usually only want a part of the business. In this field, you are most likely to sell your business to another practitioner who is either new to the field, new to the area or wants to expand his target markets.

Buyers usually don't fork over the asking price in one cash payment; they want the business to be able to earn more than enough money to make the loan payments. They want a high return, low risk, satisfying lifestyle and something that's affordable. Make it easy for them. Help them deal with the uncertainty. Provide understandable information, point out business strengths, answer questions and help them answer questions they're getting from the significant people in their lives.

I realize this process may seem overwhelming and you may be uncertain if all this work is worthwhile. But if you have built up a thriving business, you owe it to yourself to attempt to sell it and recoup some of your investment of time, energy, money and reputation.

Regardless of where you are in your practice (just starting out or nearing retirement), begin organizing your business now so it will be easier to sell at any time. Establish a clear system for documentation of your client files and financial records. Analyze your business using the eight factors highlighted below and clarify your goals and business vision. Start implementing changes now: capitalize on your strengths and do whatever is necessary to eliminate (or at least abate) your limitations. The effort you invest can only enhance your overall success.

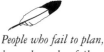

People who fail to plan, have planned to fail.
— George Hewell

Four Ways to Leave Your Business

The four most common ways to leave your business are: transfer ownership to a family member; sell your interest to a co-worker, key employee or all employees; sell to a third party, such as a competitor or someone interested in entering your field; and liquidate by selling off your assets, usually at "fire sale" prices.

In deciding which method to use, consider the following elements: minimizing risk, exercising control, achieving personal objectives, assuring payment, maximizing flexibility in structuring the deal, and fixing value. Your needs in each of these elements will determine your best selling strategy.

Transfer ownership to family member:

The down side to this method is that it simply might not be an option, it could increase family tension and it might stir resentment from the non-family members in your business. The benefits include being able to exercise more control, particularly in terms of setting a monetary value on the business and the repayment schedule.

Sell to a co-worker, key employee or all employees:

The down side is that you will not have control of the quality of services provided once you are gone. Yet this method significantly reduces your risks and you can increase the likelihood of retaining the same quality and degree of success if you have a staff person buy into your business while you are still active. In effect you are pre-qualifying your buyer through on-the-job training and observation. You can even establish a fund within the operation of the business to go toward the eventual purchase price.

Sell to a third party:

Selling to a third party (e.g., a competitior or someone interested in entering your field) is the preferred method when the business is too valuable to be purchased by anyone other than someone with access to a lot of capital. This is most likely to be your best avenue if you have a sole-practitioner business.

The down side is that the buying party inherently has more bargaining power (compared to other options), you can't be certain if the buyer's style and abilities will fit well with your current clientele and staff, and you will be required to carry some (or even most) of the purchase price—which means you will still be involved in the business for one to three years. The benefits are that you will most likely get a good price and if you have any staff at all, you will be giving them the opportunity for continued employment.

Liquidation:

Liquidation or simply closing down your practice should be considered the last resort—although sadly it's the most common method chosen by the majority of health care providers.

The Eight Selling Stages

The best time to sell your practice is contingent on the readiness of your business and the readiness of the marketplace. Most businesses aren't in a position to be sold because they aren't set up for a smooth transition (particularly in terms of documentation). If most businesses were to attempt to sell they would not be able to get a good price since owners tend to maximize after-tax cash flow and minimize profitability. They set up their business structure in terms of wages and legitimate perks in a manner which optimizes their lifestyle while doing the best they can to reduce taxes.

The Eight-Stage Selling Process

I   Review your motives for selling your business and consider the alternatives.

II   Analyze you business to determine if you are selling what buyers want.

III   Assemble an excellent team of advisors.

IV   Set a price on your business.

V   Prepare your business for sale and make it easy to purchase.

VI   Market the sale of your business.

VII   The closing of the business (often the supposed final step).

VIII   The transition time after the sale in which you may need to train the new buyer, continue to work in the business for a specified time or provide consulting services to the buyer.

Selling a business usually takes a lot of work and time. Most businesses take between six months and two years to sell. Using a broker helps to reduce some of your direct time and energy involved, but it doesn't eliminate it.

I Review Your Selling Motives and Alternatives

Reflect upon the reasons you want to sell your practice and clarify your goals. Determine which methods for selling your business (see above) you will use. The following exercise will assist you in choosing the best method for you. Take out some paper and ask yourself this set of questions for each method: Why does this method appeal to me? What reasons make this method appropriate? What conditions need to be present for this method to be appropriate? Why might this method not be appropriate?

II Analyze Your Business

You need to make sure your business is sellable. Put yourself in the position of a potential buyer. Why would they want to purchase your business? What exactly would they be buying? Can they work with your current clients? Analyze your business point by point to determine its scope and condition. Compile a written analysis which includes the following factors.

Company History: How long has your practice been in existence? What is the growth rate of your client base? What is your educational background?

Staff/Associates: Do you have employees? If so, what are their job descriptions and how long have they worked for you? Do you have associates? If so, what services do they provide, what financial agreements are in place, how long have they been associated with your business and how do they fit in with the overall structure of it?

Description of the Business: Summarize your business in terms of the services offered, equipment and products used, location, resale items, fee structure, client profile, position statement, competition analysis and differential advantage.

Financial Status: Figure out the true profit of your practice. Assemble the appropriate documents such as tax returns, profit and loss statements, accounts payable, accounts receivable and the current year's ledger.

Equipment: If you want to sell your equipment, check its condition. Are the items in good shape? Is it worthwhile to include them in the cost of the sale? Most equipment decreases in value over time, particularly electronics (e.g., telephones and computers). Items such as your table may cost much more to replace at current prices.

Facilities: If the buyer will be utilizing your office space, you need to check the condition of the premises, evaluate the overall appearance and have options ready for the transfer of real estate.

Overall Risk: This is what buyers use to determine the return they require on their investment and affects their pricing calculation (see step IV). The risk is evaluated from the point of view of not earning a return on the invested time and money or possibly losing their investment.

Strengths and Limitations: Ironically, this is the last step a seller takes in analyzing the business, yet it's the buyer's first step. After you have completed a detailed analysis of your business using the above factors, note which characteristics stand out most clearly. Clarify your opportunities and drawbacks. Think about your strengths as your selling points and your limitations as part of your improvement plan. Keep in mind that your practice may be sellable even if it isn't in shape to be sold right now. Reorganization and improvements can always be made.

III Assemble Your Advisory Team

Your advisory team saves you a lot of time and eliminates some of the inherent frustration involved in selling your business. This team minimally consists of an accountant and an attorney. Another member to consider is a financial planner. It's also helpful to get feedback from other practitioners who have sold their practices. I highly recommend working with a business broker. Brokers know how to organize the appropriate documentation, set a price and market the sale of your business. You can hire one to handle the total selling process or on a consulting basis.

IV Set A Selling Price

Many formulae exist for the pricing of a business, although valuing and pricing is not an exact science due to the large number of variables. It's extremely difficult to measure certain factors such as goodwill, risk, quality of staff, the ability of the new owner to work well with current clients and (if your practice is sold to an established health care provider) the cost savings by eliminating duplication of efforts and reducing potential competition. Unfortunately, very few people sell their health care practices, so we have few role models available, and comparisons with other professions/businesses aren't necessarily valid.

Ultimately the price a buyer pays is a subjective decision which is (hopefully) backed by objective information. The amount you receive depends on the value of the business and its affordability to the buyer. It's important that you are able to distinguish the difference between price, value and affordability.

Price is what someone is willing to pay for it. Value is what something is worth. This figure is derived from what the business owns, what it earns, and its differential advantage. Rarely do businesses sell for what they are "worth," particularly health care practices. This is mainly due to the high risk involved because of the personal nature of this field and the intangibles which greatly influence the success of a practice such as the marketing abilities of the owner and the clients' expectations of the types of treatments they receive.

Affordability is what the buyer is capable of paying. You may find a potential buyer who would be ideal to take over your business, agrees to your price, yet still may not be able to purchase your business because of the terms. Thus in many ways, what the buyer can afford will depend on you.

The Six Most Common Methods for Pricing a Business

Price Based On:
- Assets
- Capitalized earnings
- Integrating assets and cash flow
- Duplication cost
- Carry back
- Net present value of future earnings

These formulae aren't foolproof. The variables which affect the selling price vary significantly with each business. I highly recommend working with a business broker and an accountant to help you determine which method or combination of methods is best for you.

Price based on **assets** is done by determining the market value of the assets being sold and deducting the cost of liabilities to be assumed by the buyer. Assets include furniture, fixtures, equipment, supplies, inventory, client lists, leasehold improvements, accounts receivable, real estate (this isn't limited to owning property, it could include possessing a lease in a prime location) and corporate contracts. This is a fairly straightforward method.

Most service businesses are mainly based on **capitalized earnings**. To obtain this figure first calculate the adjusted cash flow and deduct a fair wage for the new owner. This is the base figure for this method. Next determine a fair return that a buyer should receive for investing in this business. Most buyers use a 15-20 percent figure for a low risk business and a 25 percent or higher for a risky business. Convert this percentage into a multiple by dividing it by 100. To get a selling price, multiply the base figure by the multiple.

If the business has both **assets and cash flow**, the first step is to determine the value of the hard assets. Then calculate the adjusted cash flow. Add those two figures together. If, as the seller, you want a full cash sale, this number is your selling price. If the business is in excellent condition or your selling terms include payments over several years, the amount you can ask for is the hard assets plus up to twice the adjusted cash flow.

Pricing your business on the **duplication cost** is done by taking the market value of assets and combining it with the cost for the number of years it would take a beginning practitioner to reach the same profit level. It can be rather tricky to determine the latter figure, particularly if you didn't market and build your practice on a consistent basis. Also, since the potential buyer is an unknown quantity, he may be excellent or abysmal at marketing.

Carry back is generally appropriate for small businesses. Calculate the adjusted cash flow of the business. Deduct the anticipated wages the buyer would need and the expenses required to run the business for one year. This figure gives you the cash available on which to set the sales amount. If you assume the loan to be a five-year payoff, simply multiply the cash available by five. You can add a reasonable down payment amount to this figure to get a total selling price.

The **net present value** method is wise to consider if you have built a very strong, diversified practice which includes other practitioners, corporate contracts, concessions at a health club or product sales. The technique involves the following steps: Adjust the company statements to show true present profit (e.g., add back in the perks you've taken); develop your business plan and project the growth for the next five years; calculate the profit, investments and returns for the next five years; and then discount the figures to the present using a discount rate which reflects the degree of risk as well as projected inflation. The major problems with this method are that the projections are purely speculative and the discount rate is totally arbitrary.

I recommend you calculate your selling price using all the above methods and see what the results show you. Inherent in all of these methods is the problem that they don't take into account that many practitioners will buy an existing practice simply to ensure themselves of a "job." Also, your business may include intangible assets on which it's difficult to put a price tag. These include your credibility, heart, reputation, goodwill and presence in the community. Many clients may stay with the new owner out of their respect and loyalty to you (given that you sell to a practitioner with the same commitment toward quality).

Another idea to consider is incorporating a contingency clause. As a result, you can ask for a higher price since you are minimizing the buyer's risk. Two techniques for contingent payment (after the down payment) are: the buyer makes the additional payments only if the business meets certain expectations (e.g., at least 50 percent of the clients stay), or the buyer only has to pay you a set percentage of the fees received from your current clientele.

The bottom line in selling your business is the foundation of economics—supply and demand: Is your business saleable and are there any buyers?

Buyers will test the desirability of purchasing your business. The first test in buying a small business is how the cost returns and effort required in running the practice measure against investing their money elsewhere. The biggest test is the "justification test." The buyer must be convinced that the business will be able to provide sufficient cash flow to repay the loan, support the business operational expenses, give a reasonable return on the down payment and allow for reasonable wages.

What a buyer can afford and what they are willing to pay will more often depend on the cash required than the selling price. The more favorable the terms of sale (such as no cash down, no security deposit, minimal interest, a lengthy repayment schedule or contingency terms) the easier it will be for you to find a buyer.

V Preparing Your Business For Sale

As stated before, the single biggest mistake sellers make is not properly preparing the business for sale. Preparation involves making the requisite improvements in order to enhance the likelihood of your business selling as well as assembling the appropriate documentation. Include the following in your documentation package:

1993 Business Reference Guide
Business Brokerage Press

How To Sell Your Business For More Money In Less Time With Fewer Problems
Audio Cassette
by C.D. Peterson

Selling Your Business
by Holmes F. Crouch
Allyear Tax Guides

Business Sale Documentation

- Opening Proposal: A one- to four-page overview of the company history, mission statement, brief business description, summary of assets, financial history, reason for sale and pricing terms.
- Samples of Promotional Materials.
- Detailed Business Description.
- Names of All Owners.
- Copy of Lease.
- Profit and Loss Statements for Past Three Years.
- Tax Returns for Past Three Years.
- Copies of Current Contracts.
- Determination of Value of Leasehold Improvements.
- List of Fixtures and Equipment with Replacement Value.
- Value of Inventory.

VI Marketing

Marketing the sale of your business includes preparation, pricing, packaging and promotion you do to bring your business and a buyer together. Accurate, organized, appealing documentation is the foundation to the successful sale of your business.

Your presentation package should include your opening proposal, samples of promotional materials and any other documents that highlight your success such as newspaper interviews.

The rest of the documentation should be provided to the prospective buyer only after they have signed a Letter of Intent to Purchase. Granted, this letter doesn't guarantee they will indeed buy your business, but it helps safeguard your business privacy by weeding out less than serious buyers.

The most common marketing methods are advertising, direct mail, telemarketing and networking. Advertising is an effective technique if the potential buyers are numerous and they are easy to reach in print (e.g., through trade journals and newsletters). Direct mail works well if you can identify buyers. It's one of the best for selling a practice because you can target specific practitioners or soon-to-graduate students. Telemarketing is an avenue worth pursuing, particularly if it's done in conjunction with direct mail. Networking is an extremely effective marketing technique. The only problem is that if you do it yourself, you lose confidentiality. Most health care providers aren't overly concerned about people discovering they are attempting to sell their practices. Although if you don't anticipate selling the business quickly, you may need to proceed cautiously, so as to not lose clients. If you desire to keep the sale of your business under wraps until the last possible moment, networking should be done through an intermediary.

Finding an appropriate buyer is crucial in this business. It's to your benefit (particularly in terms of getting paid) that the buyer can easily take over and work with your clients. This can be difficult if the techniques you utilize are extremely specialized. You need to find a buyer whose knowledge, training and personality is similar to yours. For instance, if you are a Trager® practitioner, it's wise to sell your practice to another Trager practitioner—not just any touch practitioner. If you've been in practice for many years and incorporate a variety of modalities, it's best to find another practitioner with diverse experience. If you don't match abilities and personalities, then both the buyer and seller are taking a tremendous risk because client retention will be compromised. Also, to ensure loan repayment it's wise to choose a buyer who is organized, understands business principles and is a good marketer.

VII The Actual Sale

Once you have a potential buyer you have to delineate in writing both parties' expectations regarding the selling process. Keep in mind that most buyers and sellers are inexperienced and don't know what to expect.

The next phase is to qualify the buyer. Find out where they stand financially and their sources of income. You could request a personal financial statement or a copy of the previous three years' tax returns. Realize that, as the seller, you are viewed as the prime source of financing. Seventy-five to 80 percent of businesses are seller financed, with the seller carrying one-half of the selling price. Another aspect of qualifying a buyer is to find out if there's a good fit between the buyer's goals and needs and the company as it stands. The last element of qualifying a buyer is obtaining references.

After you have qualified your potential buyer, ask for a letter of intent. This letter contains the names of the buyers and sellers, description of what the buyer intends to purchase, the date of offer, expiration date, price, terms, interest rate, repayment schedule, amount of deposit, closing date and contingencies.

The next stage centers on negotiations and documentation verification. Once a buyer submits a letter of intent, the first round of negotiations can begin. Do not be surprised if the buyer requests you sign a "non-competition" clause stating that you will not set up another practice within certain geographic limits and/or requires you to refrain from promoting your business to specific target markets for a reasonable period.

See pages 207-208 for ideas on preparing your business for sale.

Once the seller accepts the offer, she submits the rest of the documentation. The buyer then performs what is termed "due diligence." This entails examining all of the submitted information to verify its accuracy and confirm that any specified conditions are met. More negotiations may follow and the contract is drawn.

The final stage is the closing. This can be a rather stressful event, so be prepared. To ensure a smooth closing, make sure all parties understand and agree upon the terms of the sale in advance and bring copies of all important documents.

VIII The Post-Sale

In most instances sellers are required to continue involvement in the company for a short time after the official sale. This transition time allows for the new owner to be brought up to speed and provides the seller with the opportunity to introduce the new owner to the clients, suppliers and staff. It may be necessary for the seller to train the new buyer, continue to work in the business for a specified time or provide consulting services to the buyer.

• Retirement Planning •

One of the most overlooked facets of financial management is planning for the future through retirement savings. Many business owners (and employees) put off retirement planning until they feel they are "making money." Often the result is disheartening when 10 years later you find you haven't implemented a plan and will be hard pressed to have the savings necessary to comfortably retire at an age when you can enjoy it.

Have a set amount of money automatically withdrawn from your checking account on a monthly or biweekly basis and put it into a retirement investment.

Understanding the various retirement vehicle options available and incorporating a strategic savings plan is essential to good business planning (whether self-employed or an employee). No matter what amount you begin with, even $5 a week puts you that much more ahead as time goes by and interest compounds. Social security retirement income should only be viewed as a supplement to your retirement planning—not the primary source.

To be sure you're optimizing your planning strategy and following IRS regulations, check with the IRS, a pension planning attorney or a financial advisor before implementing a retirement plan.

The following is a brief overview of retirement planning options. We've been given permission by Jan Zobel to excerpt this information from her book, *Minding Her Own Business: The Self-Employed Woman's Guide to Taxes and Recordkeeping*.

Retirement Planning Options ⇜

Annuities

If you're working as an employee in addition to being self-employed, you may have a 401(k) or 403(b) tax-sheltered annuity (TSA) or tax-deferred annuity (TDA) retirement plan available to you at your job. These plans allow you to put a portion of your paycheck away for retirement while deferring tax on that income. These plans can also be set up for you as the employee of your corporation.

IRAs

Individual Retirement Arrangements (IRAs) are available to anyone with earned income (i.e., wages or self-employment income). The maximum allowable contribution to an IRA account is the lesser of your compensation or $2,000 per year. If you have a loss from your business and no other earned income for the year, your compensation amount is less than zero so you're not eligible for an IRA. The ability to put money into an IRA doesn't necessarily mean that you'll be able to deduct the contribution. Deductibility depends on your total income and whether you have a retirement plan at work.

The Roth IRA is a new plan that allows you to put money away for retirement. There is no taxed owed on the money when it's distributed to you. However, your IRA contribution is not deductible.

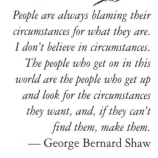

People are always blaming their circumstances for what they are. I don't believe in circumstances. The people who get on in this world are the people who get up and look for the circumstances they want, and, if they can't find them, make them.
— George Bernard Shaw

Keogh Plans

A Keogh plan is available only to self-employed people. There are two types of defined contribution Keogh plans: money purchase and profit sharing. If you have both kinds of plans, you're able to contribute a maximum of 20 percent of your net income to your Keogh. If you have only the profit sharing plan, your contribution is limited to 13.043 percent. A Keogh account can be opened with any bank, brokerage, mutual fund or other financial institution. If you have a Keogh and you have full-time employees (they work more than 1,000 hours a year) who are over 21 and have worked for you for at least three of the last five years, you must cover them under your Keogh and contribute to their retirement plan when you contribute to your own.

SEP-IRA Accounts

Similar rules for covering employees apply to the other type of retirement plan available to self-employed people: the simplified employee pension, or SEP-IRA. All employees over age 20 must be covered as long as they worked for you three of the last five years and make at least $400 a year.

The contribution to your SEP-IRA is limited to the same 13.043 percent contribution as the profit-sharing Keogh.

SIMPLE Accounts

The SIMPLE (Savings Incentive Match PLan for Employees) is designed for small businesses with employees that want to set up a retirement plan for their employees that is easier and less expensive to administer than a 401 (k). Under SIMPLE rules, the employer is required to match employee contributions or contribute 2 percent a year to the account of any employee who earns $5,000 or more during the year.

• The Canadian Supplement •

This supplement appears courtesy of M.A. LaBrash and is written to assist Canadian therapists in understanding their bookkeeping. To receive information on other business publications for Canadian therapists, contact the author at 438 Annie Street, Sudbury, Ontario P3E 2Y9. This section presents general information only and tax laws are subject to change. Readers are therefore advised to consult their accountant or financial planner for specific advice prior to making any business decisions.

Claiming Your Business Expenses ⁓

Any reasonable expense that you incur in order to earn business income should be treated as a potential deduction. In your therapy practice, you will find that many expenses can be fully claimed in the year of purchase.

Fully Deductible Expenses

- Business rent.
- Advertising and marketing costs.
- Professional fees, accounting, legal, business licenses, dues.
- Professional insurance.
- Interest on a business loan.
- Motor vehicle expenses where the vehicle is used for earning income.
- Office supplies of a current nature (e.g., pens, toner and paper).
- Treatment supplies of a current nature (e.g., oils and disinfectants).
- Professional reference books.

Expenses That Are Not Fully Deductible ⁓

Not all expenses are fully deductible. For instance, only 80 percent of business meals and entertainment are deductible and the claim must be a "reasonable" amount. Convention expenses are another example. You may claim the cost of not more than two conventions per year, and they must be held within the geographical boundaries of where the sponsor of the convention normally does business.

Other business expenses may have a personal-use component, such as a car that is used for pleasure as well as to earn income. In this case, only the business-use component is deductible. You must keep a log book in order to justify your calculations. For instance, if you are using a car for both business and pleasure, your log book would contain the date, destination, purpose and number of kilometres driven for each business trip. You also need to know the total number of kilometres you put on the car in the same period. Once you have these numbers, you can calculate the business-use percent.

Example

Total kms. driven = 4,000

Total kms. driven to earn business income = 1,088

Business use percent is therefore $\dfrac{\$1,088}{4,000} = 27\%$

In this case, 27% of the total expenses relating to the car (such as gas, repairs, license) can be claimed as a business deduction.

Business Use of Home Expenses ~~~

Revenue Canada guidelines stipulate that you must meet one of two conditions to qualify for a business use of home deduction:

1. The workplace is your main place of business, or

2. You use the workplace only to earn your business income, and you use it on a regular and ongoing basis for meeting your clients, customers or patients.

This second restriction means that you cannot pull a mat or table onto your living room floor and consider that to be your "business space." There must be a clearly defined work area that is not used for any other purpose. You must also treat clients regularly at home and at regular intervals—no six-month sabbaticals.

Assuming that you qualify for home business deductions, a percentage of the following expenses may be claimed: home rent or mortgage interest, property taxes, heating, hydro, home insurance, maintenance costs and cleaning supplies. Most accountants do not recommend claiming capital cost allowance (depreciation) on your house, because of the potential for recapture of capital gains should you sell. You may not create a business loss (i.e., reduce your net income to below zero) by using business use of home expenses. Similarly, if you are already reporting a business loss for the year, you cannot use these expenses to increase your loss. You can, however, carry forward any unused deductions into the next year.

To calculate your deductible, first determine the square area of your treatment space compared to the whole house. Common areas such as bathrooms and hallways can be omitted from the calculation. For example, suppose your house is 800 square feet and your treatment room occupies 120 square feet (excluding common areas). The work space is therefore occupying 15 percent of the house, so 15 percent of the total home expenses can be claimed.

Capital Cost Allowance ⁓

Some business expenses fall into the category of assets and need to be depreciated. An asset is real and tangible property (such as a bodywork table) that is expected to provide benefit to your business over a long period of time and not just a few weeks or months. The cost of an asset cannot be fully claimed in the year of purchase, but must be written off gradually. The amount that you claim each year is called capital cost allowance (CCA).

Capital cost allowance rates vary from four to 100 percent, depending on what class the asset belongs. The various classes and rates are set by Revenue Canada and may be found in the Business and Professional Income Tax Guide. For example, a massage table belongs to class 8, which has a rate of 20 percent. Fixtures and furnishings are also grouped in this class. Computers, printers and system software are in class 10 with a rate of 30 percent. Linens and computer application software are in class 12 with a rate of 100 percent.

In the year of purchase, the CCA rate is applied against one-half the purchase amount (instead of the whole amount). For example, in the year of purchase, the CCA claim for an $800 massage table is $80 ($800/2 x 20% rate for class 8 assets). This leaves an unclaimed balance at the end of the first year of $720 ($800 - $80). In the next year, the deduction will be $144 ($720 x 20%), and so on for subsequent years, with the unclaimed balance declining over time.

For the first year of a new business, where the fiscal period is less than 365 days, you must prorate any CCA claims you may be making.

The GST and Therapists ⁓

The Goods and Services Tax (GST) was implemented by the Federal Government in January 1992. The effect of this tax was to raise the cost of many goods and services by seven percent. Some services which had been tax-free became taxable, including therapy services. However, not every therapist has to charge the GST. For those with a combined gross business income of less than $30,000 per year, GST collection is optional. Once the $30,000 mark is surpassed, GST collection becomes mandatory.

Scenario One

Leon sells Chinese patent remedies as part of his practice as an acupuncturist. Last year he sold $10,000 worth of products and made $22,000 doing acupuncture treatments. Since Leon's combined business income is now $32,000, he will have to register to collect the GST.

Sometimes a therapist will be making over $30,000 in gross business income but from a mix of taxable and non-taxable activities. In this case, GST registration is still mandatory, except that the tax will be collected only on the taxable services (which may be less than $30,000 annually):

Scenario Two

Susan began working this year as a chiropractor and registered massage therapist. She grossed $45,000 in her first year from chiropractic services and $15,000 from massage services. Since her combined gross business income is more than $30,000 for the year, Susan has to register to collect the GST. However, she doesn't have to charge the GST on chiropractic services because chiropractic is tax exempt. But she does have to start charging the GST on massage.

You can show the GST separately on your client receipts, or include the tax in the cost of your treatments. If your fees are GST-included, you must state this either on the receipt, or have signs posted in your clinic to that effect.

Even if you are not charging the GST, you pay it on most business expenses. You may therefore want to charge the tax in order to be able to claim input tax credits. The GST you pay out is subtracted from the GST you collect, and you remit the balance (or can claim a refund).

Small businesses with annual taxable sales of less than $500,000 can use the simplified method of calculating input tax credits (GST you paid out). Add all GST-included business purchases for the reporting period, multiply by seven, and divide by 107.

For Example

Taxable expenses for a three-month period: $3,239

$$\text{Input tax credit} = \frac{\$3,239 \times 7}{107} = \$211.89$$

In other words, during this these three months the therapist paid out a total of $211.89 in GST on business purchases.

To determine how much GST was collected over the same period, multiply total tax-included treatment income by the same fraction, 7/107.

For Example

Total tax-included treatment income: $8,450

$$\text{GST collected} = \frac{\$8,450 \times 7}{107} = \$522.80$$

You may also add a column to your cash book to keep track of the GST you charged and collected on treatments. If this is the case, simply total the column. The difference between the GST collected ($552.80) and the GST paid out ($211.89) is either your remittance or your refund. In our example, the therapist would remit $340.91 ($552.80 - $11.89).

An even simpler method of calculating your GST remittance is to use the Quick Method. This method is available as an election for small businesses with annual taxable sales of $200,000 or less (some types of businesses, mostly financial and legal, cannot use the Quick Method). To use the Quick Method, simply multiply your tax-included income by five percent to determine the amount of GST to remit.

For Example

Total tax-included treatment income: $3,860
GST remittance = $3,860 x 5% = $193

GST returns must be filed for each reporting period, even if there is no GST owing. For information on registering for the GST contact Revenue Canada—Customs and Excise.

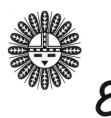

8

Therapeutic Communications

• Communication Fundamentals •

The way people talk with each other in daily life is often more traumatic than therapeutic. Good communication is the foundation of healthy relationships and thriving practices. Regardless of the type of technical work you do, it's done in relation to another person. Excellent communication skills are vital in the health care field. When you are with a client, you need to listen with all of your senses. Likewise, when you are promoting your business, you must be able to clearly explain what you do.

Some of the major benefits in honing your communication skills include: improved results for your clients, time saved in resolving any misunderstandings, improved cooperation and teamwork, increased productivity, reduced stress and increased satisfaction. Good interactions enhance the levels of connection and trust.

The purpose of this chapter is to highlight key concepts and explore communication nuances as they relate to the health care field.

Good communication is a two-way process that involves an exchange of ideas, emotions and attitudes. The ultimate goal of communication is to elicit some type of action. The communication skills necessary in effective therapeutic relationships are the ability to establish rapport, listen to a client's answers, effectively utilize communication technology, be patient, make astute observations, elicit information, ask open-ended questions, gain cooperation, conduct excellent interviews, ask for input from the client, assert boundaries, use active listening techniques and show genuine concern.

Some practitioners have a solid client base of people who receive regular treatments or come in for preventive checkups, while others desperately strive to fill their appointment books. If you are inclined to chalk it up to the ability of the practitioner, think otherwise. I've experienced superb treatments from struggling health care providers. One of the common threads of booked practitioners is that they take the time to establish a strong relationship with their new clients through their verbal communications and written documentation.

10 Keys for Excellent Communication

1. The most important thing to remember is that people act and react in order to fulfill needs. When you better understand their needs, you are able to create a better strategy for improving communication.
2. Take into consideration the person's natural tendencies and capacities. For example, if someone prefers to see things in writing, don't expect him to be very responsive to verbal communication. Also, if you are talking to someone who doesn't speak English well, avoid using polysyllabic words, rapid speech and colloquialisms.
3. Be considerate of the other person's mental, physical and emotional state; particularly if he is under a lot of stress.
4. Communicate on an equal level. Don't act superior or inferior.
5. Be honest.
6. Know her opinion of you. If someone fully respects your expertise, it isn't necessary to take the time to build up your credibility. If she doesn't know you, you need to take the time to build rapport and trust.
7. Have good timing. As "they" say, timing is everything!
8. Separate your emotions from the facts. It's difficult to have clear communication when you are coming from a reactionary position.
9. Ask questions.
10. Listen. Listen. Listen....

Seek first to understand, then to be understood.
— Stephen Covey

First Impressions

Your first interaction with a person sets the tone for future communication. You only have between four and 20 seconds to make that vital first impression. The elements of a first impression include characteristics such as: your appearance, facial expressions, body language, what you say, what's not said, your ability to gain rapport, your energy level and the actual message. An incredible amount of information is exchanged and many judgments are formed in just a few moments.

Frequently people alienate many new and potential clients because they don't present themselves positively and professionally. They don't take the time to develop even a rudimentary introduction, let alone a powerful one. When you aren't worrying over what to say, you can focus on being with your clients and listening to them.

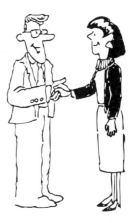

Do your best not to prejudge yourself or your clients. This prejudice can substantially alter your first impression. Focus on building rapport. Your confidence in yourself and your abilities increases the comfort your clients experience.

Building Rapport

Rapport is the bond that develops between you and clients; it's based on mutual trust and accord. You develop this by being open and demonstrating concern. Some techniques for developing rapport are: correctly pronounce clients' names, smile, shake hands, maintain good eye contact, allow ample time for clients to talk, speak with enthusiasm and conviction, be punctual, listen and ask a light personal question about the client's family, hobby or job.

See Chapter Nine,
pages 312-313
for details on developing a
self-introduction.

Neuro-Linguistic Programming

The three most common ways for people to communicate and learn are visually, auditorially and kinesthetically. People utilize all of these methods to process information, with one being dominant. You can dramatically enhance relationships with clients, as well as the therapeutic results, by communicating in your client's preferred style. The extra effort is definitely worth it!

Visual thinkers view the world in pictures, talk a little faster than average and use sighted phrases such as: "I see." "Clear-cut." "See what I mean?" "Plainly sees" and "Appears to me." When asked a question that requires reflection, their eyes tend to go up. They enjoy charts, diagrams, brochures, pictures on the walls and coloring the pain areas on anatomical illustrations. They want you to demonstrate what you tell them.

You can handle people more
successfully by enlisting their
feelings than by convincing
their reason.
— Paul P. Parker

Auditory people prefer to discuss things and are highly sensitive to noise distractions. They enjoy going into exquisite detail about their physical condition or wellness goals. They prefer oral intake interviews over filling out forms. Auditory learners speak in a rhythmic manner and use the following types of phrases: "Clear as a bell." "Describe in detail." "Inquire into." "Play it by ear." and "Squeaky clean." People who are auditorally dominant tend to look sideways when thinking. Anticipate auditory preferences by keeping a wide selection of music, make sure the treatment room is well insulated and engage in conversation. You can also be creative and install a cascading water fountain in the room.

Kinesthetic learners often employ a slower rate of speech, their eyes tend to look down when eliciting memories they and use sense-oriented phrases such as: "Boils down to." "Slow as molasses." "Control yourself." "Slipped my mind." and "Start from scratch." Kinesthetic clients like to touch items (e.g., skeletons and anatomical models) and experience sensations (they respond well to stretches and exercises).

Embedded Commands

You can enhance understanding and impact with embedded commands. The strategy is to begin as many sentences as possible with the word "you." When you say "you" people pay attention because what you say relates to them. Incorporate expressions such as "you'll notice," "you'll discover," "you'll find," "you'll receive," "you'll experience," "you'll see," "you'll smell," "you'll touch" and "you'll feel."

Listening Skills ~~~

More than half of all communication time is spent in listening, yet very few people have received listening skills training. Somehow, it's expected that people naturally know how to listen well. Actually most children are raised with the antithesis of listening; they are constantly bombarded with statements like: "Just ignore him." "Pretend you don't notice." "I didn't mean what I said." "Don't take everything so seriously." Unfortunately, the educational system tends to reinforce poor listening skills. By the time people reach adulthood they've mastered the art of not listening.

Listening goes beyond hearing. Hearing is simply the physiological process by which the brain interprets information received through the ears. Listening involves taking the time to understand and interpret heard information.

Listening Checklist

- Find an area of interest.
- Be determined to get value.
- Judge the content—not just the delivery.
- Delay any evaluations on your part.
- Allow clients to tell their stories.
- Be patient.
- Listen for ideas.
- Don't interrupt.
- Actively work at listening.
- Wait until the client is finished speaking to offer feedback.
- Periodically recap to yourself what you've heard.
- Resist distractions.
- Keep your mind open—avoid defensiveness.
- Take responsibility for what you're hearing.
- If you aren't certain you understand what you've heard, ask questions or rephrase what you think you heard.

For more information on enhancing communication skills, I recommend exploring neuro-linguistic programming (NLP). Numerous authors have published on this topic; Richard Bandler is the most prolific.

Active Listening

Active listening involves all of the senses. An active listener conveys interest with non-verbal communication (e.g., posture, movement, eye contact and gestures) and avoids distractions such as fiddling with a pen, playing with hair or reading ahead on an intake form. The active listener also pays close attention to clients' verbal and non-verbal communication.

Reflective feedback is one of the most common techniques for enhancing communication. This involves restating the feelings, concerns or content of what the client has said. An active listener allows clients to relate their stories without interrupting and then responds by asking further questions or rephrasing what was heard. For example, a client claims to be experiencing pain in her right shoulder. An active listener would explore that pain with the following: "Tell me a bit more about the pain." "How does this pain inhibit your activities?" "What I hear you saying is that the pain..."

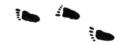

Listen long enough and the person will generally come up with an adequate solution.
— Mary Kay Ash

• Client Interaction Policies •

Client policies are about setting boundaries that encourage trust, safety and comfort. Policies explicitly define the parameters of expectations for both clients and practitioners. They make running a business easier, circumvent potentially awkward situations, provide means for conflict resolution and demonstrate professionalism.

Policy statements can be designed in various formats. They can look like a letter, a page with bulleted items or a combination of the two. The major areas to cover in your policies are finances, communication, scope of practice, etiquette and personal relationships. Written policy statements set a professional tone, even if you don't have specific policies for every situation.

Periodically review your policies, delete ones that are no longer appropriate and add ones to further clarify your requirements. Discuss your specific policies with colleagues before printing your updated policy statement.

Refer to pages 225-226 for a Sample Client Interaction Policy Form.

The main caveat with policies is: Don't have a policy you won't enforce. If you alter a policy for a client either on a one-time basis or if you change that specific policy permanently, make it very clear to the client what you're doing and that all other policies still hold.

Finances

When creating your financial policies include the following: your fee structure; sliding scale schedules; package plans; credit terms; insurance reimbursement; product guarantees and returns; bounced checks; gift certificates; and barter.

Fee Structures vary greatly depending on the type of work you do and where you are located. Once you have determined your fees, it's important to communicate the following to your clients: your basic session rate and duration of the session; other alternatives such as longer sessions; options for other services (e.g., hydrotherapy, paraffin treatments, acupuncture, aromatherapy); and types of payments accepted (e.g., cash, check, credit cards).

See Chapter Five, page 99 for more information about sliding fee scales and for specific suggestions for package plans.

Sliding Fee Scales can be awkward. It's tough to set one up in advance of the first session unless a client has said something to you while booking the appointment.

Package Plans encourage people to receive treatments more often and infuse extra income into your bank account.

Credit Terms are rare in service professions. The three most common reasons for extending credit are: the fee needs to be billed to a third party such as an insurance agency, attorney or a client's employer; a client forgets his checkbook; or a client has cash flow difficulties.

On billing to a third party have the client sign a statement saying that if a claim isn't paid within a specified time (e.g., 60 days) or if the claim is denied that the client is responsible for payment. For those with a cash flow difficulty, create a formal IOU with a payment schedule. Let's say a regular client recently got laid off from work. She has another job lined up, but won't be starting for two months. She wants to continue receiving her biweekly treatments but is unable to afford them and doesn't have anything to barter. Ideally she would pay a nominal fee with each session, but that might not be a viable option. Together, create a written agreement for payment that both parties sign. It might read as such:

IOU

I, Darlene Dunning [client's name] agree to pay the sum of $50 per session for each acupuncture treatment I receive between May 1, 2001 [today's date] and July 11, 2001 [the week after her job resumes] in the following manner: Beginning July 14, 2001 I, Darlene Dunning, pay the sum of at least $20 every two weeks until the entire amount is repaid. This amount is in addition to any charges for treatments received after July 11, 2001 (which will be payable in full at time of service).

In the event of nonpayment I, Darlene Dunning, agree to pay reasonable attorney's fees and costs for making such collection.

Insurance Reimbursement is a time-consuming, detailed process. Many health care providers prefer not to deal with it at all, some may help clients by filling out the forms (but require payment at time of service) while others will do direct billing. If you do direct billing, keep in mind that it could take 90 days to receive payment (even longer with personal injury lawsuits). Whichever method you choose, clearly state it in your policies.

Product Guarantees and Returns instill consumer confidence. Check with your suppliers to ascertain their return policies. Your customers may need to return defective or unwanted goods to the manufacturer. I recommend offering a money-back guarantee on all services and products. Of course, to take a stand such as this you need to carry quality products. You may want to include a time limit on returns, such as within 10 days of purchase.

Bounced Checks happen to the best of us. Unfortunately, as the recipient you have to deal with the repercussions and hassles. In most states you can go to the bank where the check is drawn and obtain preferential status in getting the check cashed as soon as funds are deposited into the account. Many businesses charge a fee (ranging from $10 to triple the check's amount) for bounced checks to cover their financial institution's charges and time involved in settling the account. Please note that this fee can be contested if it isn't stated in your policies.

Gift Certificates can be handled in many ways. Some people advocate putting a three-month expiration date, others say six months or a year and some recommend no date at all. There are pros and cons for all three options. Whichever you choose, make the conditions clear. I also suggest that the certificate be transferable.

Barter is one of the most commonly misused and abused areas of financial management. Although it isn't necessary to include barter in your written policy statement, it's important to set guidelines ahead of time for the types of bartering and the amount of bartering you allow. Keep accurate records particularly if you aren't doing a direct trade.

Honor is the capacity to confer respect to another individual. We become honorable when our capacities for respect are expressed and strengthened. The term respect comes from the Latin word respicere, *which means "the willingness to look again."*
— Angeles Arrien

Communication

General Interactions relate to your verbal and non-verbal communication. This mainly pertains to the environment you create, the language and terminology you use with clients, your attitudes about your clients, the types of questions you ask, the degree of honesty and self-disclosure you require of your clients, and your physical space boundaries.

Confidentiality must be maintained in a therapeutic relationship to promote an atmosphere of safety. Most people are clear about major confidentiality breaches such as sharing important personal information about a client with a third party. It is those subtle situations where it can be easy to cross boundaries. Consider the following scenario: Kelly referred her friend Terry to you for massage. Kelly very innocently (and with good intentions) says, "Well, how did things go with Terry?" You can avoid unethical behavior by saying in a light-hearted manner, "You know it's against my policies to discuss ANYTHING that happens within a session to anyone else. I'm sure Terry would enjoy talking with you about his massage."

Availability to your clients includes your hours, location (e.g., do you also work with clients at their business or home?) and the time allotted before and after sessions to answer questions or offer support.

Follow-up tends to be a weak area in most practices. While it's a good idea to place appointment reminder calls, it's important to find out if your clients want you to call them, when they prefer to be contacted and where they want to receive the calls. Some health care providers call new clients within 48 hours of their first session just to check in with them. Others also like to call clients who've experienced a major shift during the session. Regardless of the type and frequency of follow-up, always discuss it first with your clients.

Common sense is not so common.
— Voltaire

Scope of Practice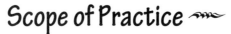

These statements define the type of work you do and assist your clients in knowing what to expect. Consider prefacing your policies with a short paragraph describing your work, the types of clients you work with (or won't work with), your training and background, any conditions that are your specialty and your procedures. Often these do not lend themselves to precise policies, yet are vital in setting the tone for a safe, enjoyable experience for both therapist and client. Some specific scope of practice policies cover draping, diagnosing and charting.

Etiquette

This topic concerns behaviors that generally fall under the heading of good manners. Policies need to address the following: late clients; clients who cancel appointments with less than 24 hours notice or don't show at all; hygiene (e.g., bathing and perfume); and personal habits such as smoking on the premises, eating prior to a session or arriving in an altered state.

Personal Relationships

Dual Relationships continue to be one of the most talked about subjects. Some people claim they should be avoided at all costs. But let's be real: they happen. It's usually not a question of whether you'll have them, but how you'll handle them. And here is where policies come in.

Dual Relationships Defined
A relationship between a practitioner and client that goes beyond the context of a therapeutic interaction (such as social, business, familial or political).

Think about who your first clients were—most likely friends and family. Many people find that at some point it becomes awkward juggling the roles of being a relative or friend as well as a health care provider. When I was in practice, one of my clients was my best friend. We had absolutely no problems for several years. Then the roles started blurring. We began chatting too much during sessions and discussing what occurred during a treatment when we were in a social setting. I created a simple ritual to transition our roles that proved to be extremely effective. Right before going into the treatment room, I would take a big step to the right and say, "Now I am your therapist and not your friend. And you are my client." After the session was over I would take a big step to the left and say, "Now we are no longer therapist and client, but friends." That simple statement with the physical movement did the trick.

Some people have very stringent policies about not working with friends or family members. There is no right or wrong here, although it's much easier if you don't have to accommodate dual relationships. You are the only one who can gauge your ability to keep clear boundaries. Even if you can work effectively in a dual relationship, you need to ask yourself if the other person can manage multiple roles.

Another aspect of working with family and friends is that they are more likely to test your policies and limits—although not always on purpose or consciously. Having clear policies makes enforcement less awkward.

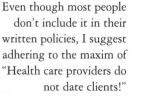

Even though most people don't include it in their written policies, I suggest adhering to the maxim of "Health care providers do not date clients!"

Sexual Activity in a therapeutic context is never appropriate (unless you are a licensed sex therapist). Sexual inappropriateness on behalf of the client or health care provider is not always easily defined. In addition to being clear with your own boundaries it helps to set guidelines for your clients that include interactions and scope of practice.

Client Policies

- List your client interaction policies for finances, communication, scope of practice, etiquette and personal relationships.

- Specify what your clients can expect of you.

- Clarify how you will handle the "bending" of policies (e.g., a client forgets her checkbook or a client thought you were going to bill the insurance company).

Sample Client Interaction Policy Form

My requirements of clients:
1. Sessions begin and end at scheduled times. Sessions begun late due to the client arriving late end at the appointed time and are full price.
2. Be present (not under the influence of alcohol or drugs).
3. Clients provide a health history and update when necessary.
4. If cancellation is necessary, please give 24-hour notice or you are charged for the appointment unless it can be filled. Emergency cancellations are determined at the practitioner's discretion.
5. Payment is expected at the time service is rendered.
6. On out-call appointments if a client does not arrive within 15 minutes of the appointed time, he is charged for the appointment.
7. Sexual harassment is not tolerated. If the practitioner's safety feels compromised, the session is stopped immediately.
8. This office is a non-smoking environment.

For touch therapists also include:
9. Be clean, having showered the same day as the treatment.
10. Do not eat a heavy meal less than two hours prior to the treatment.

What clients can expect from me:

1. I provide my clients with a competent and professional session each time they come for an appointment, addressing the client's specific needs for that session.
2. I am available to my clients between the hours of 8 a.m. and 6 p.m., and clients may reach me through my answering service on a 24-hour basis.
3. I return calls within 24 hours unless I am out of town.
4. Clients are treated with respect and dignity.
5. I charge a fair price for my services and offer a sliding fee scale when appropriate.
6. Payment is due at the time of service unless other arrangements have been made prior to treatment. I accept cash, checks and credit cards.
7. I do not provide direct billing for insurance. I will gladly assist clients in filling out the appropriate forms.
8. Appointments are confirmed the day before the session.
9. I perform services for which I am qualified (physically and emotionally) and able to do, and refer to appropriate specialists when work is not within my scope of practice and/or not in the client's best interest.
10. I keep accurate records and review charts before each session.
11. I customize my treatment to meet the client's needs.
12. I stay current with information and techniques by reading, receiving regular sessions (of the same service I provide) and taking at least one workshop per year.
13. I respect all clients regardless of their age, gender, race, national origin, sexual orientation, religion, socio-economic status, body type, political affiliation, state of health or personal habits.
14. Privacy and confidentiality are maintained at all times.
15. If I need to cancel an appointment, I do so within 24 hours whenever possible. If an emergency arises and I cannot keep an appointment, I provide a 50 percent discount with a client's next session. For non-emergency cancellations of less than 24 hours, the next session is at no charge.
16. My equipment and supplies are clean and safe.
17. Personal and professional boundaries are respected at all times.
18. If a client is dissatisfied with a treatment, and no other arrangement can be agreed upon, a 50 percent refund of the treatment is honored.
19. Clients may return for refund any unused products (in saleable condition) within 10 days of purchase.

For touch therapists also include:

20. Clients are draped with a sheet or towel at all times during the session. Only the parts of the body being worked on are exposed at any time. The genitals are never exposed or massaged.

• Telephones:
The Client Connection •

Telephones are an integral part of our lives. They are the key to nearly instantaneous communications. Next to your hands, the phone can be the most important tool in your business—or it can be an obstacle. This section covers techniques for improving your effectiveness on the telephone, choosing proper equipment and dealing with inappropriate callers.

Phone Etiquette

Every time you answer the telephone, you create an impression. The question remains what that impression will be. Within the first few seconds of a conversation you convey how you feel about yourself, your practice and the caller. Just because the caller can't see you doesn't mean that she can't sense the attitudes you convey through the tone of your voice and the words you use.

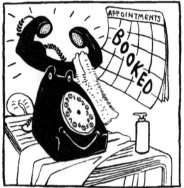

Communication is approximately 10 percent content, 35 percent voice and 55 percent non-verbal information. Given these statistics, it's easy to see why so many miscommunications occur over the telephone—more than 50 percent of the information is lost.

Illustration by Beth Grundvig

Without visual cues it can be quite difficult to determine the intent of someone's statement. For example, a caller might possess a sardonic sense of humor and you could be offended by a remark that would have been humorous with visual cues. Some guidelines to keep in mind when using the telephone are:

- Above all, be prepared logistically and mentally. You don't want to keep callers waiting while you search for supplies or information. Store needed provisions (e.g., paper, pen and appointment book) within reach and be knowledgeable about your practice.

- If you work with others, you must be aware of everyone's basic schedule. It's crucial to eloquently describe in 30 seconds or less the offerings of your practice, your policies and the type of work each practitioner does. The caller may be a potential client, so you need to immediately inspire interest.

- Answer the phone promptly: after two rings, but before five rings. By picking up right at the first ring, you may give the impression that you have nothing else to do but sit idly by the phone. Also, most people don't expect someone to pick up the phone right away, so it throws them off balance.

  If you wait too long to answer the phone, the effect is usually negative. The caller gets impatient or anxious about the machine that is sure to pick up...then you answer in person.

See Chapter Six, pages 108-110 for more information on telephone systems.

- Greet the caller courteously. Your tone sets the stage for the whole conversation. Before you pick up the phone, be sure to smile. It sounds hokey, but smiling makes a difference in your vocal quality as well as your attitude. You never know who is on the other end of the line (unless you have Caller ID).

  For instance, I was at home writing an article on telephone communications and it was late on a Saturday afternoon. I had received six or seven unsolicited sales calls in less than an hour. Lo and behold: the phone rang again and I must admit I wasn't my most "professional" self when I answered the call. After all, it was a weekend and this was my personal line. Well, it was a school owner wanting to schedule me for a seminar. He thought he was dialing my business number. I was able to recover the conversation (after all, I wasn't rude—just not at my best), but it took a little while to change the tone.

- Identify yourself and your company. Never assume your voice will be recognized. Also, ask to be of service. When you answer the telephone, your greeting might be like this: "Good morning. Thank you for calling The Northwest Health Center. This is Nancy. How can we assist you?"

- Speak in a clear and friendly manner. Personalize the conversation whenever possible by using the caller's name. Listen, give feedback and mirror language patterns.

- One of the most important techniques for improving telephone communications is to keep down background noises. Don't drink beverages, eat food or chew gum while on the phone. Also, if you listen to music or watch television, be sure that the volume controls are close to the telephone: turn off the sound **before** you answer a call.

  If you work out of your home and children or animals are present, you need to create a sound-proof environment around the phone. Your credibility as a professional can be adversely affected if your dog barks or children holler while you're talking with a potential client.

- Most people dislike being put on hold, so avoid it whenever possible. If you must put someone on hold, follow these guidelines:

  1. Get the caller's name before asking to "please hold." When you return to the caller, address the caller by name.

  2. Be specific about how long you expect to be on the other line. If it goes longer, check back in to let the caller know she is not forgotten. Even 30 seconds can seem like a lifetime when you're in telephone limbo.

  3. Always ask if the person would prefer to be called back.

  4. Give the first caller preference.

- Always follow through. Keep any promises you make to your callers. This is why it's imperative to take notes. Return all calls within 24 hours unless other arrangements have been made.

- An effective response to a potential client who asks for prices immediately is, "Before I can anwer that, please tell me what you are needing?" It's vital that you understand their needs so that you can clearly guide them.

Screening Clients ∾

Some people are at ease talking on the telephone while others freeze. Consider developing scripts so that everyone who answers your phone knows how you want callers to be treated, the information you want to obtain and give, the image you desire to portray and policies for handling specific issues. Topics to cover include: prospective clients; cancellations; re-scheduling; follow-up visits; disgruntled clients; fees; setting an appointment for a minor; scope of services; clients with special needs (e.g., people with disabilities); insurance reimbursement; and clients who want to speak directly with you. Rehearse the scripts and role-play scenarios.

Conduct preliminary interviews with all potential clients when they call to schedule an appointment (either by you or trained staff). Find out the reason for calling and the expectations. This assists you in determining if you are the appropriate provider for the caller and qualifies them (sometimes ending relationships with clients you don't want can be harder than obtaining new clients).

See Appendix A, page 407 for a New Client Checklist.

Design a questionnaire to ensure you get the information desired, disseminate your client requirements (e.g., prices, scope of services and cancellation policy) and determine if a client has special needs (e.g., assistance getting in and out of a wheelchair). If your files are computerized, you can create a new client account and directly input the information.

If you are unable to talk with the potential client initially (e.g., you have a client in the next few minutes or someone else took the call), place a personal confirmation call as soon as possible.

Inappropriate Calls

Receiving inappropriate calls can be a source of immense discomfort for anyone. Unfortunately, many practitioners—particularly massage therapists—still get calls from people who are ill-informed about the nature and scope of health care services. Sometimes people are indirect about wanting sexual services. You can often determine inappropriate callers by their tone of voice, ackward periods of silence, calls placed late at night and them wanting late night appointments. A common tip-off for massage therapists is when a caller requests "full-body massage."

When someone calls requesting sexual release, you have two choices: you can get upset and hang up the phone, or you can use it as an opportunity to educate the caller. Too many practitioners take these calls as a personal affront.

If you receive this type of call, stay centered in your professionalism. If people want genital release, that's their prerogative, but they do not have the right to expect it from you or any other health care provider. Tell them that is not what you do, give a brief description of the services you do provide, and let them know that a legitimate practitioner does not perform that kind of work. You might also say something along these lines: "Because prostitution is not legal in most states, and prostitutes need some way to let others know how to reach them, they tend to put advertisements under massage or touch therapy. This is changing as the general public becomes more aware of the therapeutic practice of massage. If you would like further information about the therapeutic benefits of massage, I'd be happy to speak with you about it or send you a brochure."

This gives the caller the opportunity to learn more about massage or gracefully remove themselves from the conversation. Remember, these callers are human beings. Just because they want something you don't offer doesn't mean they might not want a legitimate massage in the future or don't have friends who want a professional massage. Besides, these are the people we **really** need to educate. They are the ones perpetuating the myths about massage and the whole healing arts field. You can transform a potentially negative experience into a positive one by acting professionally and keeping perspective.

Machines vs. Humans

The most common mismanagement of resources concerns the actual answering of the telephone. Since many practitioners are in sole practice and don't have a receptionist, they rely on an answering machine to take messages. These machines serve a good purpose, but are generally not well-suited for this field. Most people prefer talking to another human being. They may have questions, particularly if they aren't current clients, and a machine can't handle that.

My Receptionist
is a nationwide appointment service designed for touch therapists. 800-686-0162

The other main drawback relates to scheduling. For example, imagine that you are working with a client and the phone rings. Someone wants to schedule an appointment right away. You have the next hour open, but by the time you are finished with the current client and listen to your messages it's too late for the other person to come into the office. A prospective client may have called the next available health care provider while you were busy. If you had an appointment service, that person could have scheduled an appointment and been in your office by the time you were done with your current client. An appointment service is similar to an answering service, plus they book clients.

Appointment services range from $45 to $100 per month and are well worth the money! All it takes is one to three sessions to pay for this service, which could easily be done by attracting just one new regular client. Of course, you're best off researching the different services. After you've chosen one, explain the work you do to the receptionists, furnish them with brochures and then give them a complimentary session. The receptionists can help turn an inquiry into a client.

Communication Systems

Imagine what your practice would be like without a telephone. How would clients book sessions? How would you confirm appointments? Even though the telephone is such a vital part of business, most people don't spend much money on their communication system.

Evaluate your needs and purchase a telephone with the appropriate features, especially one with high-quality reception and volume control. Some other options to consider are a clock, an alarm, memory, automatic redial, battery backup, multiple lines, conference calling, a speaker and, most importantly, a mute button. Choose a desired service available through the telephone company.

Refer to Chapter Six, pages 107-119 for more details on technology.

Improving Communication Effectiveness ~~~

In addition to allotting financial resources for equipment be sure to invest the time to improve your telephone effectiveness: Dress as if the caller could see you, get feedback from others, notice how others handle themselves on the phone, purchase appropriate equipment, practice and role-play, vary your "script" and follow the telephone guidelines established previously in this chapter. Utilize the telephone wisely to build your practice. Keep in mind that every time you answer the phone you have the opportunity to gain or lose a client.

We can't eliminate the inherent communication problems associated with telephones, but we can reduce distractors and increase rapport by incorporating these techniques:

Telephone Tips

- Be prepared.
- Greet courteously.
- Ask to be of service.
- Avoid putting people on hold.
- Smile while talking.
- Answer promptly.
- Identify yourself.
- Speak clearly.
- Take notes.
- Follow through.

• Client Files •

Client files serve three major purposes. The first is record keeping and the IRS. When you are in a service industry, basically the only way you can document your "work" is to have client files. The rudimentary information to include in each file is the client's name, address, phone number, session dates and amounts paid. Secondly, up-to-date files keep you well-informed of your client's needs. It isn't wise to rely only upon your memory for details regarding your client's history or treatment plan. The third purpose for keeping accurate client files is insurance reimbursement. Many insurance companies will not pay for maintenance care. "Reasonable and necessary" is the term used to validate a treatment modality. Thus if a health care provider can show proof of an injury or condition (reasonable) and substantiate the success of treatment (e.g., a decrease in symptoms), the care is considered curative (necessary) not palliative.

See Appendix A, pages 397-410 for Client Forms.

Some health care providers have clients sign contracts, waivers and request they fill out evaluation forms after each session.

Charting is a vital activity in a health provider's practice, regardless of whether the files are mainly for your benefit or for insurance billing. Documentation provides historical perspective, protects you in case of legal actions, demonstrates professionalism and proves progress. Some insurance companies will not honor your malpractice coverage if you don't keep detailed records.

Set it up so that your client files are useful. Make notes after each session (it can even be a visual record, such as shading a section of a drawing), include anything unexpected that may have happened during the session, things you want to follow up on, specific techniques you want to include next time, and anything else that you feel is important to remember. You may want to know personal information such as the client's birth date, family details (e.g., names of spouse/significant other and children) or the types of personal growth work the client has done. It's also helpful to know how they found out about you so you can focus your advertising.

Be sure to honor confidentiality. Although you want your files to contain accurate and thorough information, your treatment records should only include information as it relates to the treatment.

Review your files immediately before you work with each client. This assists you in being more focused with all of your clients. A client's faith and respect in you can really erode if you don't "remember" what occurred during his last session (even though you may have seen 50 other people since then). So it's best to be prepared.

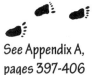

See Appendix A, pages 397-406 for sample client forms and a Sign-In Sheet.

Many types of client files have been developed over the years. You may want to use "ready-made" forms, adapt them, or totally customize your own forms. The fundamental facts to be sure to include on your client information sheets are: the client's name; address; phone numbers; medical history; chief complaints; current medication; and reason(s) for using your services.

Some practitioners also include an explanation of the range/variety of service and techniques they offer and list some of the benefits of their services on the top of their intake forms. Other practitioners incorporate a type of disclaimer. For example, many massage therapists put a statement that massage is clearly non-sexual. You must decide what purpose your client files are going to serve and choose the appropriate forms. As you and your needs change, so will the forms you use.

Charting client history, assessment notes and treatment plans is much more easily accomplished if you use standardized forms. SOAP (Subjective, Objective, Assessment, Plan) charting is the most widely used format for documenting treatment sessions in the health care field.

In addition to client files, it's recommended that you have a sign-in sheet at the front desk. This form is for your protection—it verifies the client was at your office. Keep this sheet simple and don't risk breaching confidentiality by requesting personal nformation such as "reason for visit."

SOAP Notes

Subjective

A description of the symptoms and complaints discussed by the client (or the referring primary health care provider) that is inscribed using the client's own words. Key words are symptoms, location, intensity, duration, frequency and onset.

Objective

An account of your observations and results of tests you administer.

Assessment

A record of the changes in the client's condition as a result of treatment.

Plan

A list of recommended action.

For more detailed information on SOAP charting, refer to the book, *Hands Heal: Documentation for Massage Therapy* by Diana Thompson Howling Moon Press

After the client has completed the appropriate forms, review them with her. Before each session ask the client if there are any changes or additional information that needs to be included on the form.

• The Ultimate Interview •

Interviews are pivotal in creating lasting, healthy relationships between practitioners and clients. Information is gathered, rapport is built and ideas are shared in interviews. Ideally, they occur at regular intervals. The most extensive one is the initial interview.

The foundation for the ultimate interview is good communication skills; the primary facet is the ability to listen. The initial intake interview sets the tone for your working relationship. This is not simply about obtaining a client history; it's an opportunity for clarifying boundaries, explaining procedures, defining scope of practice, determining the course of treatment, stating policies, setting realistic goals, designing a treatment plan, educating clients and creating a climate of trust.

Time ⁓

Practitioners often do not allot sufficient time for their interviews (even those who can bill for office visits), particularly the initial intake interview. Although a thorough intake interview requires between 20-60 minutes, it's time well spent. Consider that it takes approximately six times more money and three times more effort to get a new client than to keep one you already have. So, an extra half-hour is a minor investment on your part.

Not all practitioners control their schedules. For instance, those who work in a spa setting may need to be extremely creative in doing their interviews. I think the major reason most spa therapists do not work consistently with many local clients is that they tend to only do cursory intake interviews.

Allow ample time for your clients to fill out forms and ask questions. Never rush them. Keep in mind that your clients may not have the awareness or the vocabulary to accurately describe their conditions and goals. Also, tell new clients that their first visit will take approximately an extra half hour to do the interview plus the time for the treatment.

Artful Phrasing ~

Ask questions that require thought and explanations rather than a simple "yes" or "no." These open-ended questions encourage participation and self-responsibility. One of the most frequently asked questions in an intake interview is whether the client has experienced this type of treatment; for instance, "Have you ever been hypnotized before?" Two problems are inherent in this question. First of all the scope of hypnotherapy isn't clear. A client could have listened to self-hypnosis tapes, but never visited a professional hypnotherapist. Secondly, the question only calls for a one-word answer. A better series of questions would be as follows: "What is your experience with hypnotherapy?" "How often have you received hypnotherapy sessions?" "When was your last hypnotherapy session?"

Deftness at artful phrasing and leading questions is a skill that is honed over time. Mainly it involves forethought and lots of practice. Whenever you need to ask a question, phrase it in such a way that the answer will not be monosyllabic, but gives you accurate, detailed information. Develop questions that inspire clients to think and help them connect daily activities and previous injuries with current conditions.

Getting feedback from clients is a major area where communication flounders. Many people do not know how to get their needs met, so it's imperative that you (as the health care provider) be conscious of this deficiency and direct your questions in ways that foster good communication.

Incorporate the phrases "how much?" "how long?" and "what is the level of intensity?" into your questioning routine. Let's say you are a shiatsu practitioner working with a client and you sense that the pressure may be a bit too much. If you ask, "Is this pressure okay?" the response will most likely be "yes" or "I guess so" (possibly with gritted teeth). Yet if you ask your client to rate the pressure on a pain scale (after agreeing upon what the numbers mean) you will get a much more accurate response.

Demonstrate your concern for your client's comfort and well-being. Consider the following example that frequently occurs during a session: You sense your client is getting a bit chilly. Instead of asking, "Are you cold?" or "Would you like a blanket?" ask "Would you like a blanket on your feet and legs or would you prefer to be fully covered with a blanket?"

Suggested Interview Questions

- How are you feeling today?
- Tell me about your physical/emotional condition.
- Describe your specific pain or discomfort.
- How long have you been experiencing this condition?
- When was the onset of this condition?
- What is the intensity and frequency of this condition?
- What causes you stress?
- Where in your body do you feel stress?
- What activities aggravate this condition?
- What actions relieve or reduce the discomfort of this condition?
- What are your long-term wellness goals?
- What do you want to achieve in today's session?
- What kind of mobility assistance might you need from me?
- Have you ever seen a [your profession here] before?
  If so, what were the results?
- Are you currently under medical/therapeutic treatment? If so, for what condition and what medications/supplements are you taking?
- What products have you used to address this condition?
- What questions do you have about my services?
- What are your concerns?
- What are your expectations about my profession or me?
- What can I do to make this session effective and enjoyable?

Of one thing I am certain, the body is not the measure of healing—peace is the measure.
— George Melton

Educating Clients

One of the chief complaints of the health care industry is that the providers (particularly medical doctors, chiropractors and dentists) don't take enough time to explain to their clients what is wrong with them and what they plan to do to help them get better.

Educating clients so that they can understand the cause of their pain or concern and the methods by which it can be alleviated allows them to become better informed so they can assume responsibility to help themselves get better and stay well.

Education encourages the client to become an active participant in the therapy process by taking responsibility for their own care. It also enables them to become salespeople for your office.

Education plays a vital role in therapeutic relationships. Your work is more than the therapeutic interaction, it's broadening your clients' knowledge. This can be done in many ways: describe what you're doing and why; show videos; provide reading materials (including your newsletter); and assign homework.

Interview Stages ⚮

Interviews consist of four major stages—initiation, exploration, planning and closure.

The initiation stage is where you introduce yourself, establish rapport, discuss the client's general issues and expectations, describe what you can do, review your policies and explain procedures. Knowing what clients expect improves treatment results and client satisfaction.

I think the one lesson I have learned is that there is no substitute for paying attention.
— Diane Sawyer

The exploration stage encompasses reviewing a client's history, performing a physical assessment and determining the treatment course of the specific session. The flow of the exploration stage varies depending upon the actual type of service you provide and your environment. Ideally, in your initial session you would review the client's intake forms, clarify any vague responses, get a sense of the client's general well-being goals and specific goals for receiving treatments, administer some type of assessment (e.g., range of motion, visual observations and palpation), determine the course of action and modalities to use for the current session, and then do the actual treatment.

Planning is the stage that the practitioner and client create together. Long-range treatment plans are *the key* to having clients who receive treatments on a regular basis. Treatment plans are blueprints to follow while working with any specific client. Long-range treatment plans also serve as a reminder for the client to take responsibility for his goals.

The plan is based upon all the information gathered in the initiation and exploration stages of the interview as well as the session. It may seem awkward to break up the interview with a treatment, but it's the only way you can accurately develop a long-range treatment plan. It's difficult to evaluate a client's condition until you've given a treatment. Also, during the session clients often discover unsuspected problems or remember previous physical/psychological trauma. This information can be crucial in designing the treatment plan.

Some items to include in the plan are: the client's short-term and long-range well-being goals; indications and contraindications; treatment frequency; specific modalities to be used; homework; and possible referrals to other health care providers.

Create a vision with your clients so they can experience themselves having attained their goals. This makes the treatment more powerful and inspires clients to take an active role in their well-being (e.g., do homework assignments and use products). This can also elicit secondary goals.

The tricky part to designing a long-range treatment plan is setting realistic goals. Many people do not know enough about themselves or your services to gauge the potential outcomes. Begin by discussing general goals and letting them know which conditions can be successfully addressed by your services. Create short-term goals (for individual sessions and the next few treatments) and long-term goals (covering periods of three, six, nine and 12 months). The difficulty here is that unless you are a primary care provider you can't prescribe—but you can describe. Make sure you are clear about the proven benefits of your work, as you can safely make those statements. It's best to let your clients determine the treatment frequency. You can provide them guidelines such as: "Other clients with similar goals obtained their desired results by coming in twice per week for 2-3 weeks, then once per week for three months, and tapering off to a minimum of twice monthly." or "If I had a condition like this, I would..." A statement I often used in my massage practice was, "I recommend massage as often as you can afford physically, time-wise and financially."

Update long-range treatment plans after each visit. Make notes for subsequent sessions, taking into account any changes in your client's lifestyle and treatment results (e.g., what worked and didn't, the areas or modalities you didn't cover and what you want to include next time).

All too often, practitioners omit this stage, particularly with clients who have been receiving regular treatments or clients who are very educated about and involved in their own wellness. Keep in mind that most people want objective evidence that they are reaching their wellness goals. I know I appreciate it when a practitioner looks at a chart and tells me the specific changes and progress I've made *since* the last session and where I'm at in relation to my long-term goals.

Closure is the final interview stage. This can be done fairly quickly with the first session since you have spent a significant amount of time designing the treatment plan. Give a very brief overview of what took place, highlight some of the client's major goals, assign homework, give the client an opportunity to ask questions, make any necessary referrals and schedule the next appointment.

Subsequent Sessions

The first time you work with a client, the interview process is usually more extensive than in subsequent sessions. You can retain the quality of your interviews even though the time spent is reduced, by making sure you include all four stages each time you see a client.

The initiation stage involves actions to continue building rapport such as greeting each client appropriately and engaging in light chit-chat.

The exploration stage encompasses reviewing the client's files, discussing any changes that may have occurred between sessions, documenting observations, setting treatment goals and determining the course of the specific session.

Planning is usually done by the practitioner and includes updating the long-term treatment plan and making notes for activities and modalities to incorporate into the next session.

Closure tends to take longer in subsequent sessions than with the first visit. After the treatment, review the session with your client (this doesn't need to be lengthy

It is what we think we know already that often prevents us from learning.
— Claude Bernard

Some patients, though conscious that their condition is perilous, recover their health simply through their contentment with the goodness of the physician.
— Hippocrates

and can be informal). Summarize what you did, address issues that might have surfaced and answer any questions. Briefly review the client's long-term goals and make any appropriate recommendations and homework assignments. Finally, ask when she would like to schedule the following session.

Client Compliance ᴀᴀᴀ

Many health care providers complain about a lack of client compliance (e.g., clients don't do their homework, make no lifestyle changes, don't use appropriate products or fail to return for follow-up sessions). Although you can't force someone to comply with your recommendations, your communication skills can increase the odds.

Every person who ends up buying into your idea does so by changing it into his idea (even if it still looks a lot like your idea).
— Tom Peters

First of all, recognize the factors that prevent full compliance: lack of discipline, time restraints, insufficient funds or insurance coverage, social pressures, beliefs and work obligations. Explain why it is in their best interest to adhere to your recommendations, clarify the instructions and discuss ways to overcome barriers. Have clients repeat instructions or perform exercises/stretches to be sure they understand them. Give them printed reference material to take home. The most important aspect is gaining your clients' concordance about their treatment plans and assignments.

Honing Your Skills ᴀᴀᴀ

Interviewing skills take time to develop. The best way to sharpen your interviewing skills is to practice by getting together with two other colleagues and simulate intake interviews. Allot at least three hours for this activity. Run through an interview (without doing the treatment). One person is the health care provider, one portrays a client and the third person is the observer.

At the conclusion, the observer reports on what she noticed in terms of the overall flow, the client's apparent comfort level, types of questions asked, body language, what worked and what didn't work. The client shares his reactions to the interview and then the practitioner discusses what she experienced. Run the simulation three times so that each person gets to play every part. After all three rounds are completed, create an action plan for incorporating any desired changes.

Other techniques to improve communication skills are to read books, take seminars, post reminders to yourself about areas you wish to improve (e.g., ask open-ended questions, don't interrupt and suspend judgments) and ask for feedback from clients. Excellent communication skills evolve from a lifelong process of observation, study and experimentation. Have fun!

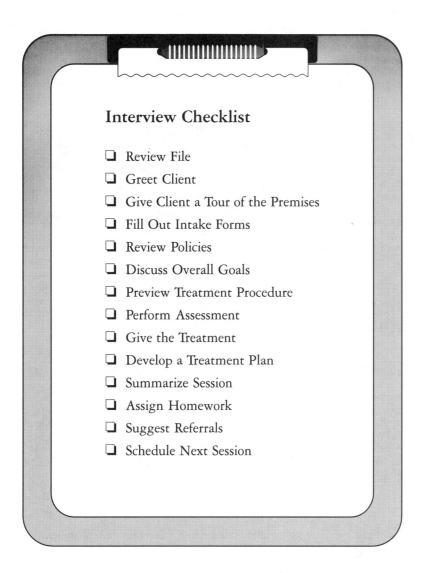

Interview Checklist

- ❏ Review File
- ❏ Greet Client
- ❏ Give Client a Tour of the Premises
- ❏ Fill Out Intake Forms
- ❏ Review Policies
- ❏ Discuss Overall Goals
- ❏ Preview Treatment Procedure
- ❏ Perform Assessment
- ❏ Give the Treatment
- ❏ Develop a Treatment Plan
- ❏ Summarize Session
- ❏ Assign Homework
- ❏ Suggest Referrals
- ❏ Schedule Next Session

• Beyond Customer Service •

Successful businesses—particularly health care practices—are built by developing strong relationships with clients. We're not talking about dual relationships here, rather the approach taken when interacting with clients. This is called relationship-based marketing and involves truly caring about your clients' welfare. In essence you become their partner in wellness. It's not about convincing or selling; rather it's about listening, planning, educating and being proactive. The time invested in developing a strong customer service action plan pays off tremendously.

Customer Service has been a popular term for the last decade; customer service workshops are offered everywhere. Whole management protocols have been built around this concept, yet very few people incorporate and demonstrate good customer service in their businesses. Customer service used to entail going beyond the expected in service; now most people don't even receive the minimum, let alone special treatment.

Baseline customer service means listening to clients' needs and doing your best to fulfill them. Offering good customer service means that you exceed clients' needs. Providing exceptional customer service means that you anticipate clients' needs.

What Clients Want		
• Convenience	• Accessibility	• Security
• Safety	• Courtesy	• Attention
• Efficiency	• Reliability	• Acceptance
• Understanding	• Compassion	• Professionalism
• Value	• Honesty	• Expertise

Baseline Customer Service ~

For health care providers, minimal customer service means that you care about your clients, you do your best to make them feel comfortable and safe, your actions are professional and you attempt to meet reasonable requests.

Facilitate clients' achieving their treatment goals: concentrate on specific requested areas or incorporate other modalities; keep accurate client files; customize each treatment; stay focused during sessions; be prompt and prepared; do good work; be a good listener; and respect clients.

According to Tom Mills of Howard Services (the company's specialty is "mystery shoppers"), nine out of ten people who have a bad experience won't tell a manager. Seven of those people won't return.

Use good-quality products: purchase a reliable, sturdy table (with side or length extensions if the table is too small for some of your clients); provide a variety of lubricants and skin care products; maintain a wide selection of music; and keep an ample supply of clean linens and accessories such as sheets, gowns, bolsters, blankets, pillows, towels and tissues.

Run your practice in a manner that demonstrates your concern: Greet clients cheerfully; have water for clients to drink before, during and after their treatment; share information and resources; send thank-you notes for referrals; adhere to a code of ethics; have an appointment schedule available; return calls within 24 hours; make confirmation calls; send appointment reminder cards when sessions are more than one month apart; call new clients within two days after their initial session; inspire trust; keep confidences; and be enthusiastic about every meeting—whether it's the first or 50th.

Good Customer Service ~

Good customer service includes all of the activities under "Baseline Customer Service" plus going the extra step to meet requests. For example, a client shows up for an appointment experiencing a headache. A baseline customer service response would be to focus attention on that condition. Good customer service would include utilizing modalities, equipment or products that are not necessarily part of your usual routine, and lengthening the duration of the session if necessary (and appropriate) until the headache is alleviated.

Good customer service requires elevating the therapeutic relationship to a wellness partnership with clients: develop a long-term wellness/treatment plan with each client; respond to requests, such as those regarding pressure or modalities; provide referrals to other practitioners who could do even more with your client; refrain from talking too much about yourself; keep conversations client-oriented; do thorough intake interviews with regular follow-up assessments; utilize appropriate equipment; demonstrate self-care techniques (e.g., stretches); provide handouts; and review client files prior to appointments.

Make your office environment comfortable and inviting: install a dimmer control for the lighting; use flannel sheets in the winter; place an oversized stepstool near the table; use clients' favorite types of products; allow clients a few minutes to just lie there before having to get up; and place a hook or shelf on the wall for clients' personal belongings. If you are a touch therapist, provide access to a shower on premises and towel off oil if necessary.

Quality is meeting customer expectations at a competitive price.
— Thad Barrington

Exceptional Customer Service 〰

Exceptional customer service does not simply involve responding to clients' needs: It requires that you be proactive—anticipating what your clients want—and making those services available. Exceptional customer service means being on the edge of anticipation. To do this, you must know your clients well. Ask clients what they want and think ahead about what they might want. If you provide what they need before they know it, your clients will think the world of you. Exceptional customer service incorporates all the activities listed above plus the following communication, session-oriented activities, practice management and support activities.

Communication: Practice active listening and encourage feedback. Your client may not know how to communicate accurately, so you may need to become a communication coach.

Mastery is not something that strikes in an instant, like a thunderbolt, but a gathering power that moves steadily through time, like weather.
— John Gardner

Session-Oriented Activities: Always review a client's chart before the session. Before you do any hands-on work, update the client's long-term treatment plan and set specific goals for the current session. Depending on the type of work you do, consider taking before and after photographs to visually document progress. If it's cold outside, warm the table with a full-length heated mattress pad and take the chill off any equipment. If you are a touch therapist, have hot packs ready and prepare a warm foot bath. If the weather is warm, be sure that the room temperature is mild and the lights are dimmed. Touch therapists can also offer clients a cool foot bath and a chilled eye pillow in the summer.

Pamper your clients with state-of-the-art equipment such as a hydraulic table, ergonomic positioning cushions and a luxuriously padded face cradle. Use fine linens, heated booties and mittens, and specialty products (e.g., aromatherapy, sports creams, custom blended oils, personalized skin care formulations and gold needles).

Provide an assortment of beverages such as juices, herbal teas and personal bottles of filtered water (with your sticker attached to the bottles). Furnish your office comfortably, including a private area where clients can put their belongings.

Appeal to your clients' senses by hanging beautiful artwork, and calm them with soothing sounds from an in-room water fountain and an excellent sound system. Take the time to research potentially effective techniques or other recommended services for specific client conditions, and prepare handouts of resources and referrals of other health care providers.

Practice Management: Ideas to incorporate excellent customer service into the day-to-day running of your practice include: place check-in calls the day after the session; return phone calls within two hours; send an anniversary card from the first appointment; give clients something for every referral—either a sample product, a 15-minute session or a free adjunct service such as a paraffin treatment; provide insurance billing; offer free treatments on birthdays; refer people to your clients' businesses; if you know a client prefers a specific time slot, do your best to keep it available; send personalized letters to your potential clients, announcing who you are and what you do; undergo semi-annual peer review; have your clients evaluate your services annually; and review all client files monthly (look for trends, note if several people are making similar requests and initiate appropriate changes).

The supplemental practice management activities include keeping in touch with announcements, holding open houses and offering discount packages.

Support Activities: Excellent customer service also encompasses supporting clients' well-being outside of the sessions. Stock books and products that can be beneficial to clients—particularly items that aren't readily available at local emporiums: books on stretching, wellness, carpal tunnel syndrome, workplace ergonomics and self-massage; stretching equipment such as exercise balls and bands; massage tools such as rollers and eye pillows; and specialty lotions, sports creams, sjin care products and aromatherapy supplies. Keep in touch by sending clients newsletters and newspaper or magazine clippings on topics in which they've expressed interest. Hold events such as monthly open houses, demonstrations and free workshops for clients and their guests.

Customer Service Action Plans

Customer service action plans grow and evolve throughout your career. The first step in developing a plan is to determine the position you desire to take and create a customer service mission statement. It might help to ask yourself what you want clients to say about your level of customer service. Survey your clients for feedback on the items they deem important.

Client Comment Cards

Client comment cards are a great tool for obtaining feedback on how your clients feel about you and your practice. These cards make it safe and convenient for clients to share suggestions, compliments or complaints.

They are easy to produce and usually cost-effective. Most people complete comment cards—whether it's for the offered premium, the opportunity to vent or simply because they want to assist you in improving your practice.

Design Tips

- Use high-quality card stock and make sure the type is large enough to read.
- Create an attention-grabbing headline.
- Mainly ask questions where the responses can be checked off or filled in with a rating.
- Ask several open-ended questions.
- Request a name, address and phone number.
- Make it a postage-paid reply card.
- Put a "Client Comment" drop box near the exit.
- Offer incentives for filling out the form.
- Include your name (or someone else in your office) on the return address.

Customer Service Action Plan

- Draft your customer service mission statement.

- Outline your goals and list the actions you commit to take.

- Answer the following questions for each activity:
    1. Is this important to my clients?
    2. How will this add value for my clients?
    3. Is this the best use of my time and resources?
    4. How will my clients know about these actions?

Customer service techniques are only powerful if your clients are aware of them. You could implement major changes, but if your clients aren't directly informed, they might never notice.

There is one caveat to customer service actions: Never implement a customer service activity that you're not willing to consistently continue. Once your clients become accustomed to a certain level of treatment, they will come to expect it and be offended if you are remiss.

Ultimately the key to going beyond customer service is to inspire your clients to move from a space of client satisfaction to one of client enthusiasm.

10 Phrases for Poor Customer Service

"I don't do that."

"Can you call back later?"

"That's not my problem."

"It's against policy."

"You don't understand."

"What do you expect me to do about it?"

"Let me put you on hold."

"I'll get around to it."

"No one's ever complained before."

"Make it quick."

• Client Retention •

Working with clients on an ongoing basis is great for your own time management as well the personal and professional fulfillment you experience witnessing positive changes in clients. A thriving practice consists of maintaining a strong client base of people who receive your services regularly, while generating a steady stream of new clients. This holds true regardless of the number of clients you have or the amount of money you want to generate. Exceptions do exist such as working in a spa or resort where there's a continuous flow of new guests, or the specific nature of a particular modality (or philosophy) that advocates working on a client only once or twice.

Unfortunately, when it comes to building their practices, health care providers often spend the majority of their marketing resources in finding new clients, instead of concentrating on keeping the ones they have. The simple steps to keep clients returning are often overlooked or ignored. Most people (particularly those that have been in business for more than two years) begin taking their current clientele for granted and focus their energy on obtaining new clients.

The core of client retention is a solid customer service plan. Taking care of oneself and doing things such as receiving your type of health care services may not be easy for the typical person. Client retention principles are founded upon making clients feel safe and welcome so they can more easily make appropriate health care decisions (which may mean not seeing you). They are not based in intimidating someone into your ordained plan. A fine line exists between supporting a client in well-being and manipulating a client into booking sessions.

Remember, on the average it costs six times as much money and takes three times the effort getting a new client as retaining one.

Preventing No-Shows ~~~

The client retention process begins before you actually see a client for the first time. This is where the pre-interview comes into play. Whenever new clients book an appointment, take the time to make them comfortable. Ascertain if they have any concerns or questions and address them. Get them involved from the beginning. Find out what they need and explain how your specific abilities can support them (or refer them to an appropriate allied professional).

Just because a new or returning client schedules a session, it doesn't mean he will show up. You can reduce the number of no-shows by incorporating the following tips into your office procedures.

Tips to Reduce No-Shows

- Send a welcome letter, your brochure and information about your practice prior to the first appointment (preferably immediately after the telephone call when session is booked).
- Ideally send a "Welcome to My Office" kit (see Figure 8.1). Items to include in this kit are: a personalized welcome letter; your specific practice brochure; a pamphlet describing (in friendly language) what a client can expect from your services, what they need to do to prepare for the session, your policies and your procedures; several business cards; client intake and health history forms; a sample gift certificate, your recent newsletter; a map to your office (if it's not already on the back of your brochure); and other promotional materials (e.g., a copy of a published interview). I know this sounds like a lot of material, but the few dollars it costs to assemble and mail this kit demonstrates your professionalism and concern about your clients.
- Confirm appointments by telephoning your clients the day before their sessions, sending reminder notes or both.
- Give clients an appointment reminder card to take home. Include your cancellation policy on this card.
- Give clients a copy of their treatment plan.
- Send clients home with assignments.

Sometimes we stare so long at a door that is closing that we see too late the one that is open.
— Alexander Graham Bell

If you follow these steps, you won't be so disconcerted if the occasional last-minute cancellation or no-show occurs. I've found that when this has happened to me—it was perfect. Either I wanted to do something else anyway or another client would call wanting to come in right away (and fill the vacant appointment slot).

Figure 8.1   Welcome to My Office Kit

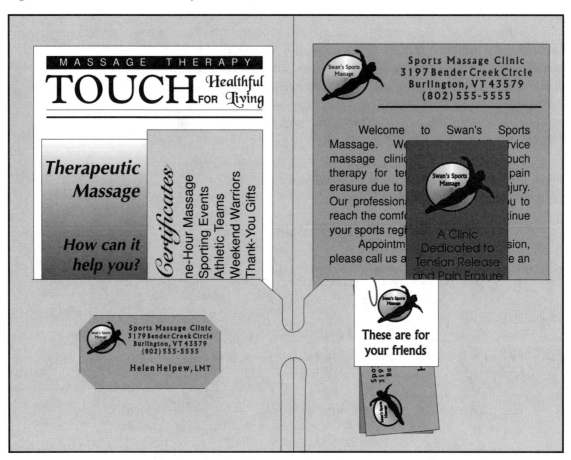

Incentive Programs ～

Incentive plans serve to reward loyal clients and to create a way to increase the session frequency for others who simply can't afford to receive treatments as often as desired. The following ideas are geared to spark your creativity. Adapt them for your specific needs and desired results.

- Offer prepaid package discounts such as: purchase three sessions and receive a 10 percent discount; seven sessions qualifies for a 20 percent discount; purchase eight sessions and receive two for free.
- Give a free session for a specific number of sessions a client receives within a certain period of time. For example, the sixth treatment is free whenever a client comes in for five sessions in two months.
- Provide a certificate for 50 percent off the client's next session whenever a client refers a new client.
- Give clients a free session for every three new clients referred.
- Give clients a half-hour session certificate for every referral.
- Give clients an adjunct service for every referral.
- Have clients sponsor a demonstration party—and thus receive at least one free session, with the potential for many more.

- Offer holiday specials: For example a touch therapist could allow clients to purchase half-hour certificates at half price with every full-hour session they purchase. These half-hour certificates can be combined for full sessions or given as gifts.
- Give a free mini-session for birthdays.
- Offer a two-for-one Valentine's Day special.

Your incentive program need not be limited to your hands-on work. For all the previous examples you can substitute products, adjunct services and seminar registrations.

These incentive suggestions serve a dual purpose—they acknowledge your current clients and many of the ideas provide a means to inspire referrals from your clients. It's wonderful to be able to combine client retention techniques with your promotional endeavors. However, do not rely on your clients to build your practice. It's not their responsibility. They may be uncomfortable telling others about your services—many consider their health care an extremely private matter.

The Client

... is the most important person in our business.

... is the reason for our work, not an interruption.

... is doing us a favor by purchasing our services and goods.

... is a feeling human being.

... is someone who wants a break—to be taken care of.

... is the person who enables us to earn an income.

... is deserving of the best service we can offer.

Transition from Student to Practitioner ∿

Client retention is also a major concern for those in the process of transitioning from being a student to a full-fledged practitioner. Shifting practicum clients to paying clients can be quite awkward. These people have been accustomed to paying a negligible fee (usually in the form of a tip) for your services. Upon graduation you may lose many of them if they are abruptly required to triple or quadruple that amount. You can ease the discomfort by devising a method for gradually bringing them up to the rates you want to charge.

For instance, let's say that you've determined your rate for a one-hour session will be $40. Several weeks before graduation, inform your current practicum clients of the rates you will be charging. Tell them that you want to acknowledge them for their support (while you were a student) by charging them a modest fee and slowly increasing the cost until they are at your current rate. After graduation you might start at $20 per session for the first three months; increasing your rates by $5 every three months until they are brought up to the rate you charge your other clients.

Recapturing Lost Clientele ~~~

At this point you may be thinking, "It's time to increase my effectiveness and work smarter by incorporating a customer service plan and a client retention program for active and new clients." Excellent plan, but what about those inactive clients—the ones you haven't seen in months or perhaps even years? You may still be able to retrieve your "lost" clients and renew your therapeutic relationships.

Kind words can be short and easy to speak but their echos are truly endless.
— Mother Teresa

Every practice experiences an ebb and flow of clients, yet many health care providers work under the false assumption that if a client doesn't return within three months, then she is lost forever. Another potentially hazardous belief for practitioners is that as long as they are attracting new clients then it's okay to become complacent with customer service and accept a high attrition rate.

Why Practitioners Lose Clients

The reasons we lose clients are numerous and may have nothing to do with us. Clients relocate, their financial situation shifts, their lifestyles change, their schedules become so filled that it is difficult to book sessions or the treatment series reaches its natural conclusion.

Then again, it may have to do with your particular kind of work, something you said or did (or didn't), your office environment or your business management.

Ninety percent of unhappy clients never return. Most won't even tell you why but they will tell 10 other potential clients. Every time the story is relayed it gets worse.

Regarding your work, clients may have gotten from your work what they intended so they don't feel it's necessary to return. For example, if the focus of your work is pain relief, once a client no longer experiences pain, he probably won't return.

Another reason for losing clients is that they may not have gotten what was wanted or needed. For instance, a client says he wants a lot of work done on his feet, yet you spend very little time there. Perhaps clients weren't asked for regular feedback, so they went elsewhere without stating complaints or preferences. Maybe the work was too challenging. Or maybe these clients are experimenting with other types of health care services.

Lack of professionalism can lead to a loss of clients. Practitioners sometimes cross boundaries or inadvertently offend. Do you greet your clients appropriately, with direct eye contact and a handshake? Do you wear appropriate attire and maintain good hygiene? Do you follow up on commitments such as researching topics and sending materials? Do you schedule ample time to see clients and regroup between sessions? Do you talk too much during sessions? Do you return phone calls within 24 hours? Do you break confidentiality by talking about other clients.

Lack of convenience or comfort are two other reasons for clients not to return. Your office may not be conveniently located for your target market. There may be scheduling difficulties due to either your hours of operation not being conducive to a certain client's schedules or because a client opted to be more spontaneous rather than planning in advance for a session (and was never able to book on short notice). There may be accessibility concerns for people with disabilities, or others who may have difficulty climbing flights of stairs. Even though you may do great work, you could lose clients to another health care provider who has better equipment, supplies, accessories or products than you do (e.g., a hydraulic table, an aromatherapy diffuser, hydrotherapy equipment, warm linens, organic skin care products, gold needles). Or there may be visual, auditory or olfactory disturbances associated with your office setting that prevent clients from returning (such as being located next to a perfumery, a music studio, a typing school, or a psychotherapist who specializes in anger release).

Financial interactions can be a source of miscommunication. There could be billing problems (particularly when it comes to insurance reimbursement). Be sure to keep track of package deals and gift certificate redemption. When questioning a client about his account, you need to be extremely careful of your wording and tone; otherwise you could easily offend.

The trouble with most of us is that we would rather be ruined by praise than saved by criticism.
— Norman Vincent Peale

You may lose a client because the receptionist or another health care provider in the office was curt, mishandled the client's records or made an error when scheduling appointments.

Regardless of the main reason people come in for treatments (e.g., pain relief, stress reduction, general wellness, relaxation, sports performance or a specific health condition), a psychological component exists. For most people alternative health care services are also a way to honor themselves, give themselves a reward or provide a time of nurturing that's just for them. It's their opportunity to be the center of the universe. If you aren't giving your full attention to your clients, you may lose them. For instance, if you allow your mind to drift during a session for too long (or too often), your client will notice the lack of connection. Are you able to leave your own troubles at the door? Also, if you answer the phone while working, you are essentially communicating to the client that she is not very important.

Reconnecting

There are as many ways to reconnect as there are to connect. Start with analyzing the possibilities behind your clients dropping you. Perform a self-inventory to evaluate your communication skills, your professional demeanor and your office operations. Identify the specific actions you take to provide excellent customer service. Pinpoint the areas most likely for miscommunication or problems. (You can also hire a colleague or business coach to analyze your practice.) This is a good time to consider what proactive efforts you can take in your practice for continued improvement. Don't be misled by the "If it ain't broke, don't fix it" philosophy. There is always room for improvement.

An error gracefully acknowledged is a victory won.
— Caroline L. Gascoigne

The best source for information about your practice is your current clients. Tell them you are evaluating your practice and would like their feedback on the following questions:

- Why do they continue receiving treatments from you?
- What do they like about you and your practice?
- What are their suggestions for improvement?

You could also assemble a focus group of current and previous clients. The purpose of a focus group is to elicit honest feedback. Ideally, the group size is between eight and 10 people and is led by an outside facilitator. The facilitator is crucial to keeping the dialogue on track and providing an atmosphere of trust and confidentiality. When you invite people to attend, tell them that you are looking for ways to improve your practice and would appreciate their input. You will fill the group faster if you provide some type of compensation and a meal or snack. Make a list of questions for the facilitator to ask (refer to your self-analysis).

The feedback you receive may offer insight into why some of your clients left and thus assist you in making necessary changes. Even if you are unable to renew many of your previous clients, these changes will help you avoid losing any more.

Let's say you discovered some things of which you were totally unaware. You could send a note to your inactive clients, saying you just want to touch base and let them know about some changes you are making in your practice (e.g., a new location, extended hours, additional services or treatment program assessment).

Another idea that helps you discover why clients don't return is to send a personal letter to your inactive clients (see Figure 8.2). The letter also serves as a way of renewing relationships.

To inspire clients to return you need to grab their attention. Send a postcard or letter with an incentive. For instance you could send a $10 discount coupon or offer a free adjunct service with their next appointment. Sometimes a simple reminder is all that's needed. A massage therapist sent me a custom-printed card that had a funny cartoon emblazoned on the front and the caption said "Remember to take care of yourself—schedule a massage today!" Right below it had her name, address and phone number. A note of caution: you can only use copyrighted or syndicated cartoons with written permission (and there's usually a fee assessed). Several companies make cards that can be used as client reminders.

You could also invite previous clients to come in for a free in-depth assessment and treatment plan (this is particularly effective if you weren't doing thorough treatment plans previously). Another idea is to create a special maintenance program and encourage previous clients to participate.

It may take several interactions to inspire a client to return. You can maintain connection by sending newsletters every quarter, mailing postcards that announce specials several times per year, holding open houses, and giving presentations. (These are also great techniques for keeping current clients and enlisting new ones.)

Many computerized clip art packages contain royalty-free images that you can use.

Kogle Greeting Cards
303-698-2583

WaterColors, Inc.
800-804-2019

Figure 8.2   Inactive Client Survey

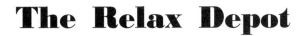

The Relax Depot

954 Miramond Way Suite #954122 • Grand Junction, CO 81501
970-555-9712 • Fax: 970-555-9713

February 2, 2001

Phyllis Forgotten
123 Prodigal Way
Anytown, CO 81506

Dear Phyllis,

Hello! It has been a while since I've seen you. You are a valued client and your satisfaction is important to me.

It is very important to establish and maintain good client relationships. Your feedback and suggestions will help me to better serve you and my other clients. Would you please take a moment to answer a few questions? Please be honest, as I desire accurate information.

1. What are the main reasons you haven't had a session lately?

2. What could have been done differently?

3. Please rate my services on the following, using a scale of 1-10 where 1 is the lowest possible score and 10 the highest:
    _____ Professional competence (e.g., the scope of services offered and your confidence in my abilities).
    _____ Session quality (e.g., the manner in which services are provided, communication and compassion).
    _____ Ambiance (e.g., room temperature, comfort of equipment, lighting and music).
    _____ Overall customer service (e.g., scheduling, attention, providing educational materials and follow-up).
    _____ Competitive pricing (e.g., are the results you receive from my services comparable to what you pay for other services, products, medications or supplements that address those same concerns).
    _____ Other (Explain): _____

4. Comments:

5. How can I encourage you to return?

Please return this to me by using the enclosed self-addressed, stamped envelope. Your answers are confidential. Thank you for your time. Enclosed is a $10 coupon toward a session to be redeemed by you or a friend.

Sincerely,

Chris Cross

Chris Cross
Enclosure

P.S. I am holding an open house on Friday, March 13 from 4-7 p.m. I will be demonstrating several self-relaxation techniques as well as displaying some nifty new equipment. I hope to see you there!

Relax Your Body Into Good Health

Remember that part of realizing how you may have lost clients is a valuable key to keep those you have from ever leaving. It's never too late to reconnect with a lapsed client. A phone call may be all that's needed. Sometimes people get overwhelmed with life and forget to take time for themselves. Others haven't made a commitment to receive treatments regularly. In either case, they may appreciate your follow-up call. It can be the ticket to their return.

• Referrals •

Clients prefer to receive treatments by someone they know. The second best option is working with professionals who come highly recommended from someone they know. Many people claim that health care is a word-of-mouth industry, but they are unaware of how to foster referrals.

Directly asking for referrals is a common and accepted form of building any service business. If you don't tell your clients you would like their assistance, they might assume you are fully booked and aren't accepting new clients.

The Direct Referral Process ⌇

The direct referral process consists of four major stages: request the referral, repeat the request, reward the referral and reciprocate the referral.

Request The Referral

Talk with your most satisfied clients and enlist their support. Ask them to tell their colleagues and friends about you. Supply them with business cards, brochures, and perhaps even some discount coupons for a percentage off an initial session (see Figures 8.3 and 8.4).

Figure 8.3

Client Referral Card

To: _____

From: _____

Give this card to a friend for $10 off their first appointment... and you get $10 off your next visit too!

Mia Lan Acupuncture
518 Broadway, Suite 3, Anytown, NJ 08413   **207-555-3271**

Figure 8.4   Sample Referral Note Card

Godiva Salon & Minispa

196 E. Maine Terrace #129
Landtown, MO 94162
(624) 555-9721

Insert
Business Card
Here

Client Referral Card

I was referred to you by your client,

_____

*I understand that I will receive 10% off
of my first appointment with you on:*

Date:_____

Time: _____ a.m.   p.m.

Repeat The Request

The next time you talk with them, repeat the request. People don't always hear things the first time. They may have been preoccupied (or if it was right after a session, they may have been too relaxed for the request to sink in). Find out if they need more promotional materials and ask them how you can make it easier for them to promote your practice. Also, send them a thank-you note even if you haven't received any referrals.

Recognize them for their intentions and support. They could be sharing information about you and passing out your cards, but you might never know it. They don't have control over whether or not the people they talk to call you to set up an appointment. Everyone likes to be acknowledged and knowing that you appreciate their efforts can inspire them to continue referring people to you.

Reward The Referral

When you do get a referral, immediately send a thank-you note. Reward the referral with something tangible such as a free session, a product sample, a plant or flowers.

Reciprocate The Referral

The last stage in the referral process is reciprocation. Whenever someone refers a client to you, go out of your way to either refer another client/customer back, use his services and products yourself, or supply the person with some type of desired information.

Indirect Referrals

Another option to cultivate referrals is to compile a list of all former and current clients, colleagues, friends and family members who value your work. Ask them to write down the names, addresses and phone numbers of people whom they think could benefit from your services. Send those prospects a personalized letter of introduction, your brochure and include a discount coupon/referral card. Keep track of which people respond to your letter. Call the rest within a month. Inquire if they received the letter and ask if they would like additional information (such as articles or pamphlets), invite them to an open house or workshop, offer a free consultation or perhaps even book a session.

Developing a solid referral process is great for augmenting your practice as long as you don't depend on it as your major source for new clients. Ultimately, when it comes to establishing a thriving practice, you are the only one who can do it. The key is to design and implement a sound customer service plan. When it comes to word-of-mouth promotion, the most important mouth is your own; you are the best advertisement for your business!

Think about the ways you can encourage referrals with new patients/clients. Chiropractic studies determined that the referrals a service provider receives are directly related to the level of enthusiasm of the patient and the efforts made by the provider to encourage referrals. The highest levels of patient/client enthusiasm tend to be after the first two to three sessions.

• Building
Professional Alliances •

Every day the health care field becomes more integrated. Providers from all realms are working together—blending philosophies as well as actual client care. You can guide the direction this takes by developing affiliations with other health care providers. Cultivating strong professional alliances provides value for you personally as well as for your clients.

One of the most important benefits is having a diverse referral base to properly support your clients' well-being. Working with other practitioners provides you with a means to get away from working alone. These associations can also supply you with new clients and offer you the opportunity to participate in case management.

Professional alliances take time and commitment. They can be best developed with a two-tiered approach. The first level is built on increasing awareness of the benefits of your specific services. The second level involves forming direct affiliations with other health care providers. It's crucial to always be working on both levels.

To see power as the ability to enhance others' lives expands society's narrow understanding of more traditional concepts of power.
— Pythia S. Peay

Increasing Public Awareness

Increasing public awareness can be accomplished in many ways—from distributing educational materials to hosting elaborate media events. One of the most effective techniques is public speaking: offer to do presentations/demonstrations for professional, business, civic and special interest organizations (such as fibromyalgia support groups). Host exhibits at health fairs and expositions. Write articles for local publications. Get interviewed by the newspaper, radio and television. Be a guest on local health-related talk shows. Find out if and when your local paper publishes a special health supplement and attempt to arrange for your interview to appear in that section.

Although these activities are geared toward increasing public awareness about the benefits of your services, they also increase your credibility and visibility.

Developing Direct Affiliations

Build your network of professional health care alliances through establishing credibility, initiating contact, forging relationships and maintaining connections. Determine your purpose, priorities and goals for developing these alliances and create an action plan. Consider how much time you want to invest, the types of professions (and how many) you want to include in your network and the levels of interaction you desire.

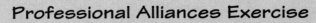
- List the types of service providers that could assist your clients in achieving their well-being goals.

- Match those categories with names of providers whom you currently know.

- Note which categories are lacking names and set goals to meet those types of practitioners.

The first step in developing professional relationships is to establish credibility. Many allied health care providers (particularly physicians) are required to obtain layers of licensure and certification. This leads them to judge competency by the number and types of certificates hanging on a wall—so some type of professional certification is helpful. Yet pieces of paper are not the only badges of credibility.

You can enhance your visibility and credibility by getting involved in the activities described in the previous section on increasing public awareness. In addition to those activities you could attend meetings where other health care providers congregate, join a local wellness organization (usually sponsored by a hospital) or volunteer your services for a charitable organization.

An interesting synergy often occurs in developing affiliations. Once the first connection is made, others occur much more easily.

If you are not well-versed in the language of professional health care providers, learn to speak it now: be aware of their philosophy, approach and terminology. While it's fine to refer to your lower leg as a "calf" when talking to the general public, you are less credible if your aren't more technical while addressing other health care providers (in those instances reference the "gastrocnemius"). Keep in mind that not everyone shares your particular approach to health care. While many practitioners believe in and specialize in prevention, others (e.g., physical therapists, general physicians, surgeons) spend most of their time working with people on the curative side of health care.

Initiating Contact

Some people prefer the front-door approach while others feel more comfortable with the side-door or even back-door method of developing affiliations. You might consider using a variety of these approaches discussed below.

Front Door Approach

The three most common front door approaches are the telephone, the mail or in person. Some people feel very comfortable just walking in and introducing themselves. This is a lot easier if your office is located close to other health care providers. In general, though, people prefer to initiate contact with a letter or telephone call. When you know the practitioner, a phone call usually suffices.

An effective technique for generating prospective alliance partners is to send a mailing to targeted health care professionals. Direct the emphasis of your letter to the benefits of the reader. First introduce yourself and what you do—include your abilities and qualifications. Focus on how you can help them, their practices and their clients. Create a separate letter for each type of health care professional you contact.

Example

Chiropractors see patients who suffer from arthritis, back pain, fibromyalgia, migraines, injuries from sports activities, job injuries and automobile accidents; psychiatrists work with people experiencing pain, stress disorders and migraines, as well as support people in personal growth and well-being; obstetricians work with women experiencing back pain, edema, hormonal fluctuations and body image issues, as well as support general mother/child well-being; touch therapists work with people of all ages providing services ranging from relaxation to injury rehabilitation. For each type of provider you contact, include examples of how your services address those specific conditions that each is involved with. (See Sample Introduction Letters, Figures 8.5 and 8.6 on pages 260 and 261)

Highlight the mutual benefits of your association. Reassure your prospective colleagues that your intent is to support and complement each other's practice, not compete for clientele. Close the letter by telling them how to contact you and that if you don't hear from them within the next two weeks, you will contact them.

Enclose your promotional material and an article that lends credence to your claim for potential benefits. You can also include a stamped, pre-printed return postcard that allows the practitioner to respond directly (see Figure 8.7, Sample Reply Postcard, page 262). After the letter has been sent you must follow up.

Side Door Approach

The side door approach is usually taken with the practitioner who keeps a buffer person—a nurse, assistant or office manager—between herself and the public. This mainly occurs with medical doctors, chiropractors, dentists and other clinicians. Always treat these gatekeepers courteously because they are the ones who will get you in the door to meet the health practitioner (and encourage patient/client referrals once a relationship is established). Be direct. Inform the office staff that you are interested in developing alliances with other health care providers.

If you are unable to make an appointment with the practitioner, ask when would be a good time to drop off your brochure. When you deliver your brochure, ask the office manager if she has any questions about your services or background and offer to demonstrate your work—for example, by teaching a five-minute self-massage routine. Give free sessions to the health care provider and the staff. This is time well invested because if you have the opportunity to demonstrate your services, and the recipient is impressed with the benefits, that person will likely be interested in building an alliance with you. Give a certificate for the session(s), and if possible, book the appointment(s) before you leave.

Another way to build alliances through the side door involves your current clients. When conducting intake interviews, ask your clients if they are working with other health care providers. If so, get their permission to send a note to those providers. This could range from a simple letter of introduction informing each practitioner that you are working with their client, to a more in-depth report with a brief description of your assessment, treatment plan and progress notes. (Note: Be sure to include your promotional literature and extra business cards.)

Back Door Approach

The back door approach can appear to be the least threatening entrance to developing professional relationships. There are various ways to enter through the back door. You can get to know other practitioners by sponsoring a talk show on radio or cable on which you bring health care providers as guests. You can also encounter health care providers by attending networking events, social engagements, professional society meetings, special interest group meetings, professional development seminars and civic functions. Research these groups to determine which ones are most likely to attract the types of practitioners you wish to meet.

An example of attending events to develop relationships—whether professional alliances or clients—happened when I did a seminar tour in Australia. One of the participants in my workshop in Brisbane was a business coach. She attended my seminar for a dual purpose: to learn new information, but mainly to get new clients. Here was a perfect opportunity: she could spend two days getting to know many people who were obviously interested in their professional development—with the knowledge that I wouldn't be there to work with them on an ongoing basis.

Forging Relationships

Your first official meeting with a health care provider sets the tone for the relationship. Be punctual and look professional. Ideally you will also be giving a session so your clothing can be a little more casual. If you are not giving a session, then business attire is appropriate. Greet the practitioner with a handshake and smile.

Briefly share information about yourself and encourage the provider to share information about her practice. Discuss ways in which you could be of mutual benefit (including reducing the demands on her time and energy) and set goals. Confer about approaches to different situations and determine how you would like to work together. Be certain to cover the preferred methods of future communication about shared clients/patients. Some people favor written correspondence only while others like to discuss cases and proactively work together to enhance clients' well-being.

Remember that a man's name is, to him, the sweetest and most important sound in any language.
— Dale Carnegie

While it isn't imperative that the practitioner experience your work, I strongly advise you make it happen. If she claims she is too busy, offer to do a modified session at her convenience. Also give a free session to the staff (see the previous section on initiating contact). Be up-front: tell her that it's important to experience your work firsthand to ethically feel good about making referrals to you. The converse is also true. For you to refer clients to her, you need to experience her work—or in the very least get a sense of her methodology and style, which can be done by assessing the person's demeanor, office environment and written materials (such as intake forms and information pamphlets).

When you give her a treatment, do an intake interview (modify it if time is limited), take notes and submit a sample of your records. This is of particular importance if you are not a primary care provider because it demonstrates your ability to do charting and follow-up. Before you leave this meeting schedule the next one—whether it's a telephone conversation, another session or a more formal face-to-face meeting. Sometimes the steps to forging a relationship take several meetings to accomplish.

Maintaining Connections ⚬⚬⚬

Maintain connections by employing customer service principles. For example: send a thank-you note after your first meeting; if they haven't used your certificate within three weeks, remind them and ask them when they would like to book the session; acknowledge all referrals; regularly submit typed progress reports (check with client first); call about dramatic results; schedule a brief meeting at least twice per year; reciprocate by sending them clients; leave an ample supply of your brochures and business cards for display in the office and distribution to clients/patients; obtain a plentiful stock of their cards and brochures; and place monthly check-in calls (instead of asking if they've run out of brochures or cards, assume that they have and ask how many you can bring by).

You want to make it as easy as possible for allied health care providers to make referrals to you. In addition to stocking your promotional material, consider printing referral pads with your contact information to give to the providers and their office staff (see Referral Pad, Figure 8.8, page 262).

Figure 8.5   Sample Introduction Letter

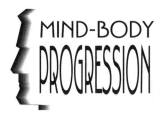
MIND-BODY
PROGRESSION

October 15, 2001

Dr. Ben Casey
123 North Swan Road
Sea City, CA 90000

Dear Dr. Casey,

I was intrigued by your advertisement in the Yellow Pages under "Psychotherapy." You appear dedicated to the health of the whole person. As an acupuncturist and Traditional Chinese Medicine (TCM) practitioner I, too, see the mind-body as so interwoven that addressing the health of one area while excluding the other is an incomplete process.

I am interested in developing a union between us for mutual referrals of our combined patient needs. I provide a complete range of services from general well-being care, stress reduction, pain relief, injury rehabilitation to illness intervention. Many of these were listed in your advertisement as well. I am also a master herbologist and have worked with people of varying ages.

Acupuncture and TCM, in conjunction with psychiatric services, can be effective treatment for patient recovery and preventive maintenance. As an adjunct to your therapy, patients utilizing my services may find a decreased need for medication, thus lowering the possibilities of medication interactions.

Many of our patients could benefit from our combined services. We tend to approach the same concept from different angles. For example, I have seen patients have emotional releases during sessions and are in need of someone qualified to counsel them. I'm sure you have patients who could benefit from acupuncture and TCM.

I look forward to meeting with you personally to discuss the possibilities. Feel free to call my office at 555-5555. Otherwise I will contact you within the next two weeks to schedule a time to meet.

Sincerely,

James Kildare

James Kildare
Enclosures

721 N. Somerset Place ❖ Arcadia, CA 91077 ❖ 415-555-5555

Figure 8.6   Sample Introduction Letter

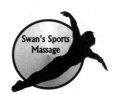

Sports Massage Clinic
3197 Bender Creek Circle
Burlington, VT 43579
802-555-5555

September 30, 2001

Charlene Goalpost, M.D.
1114 Miller Drive
Burlington, VT 43579

Dear Dr. Goalpost,

It is common knowledge that you are the finest sports physician in the area. You are blazing a needed path for more research on athletes, and I would like to offer my sports massage services to complement your work with athletic individuals and teams.

My services can assist your patients' well-being, ease your workload and contribute to your profitability. Helping athletes perform at their best and reducing the incidence of their injuries is extremely gratifying. For the last six years I have provided therapeutic massage during numerous sporting events and have regularly worked with athletes to improve their performance, minimize injuries and quicken the recovery from those injuries.

I have been practicing sports massage for the past 12 years, the last three in Burlington, and was trained at the Sports Massage Therapy Institute in Costa Mesa, California, from which I graduated in 1989.

I would like to give you a complimentary massage (or one of your patients, with your supervision) so you will know what you would be offering to your patients. Please call me at 555-5555 to set up an appointment. I will check back with you if I haven't received a call within the next two weeks.

Let's work together to keep active Burlingtonians healthy!

Sincerely,

Doug L. Gainer

Doug L. Gainer

Enclosures

Figure 8.7   Sample Reply Postcard

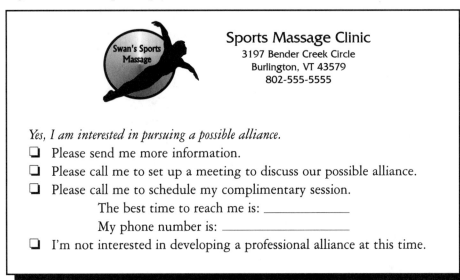

Sports Massage Clinic
3197 Bender Creek Circle
Burlington, VT 43579
802-555-5555

Yes, I am interested in pursuing a possible alliance.
❑ Please send me more information.
❑ Please call me to set up a meeting to discuss our possible alliance.
❑ Please call me to schedule my complimentary session.

The best time to reach me is: _____

My phone number is: _____
❑ I'm not interested in developing a professional alliance at this time.

Figure 8.8   Sample Referral Pad

Sports Massage Clinic
3197 Bender Creek Circle
Burlington, VT 43579
802-555-5555

Date: _____

Patient: _____
Address: _____
City: _____ State: _____ Zip: _____
Telephone: _____

Condition Related To:
❑ Auto Accident   ❑ Work Injury   ❑ Stress/Relaxation
❑ Other: _____

Body Areas To Be Treated:
❑ Neck   ❑ Back   ❑ Shoulders   ❑ Legs   ❑ Arms

Diagnosis Description & Codes: _____
_____

Duration: ❑ 8 weeks   ❑ 6 weeks   ❑ 4 weeks   ❑ other: _____
Frequency: ❑ daily   ❑ 3x/week   ❑ 2x/week   ❑ weekly
           ❑ biweekly   ❑ monthly   ❑ other: _____
Medically Necessary: ❑ Yes   ❑ No

Prescribing Doctor: _____
Doctor's Provider #: _____
Address: _____
City: _____ State: _____ Zip: _____
Telephone: _____

Signature: _____

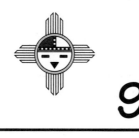

9

Marketing

• Marketing Principles •

The word "marketing" conjures up an amazing array of thoughts and feelings ranging from tremendous excitement to fantasies of instant success to studied disinterest to confusion to hand-wringing dismay. Many people automatically associate marketing with hard-sell tactics. Although effective marketing is the cornerstone of a flourishing practice, some practitioners shy away from any type of active promotion. Perhaps this avoidance stems from an innate distrust of anything that seems like "selling," is due to a lack of marketing knowledge, or simply exists because of limited resources.

One of the attractions of this field is its dissimilarity with the "typical" business world. But even the health care profession is ultimately a sales and marketing industry. Luckily, we rarely need to rely on traditional methods to promote ourselves. I believe in value-centered marketing: promoting your business in a way that reflects your personality, philosophy and integrity. Marketing is not a dirty word: it's simply sharing yourself with others so they get a sense of who you are, which allows them to make an informed choice of whether to utilize your services. It's not about coercion or pretending to be someone you're not.

See Chapter Eight, pages 252-254 for information on fostering word-of-mouth referrals.

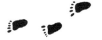

Marketing is about getting yourself known—building a professional reputation. The ultimate aim is to develop a thriving practice, and that means having a strong and continually growing clientele base.

Very few people can afford the luxury of building their practices solely by word-of-mouth. If you are very good at what you do, genuinely care about and respect your clients and charge a reasonable rate, you will ultimately develop a strong clientele base. Most of us are interested in accelerating that process and that requires marketing ourselves smartly. The best mouth is your own!

The essence of marketing is good public relations. Simply put, marketing is all the business activities done on a daily basis to attract potential clients (and retain current ones) in order for them to utilize your services and purchase your products. These activities include promotion, advertising, community relations and publicity. Marketing is about enabling your clientele to value you and your services. The biggest mistake I see people make is overextending themselves; they try to be *the* practitioner for everyone. One person cannot fulfill all the needs of every client. Effective marketing involves targeting the appropriate people and informing them of the benefits they'll receive from your services.

Marketing a service can be very different than marketing a product. For example, retailers use mass-marketing techniques such as broad-based advertising campaigns, telemarketing and in-store promotions. Service businesses usually target a well-defined market and use a more personal approach. The major portion of marketing a service business is educational in nature.

Marketing plans address the following questions: Where are you now? Where do you want to be? How can you meet prospective clients? How can you determine their needs and wants? How can you convey/demonstrate your ability to assist clients' well-being goals? There's a saying that goes, *"If you don't know where you are going, what matters the path?"* This is true in any type of planning—especially with marketing.

All too often health care providers leave their marketing to chance. They wait for people to find them—an attitude that generally isn't productive. (It's okay if you have an alternate source of income.) But then again, consider why you got into this field in the first place. What good is it to desire enhancing people's well-being if they don't know who you are? You don't have to employ the same techniques that "big business" does. You can incorporate other methods such as public speaking, visualizations and affirmations. The critical point here is to create a marketing plan with the focus primarily on low-cost techniques that build relationships.

A strange paradox of competition versus abundance exists in this career field. There truly are enough potential clients in the world for everyone, and yet not many practitioners have as many clients as they want. Part of the dilemma stems from the fact that the people are "potential" clients. You have to make them aware of you and the benefits of your services. It's not as though there are limitless numbers of people anxiously waiting for you to let them know you exist; you must create the need. Many people still don't recognize the value of complementary health care services; some of us know better.

A significant part of what you're competing with is a lack of knowledge on part of the general public, thus the necessity of including some type of direct education (e.g., writing articles, giving demonstrations, public speaking and compiling information packets) in your marketing plan. Even though competition has been historically associated with struggle and rivalry it doesn't have to be that way any more. Think of competition as a way of distinguishing yourself from other health care providers. One of the most exciting facets of this industry is that practitioners usually aren't attempting to prove that they're "better" than another—but that they're different. For this reason, marketing is vital to your career. You must sell people on your services and then on you! It's not wise to assume that you are going to attract the people who "know better," take care of themselves and use alternative health services. Such people probably already have a network of health care providers. You may need to create new markets and possibly share some of an existing market.

Don't take it for granted that people "know" what you do because you have a certain title. Define what you do. Explain the benefits of what you offer and clarify your Differential Advantage. Every practitioner is unique, and brings her experience and personality into play along with whatever techniques are employed. The power of your marketing increases with the level in which **YOU** are integrated into those marketing strategies.

Your marketing ventures can be significantly more successful, enjoyable and less risky if you participate with other practitioners in joint promotional activities. Develop a working relationship with at least two other practitioners: one person who does similar work as you but targets a different market, and another practitioner in an allied field who shares your target market. Cooperative marketing is a great solution to overcoming marketing reluctance. It provides you with the means to extend the scope of your promotional ventures. Also, some of the more dreaded aspects of marketing become less of a chore when you don't have to do them alone.

The most successful practitioners are those who incorporate their marketing activities into their daily lives. They know who they want to work with, understand how to find those potential clients through appropriate marketing techniques and attract the desired clients by being able to clearly and engagingly describe what they do. They maintain a thriving practice by being client-centered: having an inviting treatment space, using good equipment, doing thorough treatment plans, following up, and most importantly—listening and responding to each client's needs.

Everything you do makes a statement about how you feel about yourself, your clients and your practice. Thus, you are always marketing yourself—for better or worse. Marketing isn't just about the outward activities you do, such as advertising and promotions; it also incorporates the manner in which you relate to your clients, your ethics and your professional demeanor. It's important that your outward image be consistent with your vision of a successful health care professional.

The more creative and natural your marketing techniques, the more successful they will be, mainly because you enjoy doing them. No rule says that you can't have fun while promoting your business!

Stay centered in your enthusiasm about your work and the results it produces—this is what attracts people to want to learn more about who you are and what you do.

Successful marketing is based on having a clear vision for your business, defining your target markets, clarifying your differential advantage, determining your position statement, and designing a marketing plan that utilizes creative and effective strategies which reflect your values.

A popular phrase in this industry (and also the title of a book) is "Do what you love and the money will follow." Unfortunately, most people forget about the verb in the sentence: **DO**. They assume that *deciding* what to do is enough. Doing what you love doesn't mean sitting in your office waiting for the phone to ring; it implies taking action to attract new clients and actually doing your work! In other words, if you don't have a full client load, either invest that free time in educating people about your work or donate your services (do what you love)—then the money will truly come. Also, have the courage to do some of the practice building activities that you don't love.

Courage is the price that life exacts for granting peace. The soul that knows it not, knows no release from little things; knows not the livid loneliness of fear, nor mountain heights where bitter joy can hear the sounds of wings.
— Amelia Earhart

• Marketing Plan Outline •

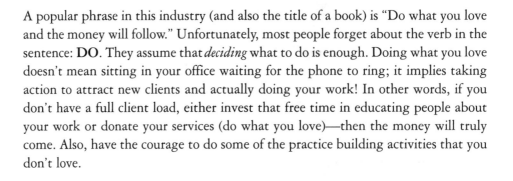

Marketing plans are internal planning documents: they keep you focused and assist you in choosing appropriate methods to build and maintain a thriving practice. The chart below illustrates the major components of a marketing plan. The subsequent pages contain exercises as well as technical information to assist you in creating an innovative marketing plan.

Figure 9.1

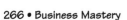

Refer to Chapter Ten, pages 371-372 for a complete marketing plan outline.

Sample Marketing Plan Outline

I **Overview (Purpose, Priorities and Goals)**
    A. Statement of why you are in this business
    B. Results you intend to create
    C. Summary of how you will accomplish your goals

II **Positioning**
    A. Differential Advantage
    B. Image

III **Target Market Analysis**
    A. Demographics
    B. Psychographics

IV **Marketing Assessment**
    A. Analysis of previous promotional activities
    B. Recommended changes for future plans
    C. Overview of competition's marketing

V **Strategic Action Plans**
    A. Promotion
    B. Advertising
    C. Community Relations
    D. Publicity
    E. Timetables
    F. Budget

• Marketing Plan Overview •

To develop effective marketing strategies you must clarify your purpose, priorities and goals and determine how to implement your marketing plan. The answers to the following questions will assist you in making the appropriate choices for your promotion and advertising campaigns.

Marketing Plan Self-Assessment

- Why are you in this business?
- What is your purpose for marketing?
- What are your priorities for marketing?
- What are your major goals for marketing?
- What are your strategies for developing and implementing your marketing plan?

• Positioning •

Positioning is a key principle of marketing. You must determine exactly what niche you intend to fill. Most businesses have weak or non-existent positions in the minds of the consumers. Prospective clients need an easy way to differentiate you from your competition; your position statement provides that information.

Positioning and target markets go hand in hand. It's difficult to explain one without the other. As a matter of fact, if you have more than one target market (which is usually wise), and they are vastly different, you may need a separate position statement for each of those target markets. To make this subject more comprehensible, I recommend that you scan both topics (this and the following one on Targeting Markets), and then study each one in depth.

Four examples of successful positioning statements are those from Avis,® Vicks,® Wheaties® and 7-Up.® Everyone knows that 7-Up's marketing position is: *Seven-Up, The Uncola.*® At the time that Seven-Up was developing its marketing campaign, a soda usually meant Coca-Cola or Pepsi. To counteract that assumption, they promoted their product as something totally "un"like competing soft drinks.

When the Vicks Company was preparing to promote its new formula, the market was controlled by Contact® and Dristan.® Instead of attempting to take away some of their share of the daytime market, Vicks created a new one. Thus, the introduction of NyQuil,® *The Nightime, Sniffling, Sneezing, Coughing, Aching, Stuffy Head, Fever, So You Can Rest Medicine.*® It took many years for them to feel confident enough to compete in the daytime market with DayQuil,® *The non-drowsy, congested-stuffy head, sore throat, coughing, aching, fever so you can get through the day medicine.*®

Avis took an innovative (and highly effective) approach. When they first started their major marketing campaign, they had to overcome two problems: another company already had a strong hold on the number one position, (can you name it?) and most people find it extremely difficult to differentiate one car rental business from another. Their solution was the slogan: *We're Avis. We're Number Two. We Try Harder.*™ This position statement distinguished Avis from the other companies and made a compelling promise to its potential customers. It was so effective that now Avis' position statement is simply: *We try harder.*®

Image plays a major role in your positioning. You need to decide the type of impression you want to give and then align yourself to match that image. For example, Wheaties is known for being: *The Breakfast of Champions.*® They back up their position statement (and reinforce their image) by putting pictures of top athletes (even Olympians) on the front of the cereal boxes.

Image Exercise

- Describe the image you wish to portray.

- How do your facilities, actions and attire align with this image?

- What changes do you need to make to alter the elements that are not in sync with your desired image?

The Differential Advantage ⁓

The next step in developing a position statement is to define your differential advantage. You must be able to describe what makes you different (unique) from all the other health care providers in your specific field. No two people are exactly alike. For instance, having been a long-time faculty member of the Desert Institute of the Healing Arts, I experienced numerous massages from students with identical training, and every single massage was different.

Reflect upon your practice. Think about what you really do: the intention of your work, the image you portray, the range of modalities you use, the specific products or other therapies you incorporate and the results your clients receive.

Your differential advantage may stem from yourself, your specialization, the range of services offered, geographic location, or a combination of all of these and other factors. In considering your differential advantage, keep in mind that what attracts potential clients are not the actual features of your practice, but *how* those features are going to benefit them.

Another way of differentiating yourself from other practitioners is through specialization. You may prefer to work on a particular condition or a specific clientele (e.g., in my coaching practice I only work with people who are committed to change).

Perhaps one of your greatest strengths lies in the actual service you offer. Do you have specialized knowledge? Are you the only one in your area who does a certain type of work? Do you own state-of-the-art equipment? Do you offer a greater range of services and products than most other health care providers?

One of the most significant yet often overlooked advantages is your actual office location. If you are situated in a large professional building, your appeal is accessibility—people can schedule appointments during breaks, before or after work, and they don't need to drive. If you do on-site work one of your major benefits is convenience—clients don't have to go anywhere or do anything but enjoy the session. If your office has a particular ambiance (e.g., a fitness motif, a clinic setting or a retreat atmosphere), expound upon those qualities.

In the factory we make cosmetics, but in the stores we sell hope.
— Charles Revson,
Revlon Cosmetics

In most instances, the strongest determining difference is you. What you do and how you do it is greatly influenced by your background, personality, education and philosophy toward the nature of well-being.

To spur your thought process for the next exercise, gather brochures about your services (in addition to yours, look at other practitioners' brochures and those published by your profession). Reflect upon the value **you** get from receiving your type of services and remember why you chose this profession for your career.

Define Your Differential Advantage

- Carefully consider the following questions:
    1. What does your business do?
    2. What needs does your business meet?
    3. What problems does your business solve?
    4. How do your clients benefit psychologically?
    5. How does your business differ from the competition?

- Write a statement that summarizes what makes you unique.

- Describe how potential clients will recognize your differential advantage.

Position Statement Examples ⚘

The following position statements illustrate the range of differential advantages from types of services, to philosophy, to specific clientele and to location. Position statements are similar to slogans—though not always so catchy.

Services

Some position statements are based solely upon the service(s) provided. This approach is usually taken when a practitioner has specialized knowledge, a unique service, a particularly clever slogan or state-of-the-art equipment.

> *"On Pins and Needles? Try Acupuncture for Relief"*
> *"We Use the Latest Advances in Dental Technology"*
> *"The Only Certified Practitioner in the Midwest"*
> *"Trained by the Founder of <insert well-known name here>"*
> *"We Use an Array of Modalities"*

Philosophy

Most health care providers have strong beliefs about the nature of well-being and their particular approach to health care. Quite often, this is the major quality that distinguishes one practitioner from another.

> *"We Treat You as a Whole Person"*
> *"Your Well-Being is Our Purpose"*
> *"The Beginning of a Healthy Lifestyle"*
> *"Helping People to Get in Touch with Their Selves"*
> *"The First Thing We Do is Listen"*
> *"Your Kids Have a Voice with Us"*
> *"Supporting You in Creating Success While Keeping Balance"*
> *"The Gentle Approach to Deep Tissue Therapy"*
> *"Our Touch Helps You Get in Touch with Yourself"*
> *"We Use Holistic Methods Whenever Possible"*
> *"Combining Ancient Healing Wisdom with State-of-the-Art Technology"*

Specialization

Some position statements are based on appealing to a target market. For example, you may prefer to only work with one gender or a specific age group. Maybe your focus is treating a specific condition or part of the body.

> *"Seniors are Our Specialty"*
> *"Woman to Woman"*
> *"Making Your Pregnancy More Comfortable"*
> *"Giving Athletes that Competitive Edge"*
> *"My Hands for Your Feet"*
> *"Helping You Overcome Your Phobias"*
> *"We Work Exclusively with ACAs"*
> *"The Specialists in Head and Neck Injuries"*

Office Location

Expound upon your location's accessibility, convenience or ambiance.

"The Healthy Coffee Break Alternative"
"Have Table, Will Travel"
"Providing All Your Health Care Needs in One Location"
"A Haven from the Hectic Workplace"
"Too Stressed to Leave Home? We Make House Calls"
"Only Twenty Minutes from Downtown, Yet a World Apart"
"A Health Oasis in the Desert"

Your Position Statement

Some people choose a position statement because it resonates with them. Others create statements to draw a specific clientele. It's best if you can do both.

To prepare for the next exercise, review your responses to the differential advantage questions and highlight the most important facets. Combine those with your image statement to formulate your general position statement. After you finish the next section on target marketing, you may find you need to create additional position statements (for each of the different markets).

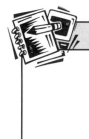

Position Statement Exercise

Write your position statement.

Evaluate it in terms of the following criteria:
- Does it convey a true benefit?
- Does it differentiate you from your competition?
- Is it unique?

• Targeting Markets •

Target markets are groupings of people who can be identified by certain commonalities. The whole concept of target marketing can seem very scary at first. On the surface, it appears to limit the pool of potential clients. Many people fear that by defining a market, they will lose business or choose the wrong one. An additional concern is that other practitioners will take anybody and therefore absorb some of their business.

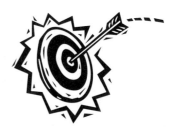

The purpose of choosing specific target markets is to make your practice more enjoyable, simplify your marketing, and increase the success of your promotional endeavors. The world abounds with opportunities and it's impossible to pursue them all or attempt to be everything to everyone. You need to decide where to focus your marketing energy and resources.

Health care is very intimate work. Think about who you want in your space. Actively seeking the type of clients you want to work with is preferred to accepting anyone who wanders through the door. My philosophy is that if I am requested to work with someone, I usually will, but I invest my marketing time and money toward attracting specific types of people.

Working with several markets is one of the best ways to avoid the potential disaster of selecting an unsuitable one. The benefits of not being restricted to only one type of clientele are manifold; in particular, your skills become well-rounded by experiencing a variety of people with their own unique issues.

Marketing Foundation Exercise

Consider the following questions:
- What types of people do you want to reach?
- What types of services would be the most fulfilling for you to offer?
- What qualities do you want your services to exude?
- What problems, conditions and issues do you want to address in your work?
- What type of environment do you want to work in?

Given your responses to the preceding questions, who would be most easily attracted to working with you?

The two most common means of market analysis are Demographics and Psychographics, which describe a person in terms of objective data and personality attributes.

Demographics are statistics such as:

- Age
- Gender
- Income Level
- Geographic Location
- Occupation
- Education Level

Psychographics (also referred to as lifestyle factors) are the major determinants in whether someone becomes a client. They include:

- Special Interest Activities
- Philosophical Beliefs
- Social Factors
- Cultural Involvements
- Health Care Needs

The more you know about your potential clients, the easier it is to develop an appropriate position statement and design an effective marketing campaign. The number of target markets you have depends mainly upon the size of your practice and the scope of your knowledge. Some target markets are more productive than others. You set yourself up for difficulty if you base your target market solely on demographics.

Connecting With the Right Clients

Some typical health care target markets are: high-stress executives, pregnant women, athletes (in general or a specific niche such as triathletes, cyclists, gymnasts), infants, children, people in self-improvement programs, pre- and post-operative recovery, people with disabilities, attorneys, seniors, the entertainment industry, natural disaster casualties, people in addiction recovery programs, patients of other primary care providers, small business owners, crime victims, students, animals, abuse survivors, computer operators, military personnel and other health care providers.

When determining the clients you want to target, ask yourself, "Who do I love being around?"

One of the vast misconceptions coursing through this industry is "people with money are a great target market." Affluence isn't a market. It's a demographic statistic only! Just because individuals have the means to easily pay for health care services doesn't mean they will ever avail themselves. If all the people who could afford your type of service attempted to book an appointment, you and your colleagues would have to work 24 hours a day, seven days a week. You need to discover what *motivates* someone to receive your services.

Still, most health care providers are not earning the incomes they desire. Obviously, the means is not a determining factor—the motive is. You must determine who the most appropriate clients are and how to communicate the benefits of your services in such a way that they are inclined to utilize them.

People want to feel special—that their needs are unique. So, even though we know just about anyone can benefit from complementary health care services, we need to find a way to communicate that in terms with which people can identify. To maximize the effectiveness of your communications, alter your language to match the style of your intended recipient.

We exist to serve the marketplace. The better we do that, the more profits we will make.
— Stephen Martin

Matching Needs and Benefits

So far we've explored potential target markets. Now it's time to look at how to analyze those markets. The first two steps are: describing each of your target markets in terms of their general needs, concerns and goals; and connecting specific benefits with each item.

Below are seven briefly described sample target markets, their concerns, and words/phrases that could address those needs. Use these examples as a springboard for analyzing your target markets. Keep in mind that the more accurate you are in

The goal is to inspire people to find out more about your services and how they can benefit by them.

identifying the needs of your target market, the easier it will be to determine the appropriate terminology.

Pregnant Women

Pregnancy is a time of great change: physically, hormonally and emotionally. In addition to being concerned about the health of her child, the mother also contends with a changing body image, fluctuating emotions, a possible reduction of activity level, back pain and edema.

When addressing these areas of concern, incorporate phrases such as: reduces edema; increases circulation; eases discomfort; soothes; enhances connection between mother and child; encourages relaxation; promotes a healthier pregnancy; reduces anxiety; relieves muscle tension and stiffness; enhances well-being; increases ease and efficiency of movement; and provides an environment for self-appreciation and nurturing.

Infants

Infants often have difficulty adjusting to being outside of the womb and the birth process itself can be traumatic. They may develop sleeping problems, colic and other ailments that can definitely benefit from complementary health services.

Even though the receiver is the child, the parents are the ones to whom you must market your services. Use terms such as: soothing; nurturing; strengthens immune system; safe; gentle; fosters easier and deeper breathing; encourages sound sleep; and promotes healthy development.

Seniors

As people age they become more concerned about their overall health and their mobility. They may be experiencing stiffness, pain and a lack of touch.

Emphasize your benefits with terms such as these: increases blood and lymph circulation; tonifies; promotes healthier, better nourished skin; improves digestion; optimizes joint flexibility; increases range of motion; offers caring and nurturing touch; maintains health; improves posture; reduces blood pressure; heightens capacity for clearer thinking; reduces stress; and relieves muscle tension and stiffness.

Athletes

Athletes are concerned with avoiding injuries, improving performance and reducing down-time due to pain or injury.

Accentuate benefits such as: increases circulation, flexibility, and mobility; relieves muscle soreness and chronic pain; improves endurance; lessens recovery time; tonifies; peak performance; reduces risk of injuries; and enhances concentration.

Entrepreneurs

Your typical entrepreneur is on the go, experiences a lot of stress, must make decisions quickly, has numerous responsibilities and "job titles," and keeps a tight schedule.

To appeal to this market, focus on the results and convenience. Use phrases such as: increases stamina; rejuvenates; relieves stress and tension; improves concentration and creativity; alleviates headaches; enhances sense of well-being; convenient; accessible; increases productivity; promotes deep relaxation; and provides an easy, affordable way to take care of yourself.

Health Care Providers

Caregivers often ignore their own well-being. In addition to the actual physical stress of their jobs, they often experience fatigue and burnout.

To best reach this market, remind them that they know the importance of taking care of themselves. Use phrases like: take time for yourself; relieves tension and stiffness; relaxed state of alertness; increases stamina; reduces injury; improves posture; enhances self-image; increases career longevity; and provides care for the caregiver.

Personal Growth

People who are actively involved in their personal growth experience this clearing physically, spiritually and emotionally. Their self-image tends to undergo major shifts.

In approaching this group, use phrases such as: tonify your body as well as your soul; soothing; reduces stress and tension; "natural adjunct" to current personal growth techniques; greater ease of emotional expression; increases self-esteem; strengthens immune system; promotes deep relaxation; encourages peak performance; and evokes a heightened awareness of the mind-body connection.

I cannot give you the formula for success, but I can give you the formula for failure—which is: Try to please everybody.
— Herbert B. Swope

Target Market Profiles

Target market profiles are statements that define your market in terms of their needs, how your services address those needs, who else caters to the target market and where they can be found. Once you've determined those components, you can choose effective marketing methods.

Create a profile of yourself as well as your clients.

At this point you may be wondering how you could possibly know this information, particularly if you are just beginning your practice or are branching out into new domains. If you don't have client files to analyze, you need to do research. (It's wise to do this anyway.) Read books and articles about your target market. Get feedback from health care practitioners as well as other businesses that cater to your desired market. Discover information by contacting organizations that deal with your target market and by conversing with people who train practitioners to work with that specific population. Talk with those who are in the know—members of your target market.

The statistics you compile are for reference only and vary according to geographic location and practitioner. Start with the general known facts about your target population and adjust them according to your own findings and feedback from others. Keep in mind that these figures are only accurate for *your* clientele. The whole purpose of creating a profile is to assist you in developing an effective, natural marketing plan. The following fictitious examples include client analyses, profiles and ideas for reaching those populations. Additional in-depth marketing techniques are explored later on in this chapter.

Massage Therapy Prenatal Client Analysis and Profile:

- Thirty percent are referred by childbirth educators, midwives and health centers.
- Twenty percent are referred by friends.
- Twenty percent were clients before they got pregnant.
- Thirty percent are referred from direct promotional endeavors.
- The average age range is between 28-35 years.
- The majority experience discomfort.
- They are all under the care of a physician.
- Seventy percent take health-related classes like Lamaze and exercise.
- Fifty percent never had a professional massage before their pregnancy.
- Seventy percent shop at The Happy Baby Boutique.
- The majority read the local *Entertainment Guide*.
- Sixty percent are professionals or teachers.
- The combined family income level is between $25,000 and $60,000.
- Seventy percent attend at least two cultural events per year.
- Sixty-five percent are interested in nutrition and shop at health food stores.
- Seventy percent receive massage once per month.
- Ten percent receive massage once per week.
- Fifteen percent receive massage twice per month.
- The majority are more motivated to receive massage in their last trimester.

By compiling this information, you could create this profile:

"My typical prenatal client is 32 years old. She has been married at least three years and already has one child. She is under the care of a physician, keeps a healthy diet, goes to Lamaze classes, exercises regularly and gets a massage once per month. She attends cultural events such as theater or concerts at least two times per year and dines out at least once per week. She shops at The Happy Baby Boutique, buys books on child care at The Basic Book Store, frequents Nature's Haven Health Food Store, reads the local weekly Entertainment Guide *and subscribes to* Parents Magazine. *Her combined family income is greater than $40,000. She holds an administrative position and works through her eighth month of pregnancy. Her major reasons for getting massage are to have an easy, healthy pregnancy and to feel better about herself—relieve her lower back pain, increase her stamina, decrease edema, improve her body image, reduce stress and enhance the overall well-being of herself and her baby."*

The prenatal market can be approached in many different ways. Before investing any time or money into a promotional endeavor, check your profile to evaluate the likelihood of success. Let's say someone approaches you with an opportunity to place a listing in a promotional piece that is being mailed to "working women" within a three-mile radius of your office. You need to obtain much more information before determining if it's worth the risk. Keeping in mind that no promotion is ever guaranteed to be successful, compare their proposed demographic and psychographic statistics with your target market profile(s) to see how well they match. You can then better decide if participation in that promotion is worthwhile.

In developing your marketing plan, prepare for potential obstacles—especially with a target market such as pregnant women. Many other people such as a partner, physician or even a mother influence whether or not a woman receives massage. Your promotional efforts, particularly your print media such as brochures and cards, need to reassure the significant people in the pregnant woman's life. The following ideas are a starting point for reaching this market.

Design attractive promotional materials. In addition to business cards and brochures, consider creating one-sided fliers that are good for tacking on bulletin boards and making informational handouts on different topics of concern to pregnant women. Print these on your letterhead or include your name, title, address and phone number at the bottom of the page.

Place your promotional materials wherever pregnant women tend to frequent: obstetricians' offices, Lamaze classes, fitness centers, health food stores, maternity shops, bookstores, childbirth centers and offices of other allied health care professionals.

Establish your credibility and build up contacts by volunteering your services (massage or other) at organizations that serve pregnant women such as health care clinics, the La Leche League and Planned Parenthood. Also, write articles on topics of interest to pregnant women and those around them, such as prenatal well-being care or the benefits of massage during pregnancy, and submit them to your local publications.

Give an instructional program that teaches birthing partners how to use basic Swedish massage strokes such as effleurage and kneading the back, legs and arms on their pregnant partners. To arrange speaking engagements contact pregnancy-related organizations, Lamaze classes, birthing centers and midwifery associations, as well as business networking groups such as Entrepreneurial Mothers. You could even get another business to sponsor a more extensive program—and handle the promotion and cover the expenses.

Establish a strong referral network of allied professionals such as obstetricians, midwives, nutritionists, other health care providers and childbirth educators.

List your name and a concise, engaging description of your practice in appropriate publications. Be sure to put these listings under the heading of "Pregnancy" or "Prenatal Care" in addition to "Massage." Some recommended publications are: the

What would you attempt to do
if you knew you could not fail?
— Dr. Robert Schuller

telephone Yellow Pages, local new age publications, newsletters directed toward pregnant women and special editions of the newspaper like its annual health and fitness guide.

Increase your visibility by participating in joint promotions. Some techniques are: include your brochures in mailings with other businesses that cater to pregnant women (e.g., maternity shops and baby stores); set up a booth at expositions such as baby shows, fitness fairs, and anyplace else that attracts your target market; and donate a few sessions as prizes at a major fund raising event. The list goes on....

Acupuncture Senior Client Analysis and Profile:

- Seventy-five percent are retired.
- Eighty percent are on a fixed annual income of $10,000 to $25,000.
- The average age range is between 65-90 years.
- Sixty-five percent are women.
- The majority eat dinner before 6 p.m.
- Sixty percent regularly volunteer for charities.
- Sixty-five percent are on a modified exercise routine: walking, swimming, golfing.
- Twenty percent live in a "retirement" community.
- Seventy percent own their own homes.
- Fifty percent listen to classical music.
- Forty percent regularly listen to a radio station that plays music from the 1940s and 1950s.
- Thirty-five percent belong to the American Assn for Retired Persons.
- The majority are concerned about their longevity and quality of life.
- Sixty percent are on a nutritional program.
- Sixty-five percent read the local *Senior World* publication.
- The majority have a lot of free time.
- Fifty-five percent attend community theater.
- The majority experience pain, stiffness and some restriction of movement.
- Sixty percent have more than one chronic medical condition.
- Seventy percent see a doctor at least once per quarter.

Given this information, the senior client profile could resemble this:

"My typical senior client is a retired 70-year-old woman. She leads a semi-active lifestyle—walks two miles at least four times per week and swims in the summer months. She is on a fixed annual income of less than $16,000 and dines out only once or twice per month. She is a member of at least one senior's club and attends four to five cultural events per year. She frequents museums, libraries and historical sites, does at least three hours of volunteer work each week and takes one class per year at the community college. She reads the local Senior World Monthly, *gets massaged every six weeks, receives an acupuncture treatment every three weeks, occasionally shops at Nature's Haven Health Food Store and takes three vacations per year. This client's major reasons for getting acupuncture are to feel better and be more energetic: enhance mobility, reduce joint inflammation, increase circulation and relieve pain and stiffness."*

The senior market is best reached through education. Create a promotional packet that contains your brochure and be sure it incorporates appropriate terminology and is printed in an easy-to-read, large-sized typeface. Also create cards, informational handouts and reprints of articles on the benefits of acupuncture and Traditional Chinese Medicine for seniors.

By the way, this packet is also useful to send with your letter of introduction to allied professionals. Place your promotional material on bulletin boards at senior centers, golf courses, wellness centers, medical supply outlets, Elderhostels, community centers, libraries, gerontologists' offices, the Department of Parks and Recreation, pharmacies, volunteer centers, fitness clubs and offices of allied health care providers.

Establish your credibility and build contacts by volunteering your services at a local nursing home, a seniors' rights advocacy association or even a senior center. Get your name in print by publishing an article on the benefits of acupuncture or by being interviewed by the press. You can also promote goodwill and gain publicity by donating treatments to major fund raising events.

Give presentations at wellness centers, community colleges, senior centers, nursing homes and other groups like civic organizations that seniors tend to join. Choose the organizations you want to develop an affiliation with and mail them your promotional packet that includes a cover letter expressing your interest in presenting a lecture or demonstration.

Also, consider teaching an extended weekly class on geriatric wellness at one of the centers or colleges. Many cities have a community cable channel. Find out if they broadcast a program designed for seniors and get yourself booked to appear on that show.

Take out listings in appropriate publications. Again, be certain to also put your name under the headings of "Senior Health Care" or "Geriatric Care" in addition to "Acupuncture." Some suggested publications are: the telephone Yellow Pages; your local seniors' publication; newsletters directed toward seniors; and special "senior sections" in the newspapers.

Another effective promotional technique is setting up a booth at events that attract seniors, such as golf tournaments, garden shows and health fairs.

You can be very creative in reaching the senior market. For example, many restaurants offer senior discounts on early dinners. You could join forces with one of those restaurants and have your cards (with or without a discount of your own) displayed on the tables at the restaurant and in return, you distribute the restaurant's coupons to your senior clients.

These examples are only a small segment of available options to reach the senior market. Whatever methods you choose to increase your clientele, take the time to establish credibility, allay concerns and build rapport.

Target Market Analysis

To clarify your target market(s), first define the demographic and psychographic factors and then identify the characteristics your clients have in common. Describe your current clients and those who are most likely your future clients:

- What is the age range and average age of your clients?
- What is the percentage of males and females?
- What is the average educational level of your clients?
- Where do your clients live?
- What are your clients' occupations?
- Where do your clients work?
- What is average annual income level of your clients?
- Of which special interest groups are your clients members?
- What attitudes and beliefs about health care do your clients hold?
- What are your clients' needs, concerns and goals?
- What is the primary reason your clients use your services?
- What are some of the other reasons your clients use your services?
- What is the average number of sessions per client?
- How many clients come in at the following intervals: Occasionally? Bimonthly? Monthly? Biweekly? Weekly? More than once per week?
- Who else services your clientele (other health care providers, vendors and businesses)?

Defining Your Target Markets

Write a descriptive profile for each of your target markets (at least three). Include a brief overview of the services you provide to each group and a detailed analysis of the characteristics of the specific clientele (e.g., psychographics, demographics, the needs and matching benefits, information on who else provides them with services and where they can be found).

Evaluate your position statement (from the exercise on page 271): Does it appeal to your target markets? Do you need to change it or create additional position statements? If so, rewrite it now.

• Assessment •

The next phase in developing your marketing plan is assessment of your previous promotional endeavors and those of your competition. If you are just starting out in practice, skip the Marketing Assessment Exercise and proceed to the competition analysis. I recommend you do these assessment exercises at least once per quarter.

Marketing Assessment Exercise

- List the marketing venues you currently employ.

- How is your business perceived by your clients, colleagues and perspective clients?

- If you offer more than one service, have you promoted each one?
  ❏ Yes   ❏ No   If no, why not?

- Have you been satisfied with the quality of your marketing efforts?
  ❏ Yes   ❏ No   If no, why not?

- What have been the results of your promotional activities so far?

- What changes would you like to see happen?

Your Competitors

The next step after assessing your previous marketing efforts is evaluating the competition. In all likelihood this won't be a straightforward task. You need to do some footwork. It can be easy to ignore this phase since many practitioners aren't willing to challenge their preconceptions about competition. Yet the more you know about your competition, the easier it is for you to determine the most advantageous manner to market your practice.

The first step is to identify your competition. Begin your research by studying the phone book. For example, you look through the phone book and discover that 40 other practitioners are listed. Of those 40 perhaps half of them appear to provide similar services as yours. Find out more about them: Give them a call, request brochures and use their services. You may discover that only four or five of these people are in direct competition with you—that is, actually offer similar services to the same market at a comparable rate. The key being the *same* target market.

Bicyclists race faster against each other than against a clock.
— Norman Triplett

Meanwhile, take note of who is advertising in other local publications (you may want to get several months worth of editions). Notice whether or not your competitors are listed in any of those publications. Some good sources for brochures and fliers are bulletin boards at health food stores, offices of other practitioners and bookstores. Ascertain who is doing what and where they are doing it. These local publications and bulletin boards may be your primary source of information about your competitors since many health care providers don't advertise in traditional ways.

Competition Analysis

Compile a profile on each of your major competitors. Include the following information:

- Name
- Location
- Length of time in business
- Description of services offered
- Manner in which services are provided
- Office hours
- Fee structure
- Clientele description
- Business strengths and limitations
- Differential advantage
- Market position
- Methods of promotion

Analyze the information you've gathered on your competition. Look for patterns and trends. Compare it to the assessment of your own business.

- How does your business compare to the competition?
- What are the strengths your business has in comparison to the competition?
- What are the challenges your business has in comparison to the competition?
- What are some steps you can take to meet those challenges?

• Strategic Action Plans •

The final portion of the marketing plan is the design of your marketing campaign. Keep in mind all important dates such as holidays, clients' meaningful occasions and seasonal events. Plan your campaigns thoroughly. Be aware that you may need separate promotional strategies for each target market.

See Chapter 10, pages 371-372 for the marketing plan segment of the business plan.

For Each Strategy, Ask Yourself the Following Questions:

- Is the strategy realistic?
- Does this strategy fit into your budget?
- What are the ramifications of spending money on this strategy?
- Is this strategy unique?
- Is the market large enough to return a profit from this strategy?
- Does this strategy relate to your other strategies?
- Does this strategy accent your strengths and differences?
- Does this strategy appeal to your target markets?
- Is this strategy directed toward your target markets?
- Are people likely to respond to this strategy?
    - If yes, why?

If your answer to any of these questions is no, alter your strategy. If your answers are all yes, it's time to put your marketing plan into action.

Implementing your marketing plan of action begins by setting up a schedule. Establish a timeline and specific deadlines for all the steps—and stay on schedule. Setting realistic deadlines and integrating your goals into the timelines so they follow a logical order enables you to stay within your time frame.

The next phase is to evaluate the results. If things are going as anticipated, review the rest of the plan to see if you can make any changes to further enhance the results. If you appear to be off target, identify the problems by asking yourself the following questions: Were the goals realistic? Was the timeline too ambitious? Did you need to rely upon too many outside factors? Did you expect more of a percentage increase than occurred? Were there any errors in your plan? Did you incorrectly add any of the numbers? Was any of your data inaccurate? Did you choose an inappropriate target market?

Once you've identified the obstacles, some possibilities for alleviating them are to change the basic goals, alter the timeline, correct the mistakes or possibly even modify the overall strategy.

In summary, when developing your marketing campaign, you must: design your strategies; determine your annual marketing budget; assess how well the plan is coordinated (see above questions); and finally put the plan into action. It's important to evaluate the effectiveness of your campaign during each phase—and make any required adjustments.

If a window of opportunity appears, don't pull down the shade.
— Tom Peters

See Appendix A, pages 382-384 for Strategic Planning Forms.

• Marketing Techniques Primer •

Now that you have clarified your purpose for being in this business; set your marketing purpose, priorities and goals; specified your target market(s); defined your differential advantage; composed your position statement; assessed your current marketing; and evaluated your competition (whew!)—it's time to determine which methods to utilize in marketing your business.

Marketing techniques can be divided into four major facets: promotion, advertising, community relations and publicity. Promotion involves the activities and materials you produce to gain visibility. The money invested is indirect (e.g., it costs money to print business cards; it doesn't cost anything to distribute them) and the activities are often free of cost. Publicity is notoriety given you or your business, usually for an event you have done or are about to do. Advertising differs from publicity and promotions in that you must pay directly for your exposure. Community relations are goodwill activities you do to create a positive public image for you and your business.

The following story illustrates the differences of these four techniques:

Figure 9.2

The Bicycle Story

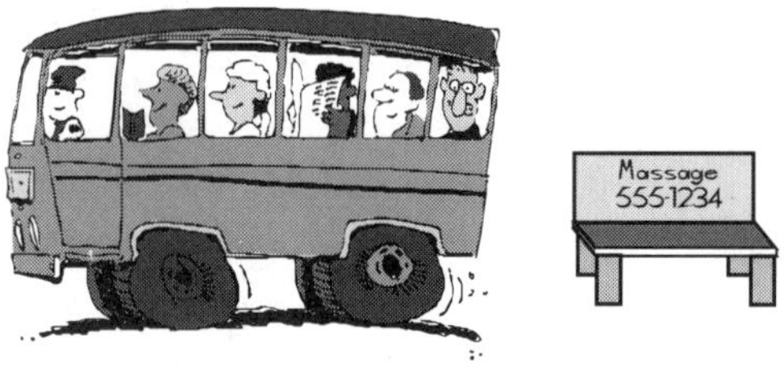

A massage therapist wants to build her sports massage practice. She places an advertisement on a bus stop bench outside the most popular cycling shop in town. That's **advertising**.

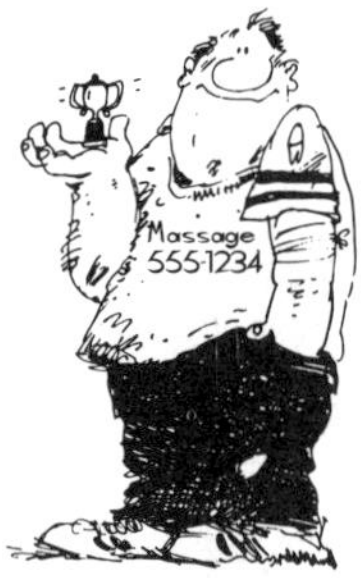

She decides to sponsor a cycling team (offers them discounts on her services and free pre- and post-race mini-sessions for major local events). She prints T-shirts with her name and number for the cyclists to wear. They wear the T-shirts while riding through town carrying a banner announcing their next big race. That's **promotion** (for both the therapist and the cyclists in this latter instance).

In their excitement, the cyclists topple three elderly gentlemen while riding through the park. A newspaper reporter just happens to be there and reports it. That's **publicity** (although not the best kind).

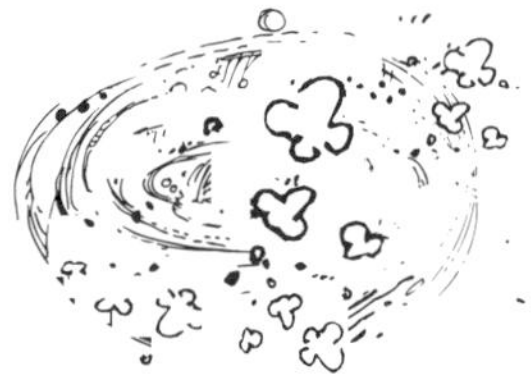

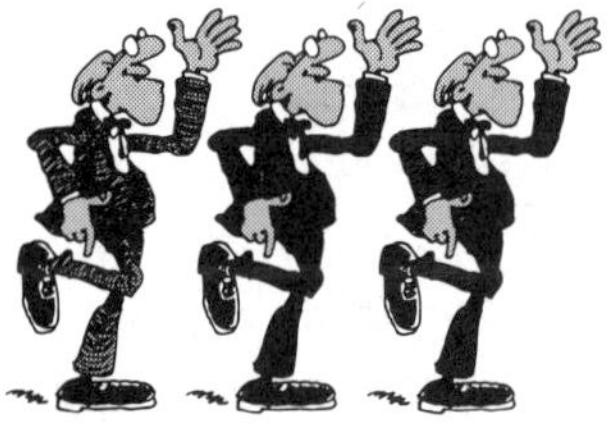

The therapist gives each gentleman a 15-minute massage. They are no longer in pain and harbor no bad feelings toward "her" cycling team. The gentlemen come to the race to cheer on the team. That's mastering **community relations**.

Establishing Credibility ⚬⚬⚬

Establishing credibility is essential to the long-term success of your practice and is the foundation of any successful marketing venture. Webster defines credible as "entitled to belief or trust; honorable; reliable." One of the best methods for establishing credibility and increasing visibility is public speaking.

Your level of professionalism plays a major role in the status of your credibility. Your actions must echo your words. Don't make promises (either verbally or in printed materials) that you are unwilling to fulfill; don't make claims that you can't substantiate. It's better to offer something and exceed it than to fall short.

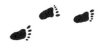
See pages 308-314 for details on public speaking.

Marketing Mix ⚬⚬⚬

Successful practitioners include a good mix of promotion, advertising, publicity and community relations in their marketing plans. Marketing your business takes a lot of time and creativity—particularly with a small practice. Don't always rely on previously used methods (even if they seemed to work), especially if you are approaching the same target group. People like and respond to variety. They don't want to see (or hear) the same thing over and over again. The other reason for altering your marketing modes is to reach potential clients that may not have been inspired by your earlier endeavors. Use an assortment of approaches in an ongoing, consistent manner. Marketing never ends; it's an integral component of your business. Plan on investing at least 15 percent of your time in marketing to maintain your practice and more to expand it. If you are just starting out, you may need to increase it to more than 50 percent.

See Chapter Four, pages 57-59 for additional information on professionalism.

The methods available for marketing your practice are vast (unless your specific profession has distinct precepts). You don't have to be a genius to develop a sound marketing plan, you don't have to go the traditional route and it isn't necessary to spend a lot of money (although it's so easy to do).

The crucial factor for selecting a marketing venue is: Does it appeal to your target market? Many years ago I heard a speaker talk about the need to learn how to broadcast on station **WIIFM** (What's In It For Me?). This is particularly true in marketing. Your marketing endeavors need to convey to the recipients exactly how your company is going to help them.

See page 367 for a sample marketing schedule.

This chapter contains numerous suggestions on promotion, advertising, publicity and community relations. The next four sections present an in-depth look at essential marketing tools, followed by information on developing joint ventures, companies that market for you and choosing a graphic artist. The chapter closes with a list of more than 150 creative marketing ideas and a sample marketing schedule.

• Promotion •

Promotion techniques and tools attract the attention of potential (and current) clients and keep you favorably established, recognized and positioned. Some of the most effective promotional techniques are: networking; holding open houses, presenting workshops and demonstrations; writing articles about your services or general well-being for local newspapers, magazines and newsletters; having booths at community events, health expos and state fairs; sending direct mail pieces and newsletters; providing your services at conventions, store openings, sporting events and at malls during the holidays; obtaining referrals; offering specials and incentives; and having professional brochures and business cards. Personalized items such as pens embossed with your name and logo, also fall under the category of promotion, even though they are commonly referred to as specialty advertising.

See Chapter Eight,
pages 244-254
for more client retention
promotional techniques.

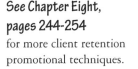

Printed Marketing Materials

High-quality printed marketing materials such as business cards, letterhead, envelopes, brochures, gift certificates, newsletters, client information sheets and fliers are essential to generate a professional image. Your visual promotional pieces reflect the character of your business. The ultimate design of your materials depends on your target market(s) and the image you wish to portray. These items don't all have to look identical (actually that's not a good idea) but the colors, designs and overall look should blend well. For your visual promotional materials to be effective, they must appeal to the clients you want to attract—which might not be the layout that you personally like the best.

Although most of your printed materials are given out by you, your friends, colleagues and clients, it's still a worthwhile idea to post your cards and/or brochures in appropriate locations. Put them in health clubs, well-being centers, medical care supply shops, health food stores, offices of other health care practitioners, bookstores and places that the people in your target(s) frequent. Your print materials should tastefully stand out (through design, ink color or paper color) when floating in a sea of other people's materials.

The first time you contact the owners or managers at these establishments, do it in person. This gives you an opportunity to introduce yourself and build rapport. Show them your materials so they can easily recognize them and hopefully point them out to their customers. After a relationship is built, it isn't necessary for you to hand deliver the materials each time; you can mail them or have a service distribute them. It's wise to visit these establishments at least twice a year to maintain connections and deliver an appropriate gift (e.g., healthy treats or a plant) once a year.

See pages 354-356
for tips on working with
graphic artists.

My own experience in preparing my printed materials leads me to recommend leaving it to the experts by hiring a graphic artist to do the job. If you are concerned about the cost, find an artist who is willing to barter services. Be very cautious about adopting a logo. Avoid using one unless you are certain that you want to live with that symbol for a very long time. People tend to remember logos and associate you with your logo even if you no longer use that particular symbol. It's much easier to change a business name or image and alter the design or style of stationery if it's without a logo. It's best to wait until you are certain it's what you want. Also, it's advisable to check to see if anyone else has the same or similar one. Contact your Secretary of State for requisite forms to trademark your logo.

You can create very attractive stationery on a computer, particularly if you purchase paper products that are specifically designed for desktop publishing. You can find hundreds of full-color brochure paper complete with matching business card stock, letterhead, envelopes, postcards and even labels. These companies also provide specialty papers to be used for newsletters, certificates, greeting cards, note cards, fliers and signs.

These paper products provide an opportunity for you to experiment without a huge outlay of money. Although my basic stationery was designed by a graphic artist and commercially printed, I often use such paper products for special announcements and direct mailings.

Business Cards

At the very least, you must have a substantial quantity of professional business cards. Choose a card that reflects who you are and captures the essence of your practice. Always carry lots of business cards wherever you go. Keep extra cards in your car (or alternate method of transportation). Be generous with your promotional materials. The whole purpose is to circulate them, not hoard them. Whenever you pass out your cards, always hand out at least three per person.

Remember that when it comes to cards, the beauty is in simplicity. A lot of controversy surrounds the amount and type of information to include on your card. Some people attempt to turn their business card into a brochure. In designing your cards keep in mind that they aren't meant for you; they must appeal to your **target market**!

Effective business cards convey the major benefits you offer in a quick glance. They should grab attention, but not be so jam-packed with information that potential clients don't feel the need to ask you questions.

The first step in designing your cards is to look at the business cards you've collected over the years (including your competitors' cards) and identify what you like and dislike. Determine the content (refer to your differential advantage exercise) using as few words as possible. Choose an appropriate image for your target market(s) that matches your other print materials. Add color whenever possible. Print them on high-quality card stock and consider using the back of your card for additional copy or as an appointment reminder. Be sure to include the basics: name, address and phone number. I'm amazed at the number of cards without phone numbers or area codes. *Always proofread carefully!*

See Chapter Five, page 79 for more information on trademarking.

Paper Direct
800-272-7377

Quill Desktop Publishing Supplies
800-789-1331

Queblo
800-523-9080

The two major *faux pas* with business cards are not having them when you need them (which is *always*), and correcting information on them by hand.

Figure 9.3   Sample Business Cards

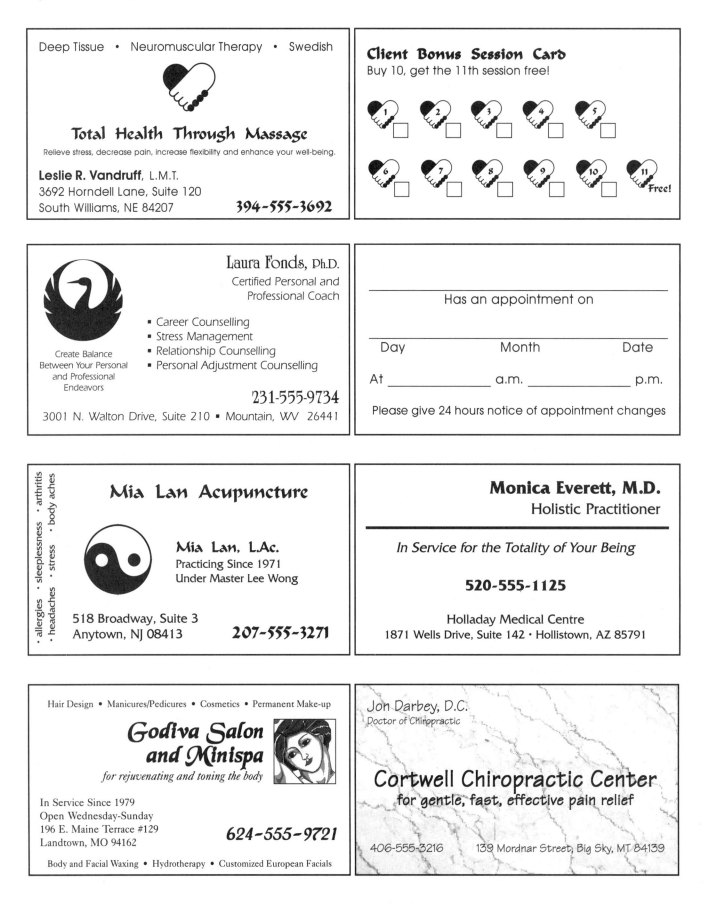

Deep Tissue • Neuromuscular Therapy • Swedish

Total Health Through Massage

Relieve stress, decrease pain, increase flexibility and enhance your well-being.

Leslie R. Vandruff, L.M.T.
3692 Horndell Lane, Suite 120
South Williams, NE 84207

394-555-3692

Client Bonus Session Card
Buy 10, get the 11th session free!

1 2 3 4 5
6 7 8 9 10 11 Free!

Laura Fonds, Ph.D.
Certified Personal and
Professional Coach

- Career Counselling
- Stress Management
- Relationship Counselling
- Personal Adjustment Counselling

231-555-9734

Create Balance
Between Your Personal
and Professional
Endeavors

3001 N. Walton Drive, Suite 210 • Mountain, WV 26441

Has an appointment on

_____
Day   Month   Date

At _____ a.m. _____ p.m.

Please give 24 hours notice of appointment changes

Mia Lan Acupuncture

Mia Lan, L.Ac.
Practicing Since 1971
Under Master Lee Wong

518 Broadway, Suite 3
Anytown, NJ 08413

207-555-3271

• allergies • sleeplessness • arthritis
• headaches • stress • body aches

Monica Everett, M.D.
Holistic Practitioner

In Service for the Totality of Your Being

520-555-1125

Holladay Medical Centre
1871 Wells Drive, Suite 142 • Hollistown, AZ 85791

Hair Design • Manicures/Pedicures • Cosmetics • Permanent Make-up

Godiva Salon and Minispa
for rejuvenating and toning the body

In Service Since 1979
Open Wednesday-Sunday
196 E. Maine Terrace #129
Landtown, MO 94162

624-555-9721

Body and Facial Waxing • Hydrotherapy • Customized European Facials

---

Jon Darbey, D.C.
Doctor of Chiropractic

Cortwell Chiropractic Center
for gentle, fast, effective pain relief

406-555-3216   139 Mordnar Street, Big Sky, MT 84139

Brochures

Your brochure is often the hub of your printed marketing materials. The purpose of a brochure is to inspire prospective clients to call you. When developing your brochure, remember that you must establish credibility and focus on the benefits a client will derive from using your services.

Techniques for establishing credibility in printed materials include providing credentials, numbers, lists, specific details, quotes, success stories, pictures and guarantees.

With unfortunate frequency, we describe ourselves (and our businesses) in terms of our features. A feature is not what attracts clients. They want to know how your services will make a difference in their well-being. A feature is a description of: your service or product; how the product was made; the training received; and the background of the practitioner and the company.

Whereas a benefit is a description of: how the client will profit from using the service and/or product; how the service/product will solve the client's problem; the differential advantage you provide; and the results that the client can expect.

One of the key elements of an effective brochure is to include at least one photograph of yourself—preferably one in which you are working with a contented client. The old cliché is true, "A picture says a thousand words."

Brochure design can be a bit complicated. As with business cards, amass other people's brochures to determine what appeals to you. Ask for input from current and prospective clients. It's usually not wise to spend a lot of money on your first brochure since, invariably, you will want to alter it somehow. You may discover that the type style doesn't work well with the paper stock, someone points out an error, the perfect way to express yourself finally dawns on you or you find something you don't like. If you plan on creating your own brochure, purchase a book on effective brochure design.

Many health care providers utilize preprinted brochures. The bright side is that someone other than you has invested the time and money to design an effective, attractive, informational marketing tool. Often the cost is significantly less than if you were to design and print your own. The problem is that they aren't personalized. You are the most important aspect of your practice and your marketing materials need to reflect that. One of the best ways to overcome the impersonal nature of preprinted brochures is to insert a panel with your specific information. Here's how a massage therapist in Tucson did it: When she purchased the preprinted brochures, she asked for the following details: the type of paper; font names; and the actual ink color name and number used for the fonts and major graphic image. She also obtained permission to duplicate the graphic image on her insert. The insert included her picture, information about her background and philosophy as well as the specific features and benefits of her practice. It was printed on the same paper as the brochure, with matching fonts, ink colors and the graphic image—it was classy.

Most practitioners design their basic brochures and purchase preprinted brochures that describe in detail the adjunct services they offer or the history of their profession.

Information for People
800-754-9790

Blue Poppy Press
800-487-9296

Hemingway Publications
815-877-5590

Whatever you do with preprinted brochures, **don't** handwrite your name, address and phone number on the back—it looks tacky! Ideally, run the brochures through a laser printer (some companies offer that option when you order their brochures), so it looks like you created the brochure. If that's not an option, print labels on a complementary colored stock and affix them to the back of the brochures.

You can usually obtain preprinted brochures through your professional association or independent vendors.

Brochure Design Criteria

- Does it easily distinguish who it's for?
- Does it identify with the target client's problem?
- Does it provide a solution to the problem?
- Does it appeal to the target client's needs?
- Does it have an interesting teaser?
- Are the main benefits listed first?
- Is it believable?
- Is it attractive?
- Is it easy to read? Does it flow?
- Does it have sufficient white space?
- Are the type sizes and styles easy to read?
- Does it have appropriate photographs?
- Is it written in common language?
- Does it establish credibility?
- Is your address included?
- Does it include a map of your location?
- Does it include contact names and numbers?
- Does it provide a call for action?

Figure 9.4.1   Sample Brochure Front

Attention getting header

Benefits listed

Call to action

Credibility

Benefits

Support information

Credibility enhanced*

Space for personalized info

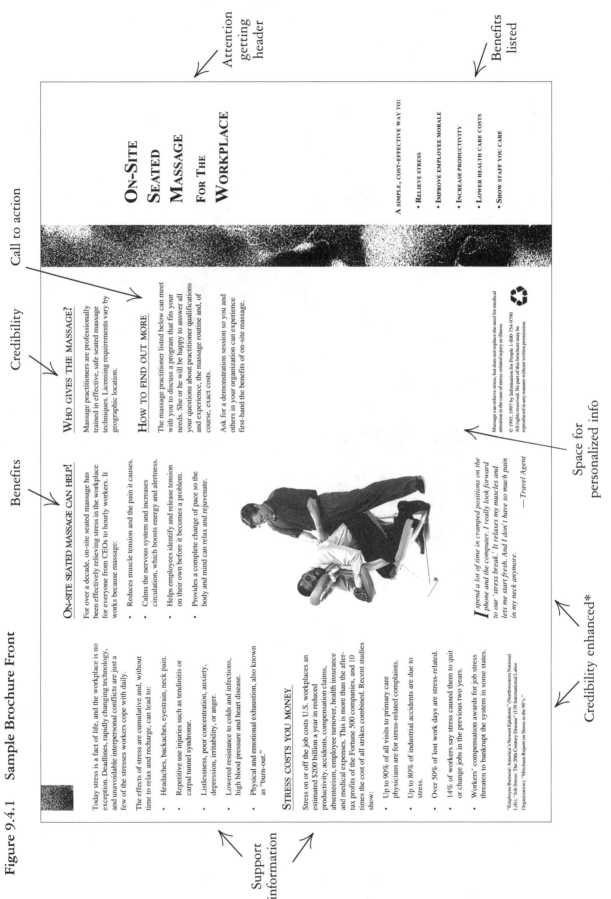

ON-SITE
SEATED
MASSAGE
FOR THE
WORKPLACE

A SIMPLE, COST-EFFECTIVE WAY TO:

- RELIEVE STRESS
- IMPROVE EMPLOYEE MORALE
- INCREASE PRODUCTIVITY
- LOWER HEALTH CARE COSTS
- SHOW STAFF YOU CARE

WHO GIVES THE MASSAGE?

Massage practitioners are professionally trained in effective, safe seated massage techniques. Licensing requirements vary by geographic location.

HOW TO FIND OUT MORE

The massage practitioner listed below can meet with you to discuss a program that fits your needs. She or he will be happy to answer all your questions about practitioner qualifications and experience, the massage routine and, of course, exact costs.

Ask for a demonstration session so you and others in your organization can experience first-hand the benefits of on-site massage.

Massage can relieve stress, but does not replace the need for medical attention in the case of stress-related injury or illness.

© 1995, 1997 by Information For People 1-800-754-9790
All rights reserved. No part of this brochure may be reproduced in any manner without written permission.

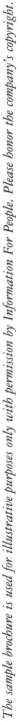

ON-SITE SEATED MASSAGE CAN HELP!

For over a decade, on-site seated massage has been effectively relieving stress in the workplace for everyone from CEOs to hourly workers. It works because massage:

- Reduces muscle tension and the pain it causes.
- Calms the nervous system and increases circulation, which boosts energy and alertness.
- Helps employees identify and release tension on their own before it becomes a problem.
- Provides a complete change of pace so the body and mind can relax and rejuvenate.

I spend a lot of time in cramped positions on the phone and the computer. I really look forward to our 'stress break.' It relaxes my muscles and lets me start fresh. And I don't have so much pain in my neck anymore.
—Travel Agent

Today stress is a fact of life, and the workplace is no exception. Deadlines, rapidly changing technology, and unavoidable interpersonal conflicts are just a few of the stresses workers cope with daily.

The effects of stress are cumulative and, without time to relax and recharge, can lead to:

- Headaches, backaches, eyestrain, neck pain.
- Repetitive use injuries such as tendinitis or carpal tunnel syndrome.
- Listlessness, poor concentration, anxiety, depression, irritability, or anger.
- Lowered resistance to colds and infections, high blood pressure and heart disease.
- Physical and emotional exhaustion, also known as "burn-out."

STRESS COSTS YOU MONEY

Stress on or off the job costs U.S. workplaces an estimated $200 billion a year in reduced productivity, accidents, compensation claims, absenteeism, employee turnover, health insurance and medical expenses. This is more than the after-tax profits of the Fortune 500 companies, and 10 times the cost of all strikes combined. Recent studies show:

- Up to 90% of all visits to primary care physicians are for stress-related complaints.
- Up to 80% of industrial accidents are due to stress.
- Over 50% of lost work days are stress-related.
- 14% of workers say stress caused them to quit or change jobs in the previous two years.
- Workers' compensation awards for job stress threaten to bankrupt the system in some states.

"Employer Burnout: America's Newest Epidemic" (Northwestern National Life); "Job Stress: The 20th Century Disease" (UN International Labor Organization); "Mitchum Report on Stress in the 90's."

The sample brochure is used for illustrative purposes only with permission by Information For People. Please honor the company's copyright.

Figure 9.4.2　Sample Brochure Inside

Descriptive text

Credibility enhanced

Features

Good use of visuals

Benefits

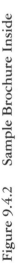

WHAT IS SEATED MASSAGE?

On-site seated massage is a short massage which:

- Comes to your workplace.
- Is given by a professional massage practitioner.
- Lasts from 5 to 30 minutes, uses no oil, and takes place with the employee fully clothed.
- Usually covers the head, neck, shoulders, back, arms and hands and can be adapted to special needs.
- Leaves employees feeling relaxed, refreshed and ready to return to work.

A portable massage chair, designed for comfort and support, is often used. It is supplied by the massage practitioner and can be set up and dismantled quickly in almost any location.

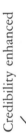

The massages helped me realize how tight and tense the muscles in my neck and shoulders were. This has helped me avoid movements and postures that cause the tension and pain.
— Medical Records Specialist

YOU'RE IN GOOD COMPANY

Here are just a few of the many organizations, large and small, private and government, that have implemented on-site seated massage programs.

ABN-AMRO BANK • APPLE COMPUTER • BOULDER COMMUNITY HOSPITAL • CITY OF ORLANDO, FLORIDA • CLASSIC TRAVEL • CYSTIC FIBROSIS FOUNDATION • H. J. HEINZ • HAWK'S ELECTRIC • MERRILL LYNCH • MOODY'S INVESTORS SERVICE • NAVY FEDERAL CREDIT UNION • NBC-TV • RODALE PRESS • SONY MUSIC • SPARTAN STORES • U. S. INTELCO NETWORKS • UNIVERSITY OF CALIFORNIA MEDICAL CENTER • WAMPLER-LONGACRE CHICKEN COMPANY • WASHINGTON STATE DEPARTMENT OF HEALTH

All our employees take advantage of it. It's economical, and I get my value out of it in appreciation alone.
— Small Business Owner

IT'S EASY TO SET UP AND RUN

- ASSIGN A CONTACT PERSON. He or she will help the massage practitioner set a schedule, publicize the program, and sign people up.
- PROVIDE SPACE. A conference room, break room, or a quiet corner is fine. After the day's sessions, the space can return to normal use.
- ENCOURAGE EMPLOYEES TO USE IT. Make sure they know you support the program. Use it yourself and encourage your managers to do the same.

If it saves even one employee from a job related injury, it's a worthwhile investment in future medical costs.
— Hospital Administrator

COST EFFECTIVE? YES!

Seated massage is quite affordable. Because it is shorter than a regular table massage, it costs proportionately less. Ask your massage practitioner for exact prices since cost varies by locale. Your minimal expenses for in-house coordination and publicity will be more than offset by these savings:

- There is no up-front investment in equipment or facilities.
- You pay only for employees who use it.
- Employees can pay part or all of the cost.
- Massages can take place on break time so no work time is lost.
- Two massages a month cost much less per employee than most other health programs.

IT EXCELS AS A WELLNESS PROGRAM

- It's CONVENIENT. No need to change clothes, shower, or leave work to participate.
- RESULTS ARE IMMEDIATE. Most wellness programs take months to show results.
- It's EASY AND SAFE. No special fitness level or training is required to receive a massage.
- EFFECTS ARE CUMULATIVE. Consistent use reinforces the benefits.
- PEOPLE ENJOY IT. You avoid two common problems: spending more selling a program than on the program itself, and then having it used most by employees who need it least.
- IT ENCOURAGES OTHER STEPS TO WELLNESS. Regular massage helps people feel better and can motivate them to take care of themselves with diet, exercise or other lifestyle changes.

We have hard deadlines and a workload that never lets up. The stress really gets to me. The break on massage day really helps, and I find that now I can relax better on my own, too.
— Legal Secretary

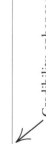

IT'S A VERSATILE BENEFIT, TOO

Once on-site massage is in place, you may find it is also a great way to recognize birthdays or service anniversaries, provide incentive awards for good attendance or an accident-free period, or give a bonus for achieving company and individual goals or completing projects.

These uses are also an ideal way to try on-site massage without an ongoing commitment.

I manage the statewide wellness program for over 100 state agencies. To any manager considering on-site massage, I say it's hard to argue against it. It has a minimal cost, the program runs itself, and employees love it.
— Program Director, State Employee Wellness Program

It's really motivational. It's a great thing the company does for employees and it gives me a positive feeling about working here.
— Data Processing Professional

Credibility enhanced*

Credibility enhanced*

Good use of visuals

Ideally testimonials should include a full name

Reducing Costs

Whether you design your own printed promotional materials or elect to utilize the services of a graphic artist, follow these tips for reducing your print media costs:

Reduce Print Media Costs

- Use interns from local colleges.
- Barter for services.
- Get at least three bids.
- Use standard size and weight paper.
- Use a photocopier for short print runs.
- Print samples before using expensive paper and ink.
- Use the printing services of trade and vocational schools.
- Reuse effective material (as long as it's not being sent to the same people).

Fliers and Circulars

Fliers and circulars are pamphlets designed for mass circulation about a specific event such as an open house, workshop or a "sale." They are usually printed (or even copied) on one side so they can be posted on bulletin boards, inserted into mailings and distributed at your colleagues' places of business. They can also be printed specifically to be used as door hangers.

One of the strongest marketing benefits of these types of promotional tools is that you determine your target (e.g., all the dentists in a three-mile radius, or people who shop at the local health food store).

Design tips include condensed information from brochures plus the following: Use an attention-grabbing headline, make it easy to respond (e.g., phone, fax and toll-free numbers) and close with a call to action such as "Call Today" or "Stop by Our Open House to Receive a Sample of Our Custom Blended Products."

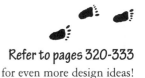

Refer to pages 320-333 for even more design ideas!

Figure 9.5   Sample Flier

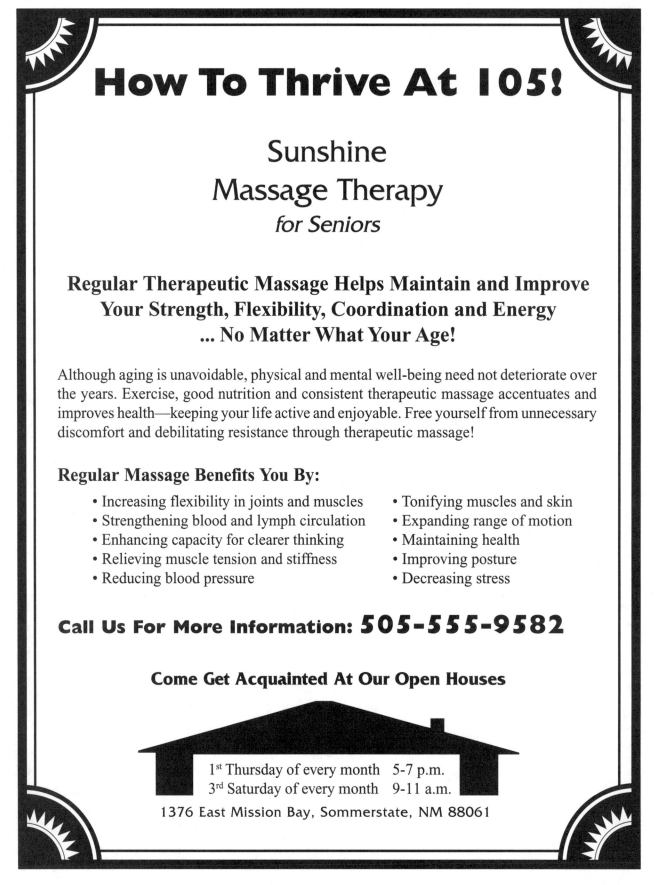

How To Thrive At 105!

Sunshine
Massage Therapy
for Seniors

Regular Therapeutic Massage Helps Maintain and Improve Your Strength, Flexibility, Coordination and Energy ... No Matter What Your Age!

Although aging is unavoidable, physical and mental well-being need not deteriorate over the years. Exercise, good nutrition and consistent therapeutic massage accentuates and improves health—keeping your life active and enjoyable. Free yourself from unnecessary discomfort and debilitating resistance through therapeutic massage!

Regular Massage Benefits You By:

- Increasing flexibility in joints and muscles
- Strengthening blood and lymph circulation
- Enhancing capacity for clearer thinking
- Relieving muscle tension and stiffness
- Reducing blood pressure

- Tonifying muscles and skin
- Expanding range of motion
- Maintaining health
- Improving posture
- Decreasing stress

Call Us For More Information: 505-555-9582

Come Get Acquainted At Our Open Houses

1st Thursday of every month   5-7 p.m.
3rd Saturday of every month   9-11 a.m.

1376 East Mission Bay, Sommerstate, NM 88061

Direct Mail Letters

Direct mail letters are simple, inexpensive and highly effective marketing tools. They are great for introducing yourself to potential clients as well as keeping in touch with current ones. They range from a formal letter of introduction to announcements to surveys. These letters are personalized; you can address specific needs in a friendly, low-pressure manner.

Make sure the letter is typed and kept to one page. Since most people are affronted by form mail, it's advisable to tailor each one for the particular individual. Do your homework and find out as much specific information as possible. Add your special touch. Consider signing your letter in an ink that's a different color than the type (I like to use a teal colored felt pen).

Research shows that sales letters garner a response rate of up to 80 percent higher than other types of mailers. The key elements to success are a great design, an excellent mailing list and follow-up.

Design Tips

- Use an eye-catching headline.
- Highlight the benefits immediately.
- Use your prospect's name.
- Clarify why you have selected the recipient to receive your letter.
- Build rapport and develop credibility.
- Keep it short.
- Use sincere, friendly language.
- Include powerful words such as "new," "free," "save," and "now."
- Use embedded commands.
- Provide a guarantee.
- Offer incentives.
- Include testimonials. Always use a full name. If possible, include a company name, title and location.
- Include a time limit or expiration date.
- State your offer in clear, simple terms.
- Provide step-by-step instructions so your readers know how to respond.
- Close with a call to action.
- Use a postscript (P.S.) at the end of the letter—next to the headline, it's the most-often read part of any letter.
- Compose the letter on a computer (or typewriter).
- Use bold type to emphasize key points.
- Print the letter on high-quality paper.
- Enclose a response card or an invitation.

Your envelope needs to motivate readers to open it and see what's inside. Printing teaser copy or an illustration on the outside helps. Also, a large or irregularly shaped envelope stands out from regular mail. If you are sending letters to general consumers (current and prospective clients) use a first class stamp instead of metered or bulk mail to increase the odds of your letter getting opened.

Figure 9.6

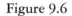

Stress Reduction Clinic
971 Montrose Canyon Way
Suite #102-A
Cleveland, OH 44114

Look Inside for 5 Easy Ideas to Reduce Stress by 50%!

Miriam Webster
129 Miracle Highway
Cleveland, OH 44114

Some incentives that inspire people to respond to direct mail letters are: free merchandise or service; free demonstration; free literature such as a newsletter, catalog or handout; technical assistance; discount coupon; free training; and a free consultation.

Response cards are very effective for generating leads and come in two major categories: Business Reply Cards (postpaid) and Courtesy Reply Cards (not postpaid). Postpaid cards get the best response (free is usually better). Keep the information clear, concise and engaging. Restate your offer and include an incentive for a quick reply. It's wise to use check-off boxes with different options—the less amount of time and energy the recipient has to expend, the more likely you are to get a response. Perhaps include "Maybe" along with "Yes" and "No" options. Put your name, address and phone number on the bottom. If possible, print the recipient's name on the top of the card.

Generate an internal mailing list. Collect business cards at networking events and your public speaking functions. Combine them with your client list.

You can develop your own internal mailing list or purchase lists through a broker. The fees for mailing lists range from $45 to $200 per 1,000 names. The major problems with purchasing brokered lists are that it's difficult to get a list of qualified prospects and the list itself may be of poor quality (outdated or contains incomplete information). Another option for mailing lists is to contact organizations and associations that serve your target markets. They often share their lists for a nominal charge—if anything at all.

An option to mass mailing is to send out one letter each day to prospective clients and other health care providers with whom you wish to develop alliances.

Follow-up is crucial. You can increase your direct mail letter response up to 800 percent by following up the mailing with a telephone call.

Figure 9.7   Prospecting Survey

Westside Wellness Center

6000 N. Windy Way • Fairbanks, AK 99710

907-555-5555

Susan Izensnow
1900 Frostbite Circle
Fairbanks, AK 99711

Dear Ms. Izensnow,

We realize that your well-being is a high priority. Your opinion of chiropractic care is important to us and finding out what how you feel assists us in meeting your expectations. Please return this survey and we will send you a free booklet titled, *Ten Things You Can Do Today to Increase Your Vitality and Longevity*.

Are you currently under chiropractic care?   ❑ Yes   ❑ No
   If yes, how often?   ❑ On a regular schedule   ❑ On an as-needed basis
      ❑ Weekly   ❑ Biweekly   ❑ Monthly
      ❑ 6 times a year   ❑ 4 times a year   ❑ Less than 2 times a year

If you are currently under chiropractic care, please describe what you like best about it:
_____
_____

What you like least about it: _____
_____

If you do not receive chiropractic care, please check which of these reasons apply:
   ❑ Too expensive   ❑ My insurance doesn't cover it
   ❑ My insurance limit is up   ❑ I don't have the time
   ❑ My course of treatment has concluded   ❑ I'm not certain of the benefits
   ❑ Not a convenient location   ❑ Hours not convenient
   ❑ Other _____

If you were to utilize chiropractic care, which of these features would be most important to you?
   ❑ Working with the same physician each time
   ❑ Flexible office hours, including evenings and Saturdays
   ❑ Honoring insurance claims
   ❑ A guarantee of satisfaction
   ❑ Other _____

Thank you very much for your time in filling out this form. Return this survey today and receive your free booklet.

Sincerely,

Thomas Moore

Thomas Moore, D.C.

P.S. If we receive your survey in the next 10 days, we will also send you a complimentary registration for one of our upcoming seminars.

Articles 〰

The written word is a powerful tool. It can immensely effect your business as well as your profession. There are over 100,000 newspapers, magazines, journals and association newsletters published regularly in North America. They welcome information that is beneficial to their readership.

Write an article on general health care, the value of your particular area of expertise, or the latest innovations in your field. Don't worry about whether or not it's written perfectly—that's the job of the editor. Another option is to hire a professional journalist to write an article for (or about) you.

Articles build your credibility. Whether or not your articles get published, use them as promotional tools. Send them to your current clients and make them available to prospective clients.

Newsletters 〰

Newsletters are used by all kinds of organizations and businesses as an effective informational marketing tool. Newsletters can provide an individual forum to communicate with your current and potential clients. Readers tend to pay more attention to a newsletter than an advertisement—and it's less likely to get tossed out as junk mail.

Good newsletters pique the interest of the reader. They balance promotional content with specific information that benefits the reader. The language tends to be more conversational in tone than a typical advertising piece or technical publication.

Marketing with Newsletters
by Elaine Floyd
Newsletter Resources

Editing Your Newsletter
by Mark Beach
Coast to Coast Books

The Newsletter Editor's Desk Book
by M. Arth, H. Ashmore & E. Floyd
Newsletter Resources

Most health care providers are multi-talented and oftentimes clients are unaware of the scope of services they have available. A newsletter gives you an ideal opportunity to educate your clients about your other areas of expertise.

Newsletters don't need to be an elaborate production to be effective. You can even create one on your letterhead. Before you decide upon the appropriate length, style, format and content of your newsletter, you must first clarify your purpose and goals for your newsletter and determine how to make it attractive to your target market(s).

Newsletters often serve many purposes: to attract new clients; encourage current clients to come in more often; bring back lost clients; inspire clients to try different services; promote products; provide information; improve client retention; build credibility; and demonstrate concern for your clients.

Examples of Newsletters I Receive

- The company that installed my phone system sends a beautiful four-page (11x17 folded in half) two-colored newsletter three to four times per year. It contains product reviews, tips on equipment care, a column on telephone techniques including telemarketing ideas, a contest, information on how to best use equipment and comments and ideas from customers.

- Along with my bill the water company encloses a two-color, two-page newsletter several times a year. It gives water conservation tips, discusses current local ecological issues and lists resources.

- My insurance agent sends out a one-page quarterly newsletter with safety tips.

The most amazing thing is that I always read these newsletters as soon as I get them. Because they're short enough and I know that I can read them in less than 10 minutes, they don't get relegated to the ever-increasing pile of "to be read soon" publications.

Several companies produce newsletters specifically for health care providers to purchase and distribute to their clients. The advantages of buying a pre-made newsletter over designing your own are a lower overall cost and time savings. The disadvantages are that pre-made newsletters lack your personal touch and you have no control over the content or layout. If the newsletter templates aren't sold in a kit, you have to hope the publisher gets them out in a timely manner. Also the information may be inaccurate or dated.

If anything is worth trying at all, it's worth trying at least 10 times.
— Art Linkletter

Two options for personalizing a ready-made newsletter to maximize the benefits are: write a column for a pre-existing newsletter; or purchase a pre-made newsletter and insert a note or personalized page. If you decide to insert a page, be sure that it matches graphically in terms of overall style and typefaces. Some newsletter publishers place a blank section on the template for personalization.

The steps involved in creating a newsletter can seem overwhelming and financially prohibitive. To lessen the burden and costs consider teaming with health care providers and people that provide products or services to the same target market. Thoroughly analyze your target market so you can determine who to include as a co-producer of your newsletter.

For example, let's say that one of your target markets is infants. Many other people service this market: pediatricians; baby food companies; specialty stores (clothing, toys); baby seat manufacturers; bookstores; massage therapists; and educational companies that publish information for the parents of infants.

Another market with a multitude of attending providers is personal growth. People in this category often utilize the services of psychotherapists, counselors and other health care providers such as touch therapists, nutritionists, holistic physicians, homeopaths, acupuncturists, chiropractors, herbalists and estheticians. They may attend workshops and 12-Step meetings. They read books on personal development and spirituality. They often shop at health food stores and natural clothing shops. And they are probably involved in some type of physical toning program such as exercise and yoga.

Some of the most popular newsletter sections are industry news, well-being tips, editorials, cartoons, product reviews, success stories and announcements.

Don't limit yourself to the obvious. Sometimes the more unique the pairing, the more effective. For example, an on-site massage therapist and a "quick-print" copy shop might co-produce a newsletter. They could utilize a slogan such as, "For people who don't have an extra hour." Also, your co-sponsors can be located in a different city. For example, a baby food company or a home exercise equipment manufacturer.

Newsletters often center on a theme, particularly when they are a cooperative venture. Several possibilities are: a "generic" well-being newsletter that appeals to a specific market such as athletes, pregnant women or stressed executives; or a newsletter that addresses specific health issues like arthritis, aging or carpal tunnel syndrome.

In terms of content, your newsletter can encompass new services, changes in hours, how-to's for stretches, relaxation exercises, specific tips on self-care, technical information regarding new research, survey results and product reviews, a detailed description of one of your services, toll-free numbers of interest, articles, new products, success stories about your clients (get written permission first), book reviews, cartoons, advertisements, specialty columns such as a question-and-answer column, a section on different health care modalities and their specific benefits, a "what's new in..." column, poems, articles written by clients, puzzles, contests, quotes, interviews, anecdotes, letters to the editor and discount coupons.

Gather information for your newsletter from newspapers, magazines, books, radio and television programs, documentaries, workshops, other health care providers and your clients. The United States government is a great source for free information. For a list of publications, write the Superintendent of Documents, Washington, D.C. 20402. Another option for material is to purchase rights to syndicated columns. Every July, *Editor and Publisher* releases its annual syndicate directory. Check your library for a copy or contact the company at 11 W. 19th St., New York, NY 10011. Oftentimes, it's fairly easy to obtain reprint rights of articles from existing publications. These are usually available at low or no cost, they provide variety for your readers and ease the load of material you personally have to generate. Call your main library or local university and inquire into accessing their computer database to search for a topic of interest. You can also do this at home if you have access to the Internet. Search for articles by subject, such as "massage" or "stress" or "nutrition" or by your target market's concerns, (e.g., arthritis). Given the myriad of publications, you'll most likely find ample material for your newsletter. After you have located appropriate articles, contact the editor of each publication to ascertain their reprint policies. If your newsletter is targeted to a specific market, contact the public relations department of other organizations that cater to that market. Those organizations might have articles of interest and most likely will gladly give them to you free of charge. If you are unable to get reprint rights for material that you want to include, you can directly quote a sentence or two. Getting other professionals that serve your target markets to write a regular column for your newsletter is another source of material.

The personal computer has allowed desktop publishing to flourish. Most people who use newsletters to promote their practices either buy pre-printed ones or create them on their own computer. But even if you don't own a computer, many graphic designers and print shops can produce your newsletter for you. If you plan to self-publish a newsletter on a regular basis, I highly recommend that you invest in a quality page-layout program such as PageMaker® or QuarkXPress.®

Sources for visuals include clip art images (either computer-generated or cut-and-paste), original drawings and photographs. If you are producing the newsletter on your computer, you can purchase various clip art packages that allow you reproduction rights. If you have a picture or piece of artwork (that you created or own the rights to), you can scan it into your computer and incorporate it into your newsletter. If you do not own a scanner, a service bureau can scan in the art, clean it up and give it back to you on a disk. Also, a print shop can place the art (reducing the size if necessary) directly on the layout sheets.

Be certain the newsletter style and colors match your image as well as appeal to your target markets. To start off consider keeping your newsletter to two pages. Either use your letterhead or some fun stationery. If you decide to publish a newsletter that is four or more pages long, I recommend you hire a professional graphic artist to create a template (a reusable design form) to use for each issue. Of course, if you are artistically inclined and possess the appropriate software and artwork packages, you can do it yourself. If you're not certain about the look you want or the number of pages, you can purchase pre-designed laser-printer newsletter paper from companies such as Paper Direct. These sheets are usually on a high-quality 11" x 17" paper, printed on both sides with a pre-set layout for columns and announcements. Most are printed in two-color ink. The major drawback to using this paper is adjusting your content to fit in their layout. But then again, that could also simplify things for you. We produce a school newsletter totally in house. We hired a graphic artist to design the basic layout and we simply place the new information within the template. We usually add a different clip art graphic for the cover page of each issue (that reflects the subject matter or season). We change the color of the paper with each issue. At first we printed them on our own copier; now that we produce more than 1,000 at a time, it's more cost-effective to take them to a printer. If you are reproducing 200 copies or less, it may be advantageous to print them on your laser printer or copier. Keep in mind that your newsletter will continue to evolve, so don't worry about it being perfect from the start.

Be Seasonal!
Change the paper color to reflect the seasons (e.g., orange in Autumn). You can also use graphic images such as snowflakes for winter or flowers for spring.

As far as technical layout is concerned, include plenty of white space. Too much type is overwhelming and unattractive. Also don't use too many different type faces. "Air out" the copy by incorporating visuals such as photographs and graphics. Pictures really do convey a thousand words. Also, keep the style consistent. Simplicity is the key. Avoid using too many lines and boxes, and make certain that your graphic images don't detract from the content. Screens (a graduated shading of ink from clear to solid) are creative tools for newsletters: they provide visual depth and can make it appear that you've used an additional color of ink. You also want your newsletter to stand out visually and tactilely. This can be accomplished by printing it on colored paper, using textured stock, or folding it so it's a different size than most mail (e.g., magazines and #10 envelopes).

Entice your potential readers to open your newsletter immediately by prominently displaying your company name and logo. If you are unsure that readers would recognize your name, highlight the newsletter's purpose or slogan. Then list the contents or use some type of teaser. Let your potential readers know why they should read your newsletter right now!

Avoid staples. Readers get annoyed by them because they must find a staple remover or resort to tearing open the newsletter.

It's wise to keep your newsletter length to six pages or less. You want to provide enough information to inspire someone to read it, but you don't want it so filled with material that it requires a significant block of time to read it. The idea is to create a newsletter that grabs your potential readers' attention so they pick it up and read it *immediately*, and to furnish readers with just the right balance of graphically appealing and interesting material so they read it from cover to cover in one sitting.

Also, leave your readers anticipating your next issue by giving them a preview. For example, say "In the next issue we will describe six techniques for alleviating headaches," or "Next issue includes an interview with Alexa Swift, a local track star who shares how she reduced her sprint time by 10 percent."

Newsletters can be published on a set schedule (e.g., monthly, quarterly, biannually) or you can simply produce them whenever it's appropriate. Oftentimes a business owner generates a newsletter when a change occurs in the company or something major happens within the industry.

Keep your newsletter straightforward and personal. Remember, it isn't a magazine or a newspaper—it's a personal communication to keep you in touch with your current clients, educate the public and promote your practice. Newsletters keep you and your clients connected.

Personalized Gift Items

Personalized gift items—also known as premiums and specialty advertising—provide a daily reminder of your business while either being passed around from person to person, landing on a refrigerator or being seen on handy items.

Premiums can be worthwhile in any business. They are fun promotional tools and often quite inexpensive. For health care providers the main focus of premiums is to develop relationships with prospective or current clients. In most instances the perceived monetary value of the item isn't as important as its use; select items that the recipients want or need.

You can give premiums as gifts at special events, whenever new clients come in for their initial visits, include them in your mailings or hand them out whenever you're so inclined. Some typical items in this category are erasers, magnets, pens, pencils, note pads, letter openers, calendars, mugs, visors, canned beverage openers, nail files, tooth brushes, bumper stickers, sports bottles and T-shirts.

They can also be used as incentives (e.g., offer a free tote bag with every $50 spent on products). In addition to the national catalogs listed in the margin, check your local yellow pages for names of advertising specialty companies. Call them and request a catalog. The variety of these items is amazing. You can get almost anything personalized with your company name or logo! Choose items that either directly remind your clients of you (or your specific services) or are of definite interest (or benefit) to the people in your target markets.

An inexpensive idea for a beneficial personalized gift item is to print labels and affix them to water bottles. You can purchase bottled water by the case (they usually come in 8- to 24-ounce bottles). Most print shops have specialty labels in different colors, shapes and designs (e.g., golf balls, hearts, stars) that you can have imprinted with your name, phone number and address. Every time your clients come in for an appointment, greet them with a smile, handshake and a water bottle. If they drink all the water before they leave, offer to refill it from your water cooler.

Booths

Another effective method for gaining visibility is to set up a booth at conferences, conventions, expositions and trade shows. You can meet a lot of people at these events. Choose shows that attract your target markets. Be creative in your choices. For instance if one of your target markets is infants, take a booth at a baby fair or even a bridal trade show—a health care booth will stand out amongst the plethora of product vendors. It's also important to establish your community presence by being part of wellness and health expos. Other factors to consider in selecting which shows to exhibit at are: who are the targeted attendees, what is the cost in terms of time and money, what other companies are exhibiting and how successful has the show been in the past.

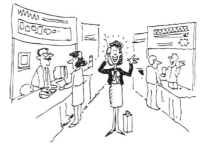

To find out which shows are happening in your community contact your convention bureau, the Chamber of Commerce and the sales directors at major hotels. Check specific trade journals and local business publications. Your library might also carry reference materials on local and worldwide trade shows.

Make sure your booth design fits your image. You can create your own or purchase a portable display. The following tips assist in making this a productive experience.

Best Impressions
800-635-2378
www.bestimpressions.com

The Drawing Board
800-210-4431

Nelson Marketing
800-982-9159

Promo Unlimited
800-748-6150

Sales Guides, Int'l
800-352-9899

Valentino T-Shirts, Aprons
& Uniforms 800-448-7017

Advertising Specialty Inst
www.promomart.com

Promotional Products Assn
www.ppa.org

Making the Most of Your Booth

- Send out invitations to prospects to attend the show and pick up a free product at your booth.
- Be sure to have ample promotional materials available. You may want to print special fliers (much less expensive than brochures) for these events.
- Display your promotional materials in such a way that people will take them. This enables you to engage in a conversation with someone and not be concerned about missing potential clients.
- Although it's great to have an elaborate booth, don't let the lack of one be a deterrent. Do the best that you can within your budget. Just be sure to personalize it somehow with plants, photographs or flowers.
- Grab people's attention with an eye-catching sign. If you are unable to hang it up, put it on an easel. Make sure the graphics and words are easily viewed from all sight lines.
- Provide ongoing hands-on demonstrations.
- Give away product samples.
- Set out a bowl or basket to collect business cards. Put a sign in front of the bowl stating, "Enter here for a free drawing of..." If possible, donate your services or products. If that's not appropriate, then give a prize (e.g., a book, a basket of healthy goodies or a gift certificate from a local store).
- Play a video tape that either demonstrates your services or gives interesting information (in an entertaining format). Be sure the tape is less than six minutes long and looped (so it plays continuously).
- Bring necessary supplies. In addition to your promotional materials, make sure you have plenty of logistical supplies (e.g., equipment, masking tape, extension cords, pencils, paper, tissues), refreshments and clothing (in case you get cold, sweaty or spill something on yourself).
- Bring a friendly, knowledgeable person to help staff your booth. You need to be able to take breaks. It's imperative that you walk around and check out the other booths. Quite often, the best networking takes place between booth owners.

Exhibitor Magazine
507-289-6556

Special Events ⌇

Marketing your practice can oftentimes appear overwhelming and arduous, yet no rule says you can't have fun while promoting your business. You can incorporate creative approaches to building your clientele. Keep in mind that the most effective means of marketing health care services is through a personal approach. Given that the majority of people become your clients out of an experience with you, it's vital that your marketing plan include informal ways for people to get to know you and your work.

Parties

A party is a fun and creative way to market your services. The best way to hold this event is to have a current client sponsor a casual in-home or in-office gathering. This approach has proven extremely effective with products such as vitamins, cosmetics, designer clothing, and of course, the most famous, Tupperware.®

This marketing strategy works because the guests feel comfortable. They are in a safe environment, the atmosphere is festive, and they can experience the product firsthand. I know a Rolfing® practitioner who dramatically increased her clientele through these types of parties.

You may be wondering how a party differs from an introductory demonstration given at your office. The major differences are in the sponsorship and the tone of the event. These parties tend to be small and intimate—five to 10 friends or colleagues of the sponsor.

People attend the party not only to find out more about what you have to offer, but also because their friend invited them. These people are usually more open to your presentation and more likely to become clients than strangers who come to an introductory demonstration they saw announced in the newspaper. Also, guests at the party expect to have fun and receive more personalized attention than if they were at a more formal demonstration.

Design the party in such a way that the atmosphere is lively and promotes involvement. The sponsor usually provides refreshments, and the first portion of the party is spent casually getting to know each other.

When you begin your presentation, give a brief overview of who you are, your training and your philosophy toward your work and health. Describe your work and do a formal demonstration on a model (preferably the client who is the sponsor). Position your table, chair or mat so that the guests can easily gather around to see you in action. Encourage people to ask questions of yourself and the model.

If you are a touch therapist, allow every participant the opportunity to experience your technique after you've finished the demonstration. This could be anything from a five-minute neck session to a three-minute hand massage—and you can do it while talking and answering questions.

If the group is playful, include health-oriented games. Offer prizes for correct answers to general health questions such as how much water the average person should drink each day, or to the first person to correctly identify a specific muscle.

Depending upon the type of work you do, you may also want to display products at the party. Be sure to describe the products, their benefits and how to use them. Do a product demonstration. If possible, use the products while working on your model. Practitioners often avoid incorporating products into these events, let alone their practices, because it reminds them too much of those aforementioned parties.

Far better it is to dare mighty things, to win glorious triumphs even though checkered by failure, than to rank with those poor spirits who neither enjoy nor suffer much because they live in the gray twilight that knows neither victory nor defeat.
— Theodore Roosevelt

If you intend to sell products at the party, you must be clear on your focus and the guests should be told ahead of time so they bring their checkbooks. Realize that most people have never seen some of the wonderful accouterments available for their health care and relaxation, and they will enjoy the opportunity to see and test these products.

The income generated by the product sales gives you immediate compensation for your time, whereas the long-term benefits are achieved by the new clients you generate from the party. As long as you keep perspective and concentrate the majority of your presentation on hands-on work, product sales can be a profitable adjunct.

Some examples of suitable products to display are: books; relaxation tools and implements (e.g., percussion instruments, massage pads); audio cassettes and CDs; hot and cold packs; ice pillows; lotions and oils; support pillows and similar ergonomic devices; stretching bands and balls; herbs; supplements; remedies; essences (such as aromatherapy) and the equipment to use with them; and self-health videos.

The first step to organizing a party is to choose an appropriate sponsor. Review your client list and pick several possibilities. The most important characteristics are that the client values your work, is fairly outgoing, is reliable and knows a lot of people.

Talk with your potential sponsors. Most clients eagerly agree to sponsor a party if you offer them some form of compensation either in services or products. I recommend giving the client one treatment just for organizing the party, and one treatment for every three to four attendees. You can also give a bonus of one session for every person who becomes a client. Be certain to tell the sponsor to limit the number of guests to approximately 15. If too many participate, the informal nature becomes disrupted and you lose the power of intimacy.

Even though your sponsors may be enthusiastic about the party, it doesn't necessarily follow that they can coordinate well. Play an active role in the party's preparation and promotion. Once a client has decided to be a sponsor, set aside at least one hour to plan the event. Choose a date and select the format. Factors that influence the choice of format include the number of prospective guests, their background, the time allotted, and the time of year the party is scheduled to take place.

For instance, if five people attend, you would be able to include more hands-on time with them than if 15 people show up. Also, if the guests are conversant with your type of services, there's no need to spend much time covering the basics—you can focus on the specific benefits of your techniques. If the party is slated for three hours, you must prepare more information and activities than if the party lasts an hour.

Be creative by incorporating the time of year into your presentation. Make it a theme party. For example, if the party takes place close to St. Patrick's Day, you can use green paper for your handouts, and decorate accordingly. If the party occurs close to Thanksgiving, include an exercise or discussion about the things for which everyone is thankful—particularly regarding their health, and discuss ways to ensure continued good health.

The secret of success is to be ready for opportunity when it comes.
— Benjamin Disraeli

After the date has been chosen and the format selected, the sponsor creates a guest list and sends out invitations that include RSVPs. The next stage is your preparation: scripting the party and rehearsing, creating appropriate handouts, assembling supplies, and supporting your sponsor.

When you script the party, designate time parameters for each segment. A sample party outline might look like this: 15 minutes informal talking; five minutes self-introduction; 10 minutes discussion on benefits of your services and description of your work; 10 minutes group activity; 10 minutes break; 15 minutes demonstration on model; 20 minutes questions and demonstrations on guests; 10 minutes break; 15 minutes additional questions and demonstrations on guests; and 10 minutes wrap-up. Your script would include more details of the actual content to be covered in each section. After designing the outline, rehearse the presentation several times, making any necessary adjustments to the script.

Handouts are an integral part of any successful presentation. Most people are visually oriented, so it's important to give the guests something to look at and hold. Design one or more handouts that are tailored to the specific presentation or to the group. For instance, let's say the guests are all co-workers at a computer data entry company. You could create a handout that shows self-care techniques for alleviating eye-strain and avoiding carpal tunnel syndrome. However you design your handouts, include your name and phone number.

The basic supplies needed for any presentation are: promotional materials (e.g., cards, brochures, gift certificates, appointment book); personal items (e.g., throat lozenges); and general purpose supplies such as facial tissue, name tags, markers, scotch tape, scissors, masking tape, glue, an extension cord, trash bags, a clock, writing implements, paper and a receipt book. I always keep a small, lidded carrying box stocked with these items. Also, you'll want to have any specialized equipment/ supplies needed for your specific presentation such as handouts, table, sheets, lubricant, music system, music, props and charts.

The final element in pre-party preparation involves supporting your sponsor. Keep in contact with this person. Check in regularly to get updates on the responses to the invitations and offer any assistance in follow-up or organization of the event. Call your sponsor to find out if any last-minute hitches have arisen. Arrive at the party at least one hour ahead of time to help with any logistical needs, arrange your equipment and supplies, display your promotional materials and products, and prepare yourself. You want to be organized and centered when the guests arrive so you can concentrate on building rapport and getting to know them.

Next is the party itself. This is the time to share your expertise, make new acquaintances, and obtain clients—all while enjoying yourself in a relaxed yet festive atmosphere.

The final activity to ensure positive results from the party is follow-up. Send a thank-you letter to your sponsor, mail notes to all guests thanking them for attending and confirm any appointments made.

These parties are positive for all involved. You get to promote yourself in an informal manner, the guests get the opportunity to be introduced to the benefits of your industry and your work in particular, and the sponsor receives free sessions.

Show and Tell

Remember "show and tell" from grade school? This was your opportunity to share something wonderful that happened to you or to show off a favorite possession with your fellow students. Most kids look forward to show and tell. I hated it at first. My family never went anywhere exciting and I didn't have any exotic toys. But that's when I discovered the two keys to grabbing people's attention: exude enthusiasm, and demonstrate uniqueness and benefits. Both elements are crucial. Who would have known back then that I was learning how to be a good public speaker? For most of us show and tell was our first experience at public speaking—only it wasn't called that. It was simply sharing, and usually it was fun.

As the school years progressed, most of us were subjected to getting up in front of a class to give reports, recite poems, make speeches and engage in debates. Often the topics were imposed on us and it was difficult to muster much enthusiasm. It's no wonder that as adults, most people dread public speaking. In fact, surveys show the majority of people are more afraid of public speaking than they are of death.

Public speaking is not just about getting up in front of 25 (or even 2,500) people and giving a formal presentation. It's about the ways you share information with others. These activities range from casual encounters such as talking with people while waiting in lines and networking at social and business functions to informal events such as holding open houses and giving parties to more formal examples such as: providing free talks at civic, professional and business meetings; doing demonstrations at public events (e.g., fairs and health expositions); facilitating workshops; and giving keynote speeches.

As in show and tell, public speaking is easy as long as you share something that excites you and can make a difference in the audience's life. As health care providers you've got it covered—you frequently witness profound changes in your clients! How can you NOT be enthusiastic about your work? When I was in practice, I was always talking with people about massage whether or not I initiated the conversation. Granted, I didn't corner people in elevators (well, hardly ever), but I wanted the world to know how wonderful massage was and how it could change people's lives. It's not necessary to become a zealot—just be open. I suggest that every day before leaving your house you remind yourself of all the benefits of your services and recall at least two instances when you or one of your clients experienced a significant change. This puts your work in your conscious awareness so that you will be more cognizant of appropriate instances in which to share about it.

One of the most successful ways to do "public speaking" is whenever you are waiting in a line start talking with people: share about your services; recommend stretches; tell them about the latest product you've discovered; and offer to show them

When you work you are a flute through whose heart the whispering of the hours turns to music...And what is to work with love? It is to weave the cloth with threads drawn from your heart, even as if your beloved were to wear that cloth...
— Kahlil Gibran

something to alleviate their pain. It may sound hokey, but if you're enthusiastic and sincere, it's the best form of education and marketing.

Educating people about your field is vital to the growth of your profession as well as building your own practice. Start where you are most comfortable (typically casual encounters or informal events). Commit to sharing about your services at least five times weekly. Once you have increased your level of comfort and confidence, you can move on to more formal presentations and demonstrations.

Formal presentations can be fun. They are not limited to traditional platform speaking. Plus, you don't have to do them alone. You can ease your discomfort and make the presentation more appealing by co-leading or holding panel discussions. Actually, in this industry the most effective presentations are informal in nature and include demonstrations and/or group participation.

How to Prepare, Stage and Deliver Winning Presentations
by Thomas Leech
American Management Association

Present Yourself Powerfully
by Cherie Sohnen-Moe
Sohnen-Moe Associates, Inc.

The Public Speaking Circuit

Many health care providers contend that the major catalyst for increasing their practices is giving "free" talks. Even though you don't get paid for these presentations, they are a superb training ground and a great way for getting new clients. I recommend approaching public speaking from two points: general education and marketing. General education public speaking involves talking to anyone who will listen. While the audience might not be likely candidates for your services, you will be raising the consciousness level—which benefits the profession as a whole.

As a marketing tool, public speaking requires finding out which groups are most likely to include your target markets as members. Utilize your public speaking time wisely by making certain that at least one-half of your formal presentations are to groups with members in your target markets. The following list contains examples of several target markets and places where they could be found (and likely sponsors of your presentations).

Target Markets for Giving Presentations

- Specific Health Concerns (e.g., fibromyalgia): Support groups, clinics, book stores, health care provider's offices and health food stores.

- People in recovery: Counseling offices, treatment centers and specialty bookstores.

- Animals: Veterinary clinics, pet stores, grooming centers, 4H clubs, dog obedience classes and county fairs.

- Seniors: Volunteer organizations, senior centers, civic groups and parks.

- Pregnant Women: Lamaze classes, the La Leche League, baby boutiques and Ob/Gyn offices.

- Athletes: Sporting events, health fairs, sporting goods stores, sports medicine facilities and health food stores.

- Attorneys: Bar association meetings, law library and legal aid department.

Research Studies

The Touch Research Institute
305-243-6781

Institute for Studies in
Chronic Pain
301- 698-0932
Fax: 301-698-9299
www.erols.com/fibrosym

American Massage Therapy
Association Foundation
847-864-0123
Fax: 847-864-1178

Blue Poppy Press
800-487-9296
Fax: 303-447-0740
102151.1614@compuserv.com

Reflexions
888-777-9911
www.reflexology-research.com

National Institutes of Health
Office of Alternative
Medicine Clearinghouse
888-644-6226
http://altmed.od.nih.gov

*The Physician's Guide to
Therapeutic Massage*
published by the
Massage Therapists
Assn. of British Columbia
604-873-4467

*Alternative Medicine: What
Works—A Comprehensive,
Easy-to-Read Review of the
Scientific Evidence, Pro and Con*
by Adriane Fugh-Berman, M.D.
Odonian Press

Getting on the public speaking circuit is easy. Contact civic clubs, professional societies, business groups and networking associations. These organizations are always on the lookout for speakers. Their members enjoy learning specific techniques that improve the quality of their lives. Indeed, any topic relating to well-being or stress reduction is in demand. Even bookstores sponsor talks regularly. The most common duration of these presentations is 20 minutes but they can range up to one hour.

Successful Presentations

The foundation for successful presentations is planning. Investing the time in planning can make the difference between a powerful, flowing, fun presentation and one that's stilted and ineffective. Planning includes understanding the audience, assessing their needs and objectives, determining the presentation purpose, researching the topic, designing the presentation and matching facilities to program requirements. It's important to evaluate and update your information and audio-visual materials before each presentation—regardless of whether you are preparing a talk from scratch or if you are delivering the same topic for the fiftieth time.

Sample Topics

Some general ideas for health care presentations are: Stress Management Techniques, Self-Massage, Stretches and Exercises People Can Do at Their Desks, Self-Hypnosis to Gain the Competitive Edge, Couples Massage, Acupressure, Peak Performance Through Proper Nutrition, Preventive Health Care, Infant Massage, Hydrotherapy, Nutrition, Movement, Dream Analysis, Aromatherapy, Healthy Baby Care, Common Use of Herbs, Personal Growth and Fitness. You can also give talks on other subjects in which you have experience or training. Some of the most enjoyable "talks" are when you demonstrate your services. You could create numerous different presentations for every example given above. You can also tie in your presentation with holidays or major events and title them accordingly. Two examples are: "Stress Deduction" during tax time; and "The Gift of Touch" for the pre-holiday buying season.

Resources

Vast resources are available for ideas on presentation topics, products to sell and handouts. Peruse your personal library. Check your books and magazines for topics of interest. Go to health food stores, book stores and libraries. Research information about your specific industry and then look at general topics such as health, wellness, fitness, stress and alternative health. You can also do extensive research at home via the Internet (beware: web-surfers can spend days sorting through the research results).

Delivery

In any presentation how you say something is just as important as what you say. Approximately 55 percent of your presentation impact comes from your non-verbal communications, 35 percent from your voice and 10 percent from the actual content. Not aware of these numbers, most people spend the majority of their preparation on the content. Power and presence are established through the mastery of body language while the energy in your voice conveys your sincerity. The methods used to communicate information often determine whether or not the information is fully received.

Incorporate activities that involve the major senses of sight, sound and touch. If you work with aromatherapy, also include smell. People like to feel as though they are being talked with directly—even if they are part of a large group. Some creative techniques for involving your audience are: have the audience participate in an activity such as stretching; lead a visualization exercise; ask questions and have the group raise their hands or stand up in response (e.g., How many of you get headaches? How many of you have ever received an acupuncture treatment? How many receive acupuncture regularly?); make specific reference to a participant or the group (e.g., "Since everyone here today either suffers from fibromyalgia or is close to someone who does, you know how debilitating pain can be."); request feedback; facilitate a question and answer format; and give a demonstration.

It's all right to have butterflies in your stomach. Just get them to fly in formation.
— Dr. Ron Gilbert

The more experiential the activity, the better. When talking about touch therapies, show the group how to do some simple techniques on themselves or each other. If the group members know each other well and aren't dressed in business suits, you can organize a massage circle. If you are including information on aromatherapy, bring some essential oils for the audience to smell.

The activities need not be elaborate to be fun and effective. For instance, you can demonstrate stretches that the audience can do with you while sitting in their chairs. You can lead activities based on popular games, such as crossword puzzles and Scrabble,® and even design a health care edition of Trivial Pursuit® or Jeopardy® that includes facts about your specific industry.

Overcoming Nervousness

Some people are fortunate in that they are naturally good speakers; they feel comfortable being in front of a group, easily relate to their audiences and can think while on their feet. Most people must develop these speaking skills. The first step is to assess your attitude. Many people are hesitant to do any type of public speaking for fear of appearing inept. The beauty of doing presentations about health and well-being is that you intrinsically know the benefits of this work. Granted, you might not know everything about a specific topic or be able to answer every question—but no audience expects that.

Toastmasters International
P.O. Box 9052
Mission Viejo, CA 92690
714-858-8255

The second step is to increase your knowledge and experience. You can take classes (through your local community college, university or a private company), read books or join a public speaking group such as Toastmasters International.

The final step is to practice. By joining a group such as Toastmasters, you get weekly practice in public speaking. You can always devise ways to weave information about your services into your topics. Another practice option is to create a support group where you coach each other on your presentations and do public speaking engagements together.

Everyone gets nervous. The difference between a good presenter and a poor one is that the good presenter knows how to manage her fears. Use the adrenaline that's pumping through your system to keep you alert and sustain a high energy level.

Tips for Alleviating Nervousness

- Before your presentation, visualize yourself having a fabulous time; being dynamic, energetic and connecting with the audience.
- Take a few deep breaths and relax your body.
- Get a touch therapy treatment prior to speaking.
- Avoid eating a heavy meal before speaking.
- Drink warm non-caffeinated liquids (e.g., lemon tea)
- Maintain good posture: unlock your knees and stand with equal weight on both feet.
- Organize your notes and audio-visuals.
- Wear comfortable clothes.
- Practice.

Developing a Dynamic Introduction ᨁ

No matter what you do in life, your ability to introduce yourself well greatly impacts your success. Because this business thrives on word-of-mouth promotion, you must be able to inspire others by the way you introduce yourself.

Actually, it's wise to have several exciting introductions down pat. The advantage is this: you may want to vary what you say and how you say it depending on the time parameters and the audience. Your introduction will differ if you are talking directly with one person rather than a group. Most likely you will use different terminology when you are talking to a group of your peers rather than a business group, or even a mixed group.

The real secret of success is enthusiasm.
— Walter Chrysler

In most networking groups you are only allotted 30 seconds or less to introduce yourself. Without a prepared introduction you probably will only say a small portion of what you wish to convey. Yet 20 seconds is ample time if your basic introduction is clear, concise and engaging.

I recommend having a memorized 20-second and 30-second introduction. I also advocate designing a one-minute and a five-minute presentation in which you memorize your opening and closing lines, and have a clear outline of the salient points you wish to cover. Conversely, I highly discourage memorizing any presentation that is over 30 seconds in length, since this puts too much emphasis on the words and not the relationship between you and your audience. Another problem with a memorized speech is that if you forget a word, or someone asks you a question, you may get totally thrown off track and not be able to gracefully recover.

Simple Yet Effective 20-30 Second Introductions

"How would you like to make your pregnancy—or that of a friend's—much more enjoyable and comfortable? This can be achieved by receiving regular massages. I am Mary Smith and I'm a licensed massage therapist, specializing in prenatal massage. The work I do with pregnant women assists them in increasing circulation, reducing edema, improving muscle tone, and easing tension and fatigue. Please feel free to talk with me after the meeting. I have cards, brochures and gift certificates available at the back table."

"Hello, I am Kerry Billings and I am a chiropractor. I've been in practice since 1985 and have recently moved to Sunny Hills. My focus is on well-being and preventive care. I have an extensive background in Oriental philosophy and incorporate that into my approach. Please call me if you are interested in more information. I do not charge for an initial consultation. I look forward to meeting with you and being able to assist you in achieving optimal health."

"Do you experience a lot of stress? Is your life filled with activities—career, family and friends? Are you involved in a fitness program? If you answered yes to any of these questions, you probably experience some form of physical discomfort—be it muscular aches and pain, fatigue, or even tension headaches. Yoga can help reduce stress, improve circulation, ease tension and improve muscle tone. I am Randy Harris and I am a certified yoga practitioner. If you would like more information on how yoga can enhance your well-being, please talk with me after the meeting."

Designing your introduction needn't be a grueling experience. You can generate and refine several introductions in less than three hours. Make it fun by getting together with several friends and all work on your introductions. The material you develop for your introduction(s) can be utilized in creating other promotional material such as brochures and press releases.

Introduction Design Suggestions

- Begin your adventure by collecting descriptive material: informational packets on your services, magazine articles, brochures from other practitioners and promotional pieces on yourself. Go through this information and highlight the words and phrases that appeal to you.
- Write a detailed statement of what you do. Be certain to distinguish the features from the benefits. Features are the descriptive characteristics about your service, your background including experience and education in this profession. Benefits are the results that a client receives by utilizing your services.
- Review your differential advantage statement.

- Write your introduction. Choose a specific audience and a time frame (e.g., a business networking meeting and 30-second general introduction). Look over all of the material you have—the highlights from your sample promotional pieces, your business description, and your differential advantage statement. Combine these to formulate your written introduction; review it, replacing any passive words or phrases with dynamic, active, present tense terms. To alleviate the habitual use of the same language patterns and vocabulary, use a thesaurus to discover different words (terms, jargon, expressions). If you are doing this exercise with colleagues, read your introductions to each other and get feedback. Repeat this process for each introduction you decide to prepare.
- Refine your introduction. The best way to do this is to practice it in front of friends (ones who will be honest with you). Get their input on the content and your delivery. If this is not feasible, practice out loud, standing tall in front of a mirror. Use a tape recorder (videotape if available) and critique the results. "All the world's a stage," and these are your lines. Remember, the more comfortable you are in dynamically introducing yourself, the greater your impact. And in this profession, first impressions have a significant influence on your success.

Networking

Establishing a strong network is fundamental for success in this field. Since so much of our business comes from word-of-mouth (referrals from clients, friends and other networking associates), it's crucial to begin fostering these associations immediately!

Networking is essentially a group of interconnected or cooperating individuals who develop and share contacts, information and support. An effective network is composed of many different types of people: individuals from whom you get information; experts whose services you utilize and can refer to others; people who keep you informed of events and opportunities; role models; those who are genuinely concerned about you, listen to you and support you; mentors; people who actively refer potential clients to you; and centers of influence.

Networking is a perfect example of the adage: the more you give, the more you receive.

Centers of influence can have a dramatic impact on your practice. These are individuals who are well-known and highly respected by your target markets. Just one word from them could inspire droves of people to flock to your roost.

Networking is a process, it's giving and receiving support. You can network informally by sharing resources with the people you contact or formally by joining one or more networking groups. It's important to remember that networking is composed of many skills that you must continue to develop and refine. The most successful networkers are those who actively support others in making connections.

Enhance your networking abilities by recognizing the vast potential for making connections for yourself and others. Whenever you meet someone, jot a few notes about them: where and when you met, who introduced you, what line of business they're in, what their interests are and what types of resources they have. Think about the other people you know to see if it would be beneficial for them to meet each other. Even if you are unable to make any connections right away, you may be able to do so in the future. You never know when a contact will come in handy.

Networking Success
by Anne Boe
Seaside Press

Build your network. Purchase a professional address book, computer contact program or card filing system for keeping track of your contacts. Include all pertinent information on each person and then keep it current. You may want to cross-index your files. When you collect business cards, always get at least three: one to file by name, one to file by business or occupation and one to give away (which ties into why you should always give out three of your cards). Become visible in your community by attending business, civic and social events, and joining professional and networking associations. Take seminars and classes. Be sure to attend various types of functions so you can widen the scope of people you meet.

Work your network. Follow up on leads and information with a phone call or note. Take the initiative. Always thank people that help you (either by giving you their time, support, advice, leads or contacts) even if you are not able to use their help or if the leads don't work out. When you are given a recommendation to utilize someone's services, tell the person who it was that gave you her name. When you give out referrals, make note of who you referred to whom. Find out if the referral was successful. Be a giver and a receiver. Maintain contact with people in your network and stay up-to-date with what's happening. People's lives are constantly changing and so are their networking needs. Given natural attrition, add at least two people per month to your active network to keep it thriving. The most fundamental element in effective networking is to follow through on your commitments.

You can make more friends in two months by becoming interested in other people than you can in two years by trying to get people interested in you.
— Dale Carnegie

Choosing a Networking Group

It's essential for your professional and personal well-being to belong to at least one networking organization. Numerous types of networking groups exist from monthly social clubs, to community groups such as the Chamber of Commerce, to weekly "needs and leads" business associations. Participate in functions where you meet people to develop mutually beneficial relationships.

To determine which organization is best for you, assess your needs and clarify your purpose and goals for networking in general. Ascertain the types of contacts you desire and appraise the assets you have to offer others. Delineate your purpose and goals for each specific group you are considering joining. You may want to become a member of one group mainly as a means for getting clients and join another association because you strongly support their goals and activities. You may decide to become part of an organization for the educational and informational opportunities or join a club to make new friends and have fun. Sometimes one organization can meet several of your criteria.

Attend one or two meetings as a guest. Get a feel for the group. Notice whether or not you share any common interests and goals. Ask to see their bylaws and mission statement. If they don't have anything written, talk to several members and get feedback on their impressions of the group's purpose and philosophy. Find out the types of businesses and professions represented by the membership. Many organizations have a substantial membership fee, so it's wise to do some research before joining to determine if it's the right group for you.

Effective networking can be exciting as well as financially rewarding! Become active in at least one business association and invest time in building your network of contacts and refining your networking skills.

Figure 9.8

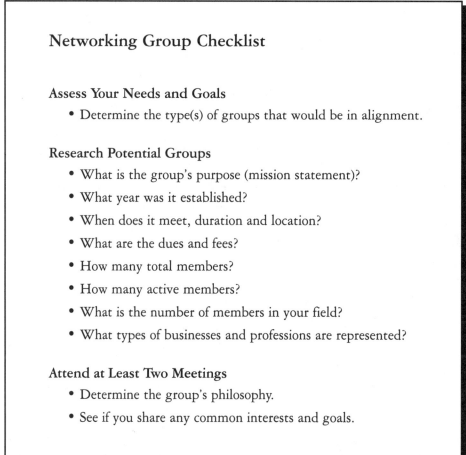

Networking Group Checklist

Assess Your Needs and Goals
- Determine the type(s) of groups that would be in alignment.

Research Potential Groups
- What is the group's purpose (mission statement)?
- What year was it established?
- When does it meet, duration and location?
- What are the dues and fees?
- How many total members?
- How many active members?
- What is the number of members in your field?
- What types of businesses and professions are represented?

Attend at Least Two Meetings
- Determine the group's philosophy.
- See if you share any common interests and goals.

Figure 9.9

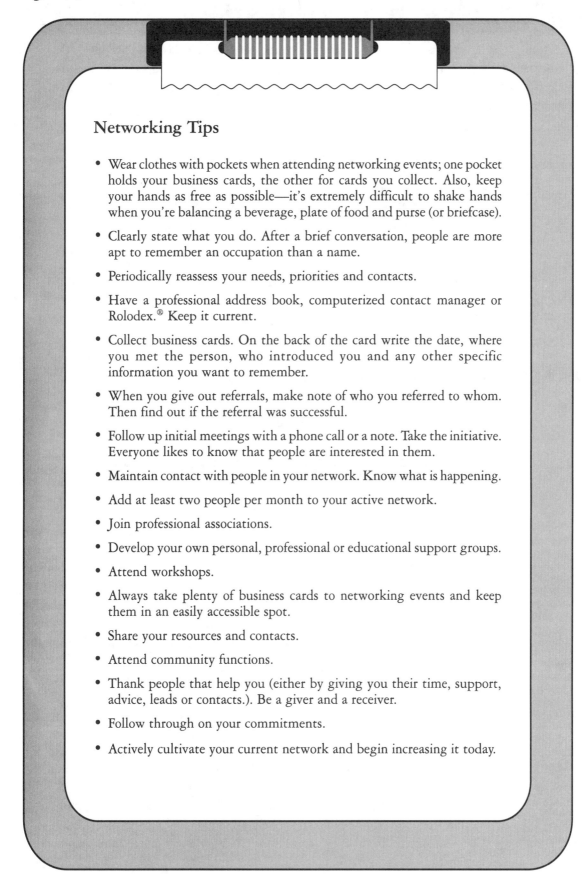

Networking Tips

- Wear clothes with pockets when attending networking events; one pocket holds your business cards, the other for cards you collect. Also, keep your hands as free as possible—it's extremely difficult to shake hands when you're balancing a beverage, plate of food and purse (or briefcase).

- Clearly state what you do. After a brief conversation, people are more apt to remember an occupation than a name.

- Periodically reassess your needs, priorities and contacts.

- Have a professional address book, computerized contact manager or Rolodex.® Keep it current.

- Collect business cards. On the back of the card write the date, where you met the person, who introduced you and any other specific information you want to remember.

- When you give out referrals, make note of who you referred to whom. Then find out if the referral was successful.

- Follow up initial meetings with a phone call or a note. Take the initiative. Everyone likes to know that people are interested in them.

- Maintain contact with people in your network. Know what is happening.

- Add at least two people per month to your active network.

- Join professional associations.

- Develop your own personal, professional or educational support groups.

- Attend workshops.

- Always take plenty of business cards to networking events and keep them in an easily accessible spot.

- Share your resources and contacts.

- Attend community functions.

- Thank people that help you (either by giving you their time, support, advice, leads or contacts.). Be a giver and a receiver.

- Follow through on your commitments.

- Actively cultivate your current network and begin increasing it today.

An effective network is composed of many different types of people. List the names (or titles) of the people who fit into each category (some names may be repeated since people often have more than one role in your life).

- Who are your sources of information?
- List the people who could be centers of influence.
- Who are the people who actively refer potential clients to you?
- List the experts whose services you use and can refer to others.
- Who keeps you informed of events and opportunities?
- List the people who genuinely care about you, listen to you and support you.
- Who are your mentors?
- List your role models.

Now that you have specified the people in your current network, review the lists. Do one or two people perform most of the roles? Are there any areas that are lacking names? Are most of the people the same "type"? How do you feel about your network?

- List the kinds of support you would like to have right now.
- What additional types of support do you need over the next year?
- Who would you like to add to your network?
- List at least 10 goals for improving your network.

Tools for Effective Follow-up And Networking

Tickler Files

Many people in all professions have found it useful to have some type of a "tickler" file. A tickler file reminds you of your commitments and assists in follow-through. Essentially, it contains 12 separate sections (one for each month) and a set of dividers numbered 1-31 (one for each day of the month). You can put these in a three-ring binder, an accordion file or hanging files. (Office supply stores carry a variety of these systems.) Place the 31 dividers in the Current Month Section. Then if someone asks you to contact them in two weeks, you go to your tickler file, turn to the corresponding date and make a note to call that person. Check your tickler file daily. Look at the current day and possibly the next two days. If you have a computer you can purchase planning software programs that include tickler systems.

The true beauty of a tickler file is not so much in recording short-term information but for keeping track of future events. For example, a client is going out of town for the summer and asks you to call back on September 12th. You put a note in the "September" section of your file. When it's the end of August and you are transferring your 31 dividers to September, you would put the note under the 12th. Using this system frees you from having to actively remember everything and helps ensure that you won't "forget" your commitments. Various computer programs do this automatically.

Contact/Referral Records

It's important to keep track of contacts and potential business resources. Use your computer contact manager or place sheets (purchase pre-designed forms or make your own) in a binder with alphabetical dividers. Each contact has a separate sheet. Some of the information to include is the person's name, company, title, work address and phone number, home address and phone number, who referred you, where you met, any personal or professional information that you want, and action to be taken. Transfer the items from the action to be taken section to your tickler file or appointment book. You might also want to list the dates and times of any actions (e.g., telephone calls, meetings) directly onto the contact form. This is particularly helpful as a document to record business interactions. For example, you get a bid for supplies over the phone and you place an order. Then you get your bill and it's for a different price. You are more likely to resolve the difference in your favor if you are able to say, "I talked with Ann Alleby on Tuesday, August 17th, at 3:20 p.m. and was told..." The fact that you kept such precise records gives you more credibility.

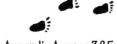

See Appendix A, page 385 for sample Contact Forms.

Contact records also serve as a reminder. Review your contacts at least every two months. You may not have needed someone's services in the past, but as circumstances change your needs may vary. Maybe you just met a person who could benefit from the services of someone in your contact files. Remember, networking isn't just fulfilling your needs but also assisting others in meeting their needs.

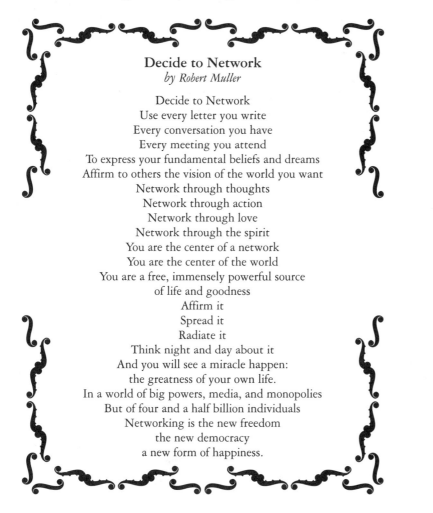

Decide to Network
by Robert Muller

Decide to Network
Use every letter you write
Every conversation you have
Every meeting you attend
To express your fundamental beliefs and dreams
Affirm to others the vision of the world you want
Network through thoughts
Network through action
Network through love
Network through the spirit
You are the center of a network
You are the center of the world
You are a free, immensely powerful source
of life and goodness
Affirm it
Spread it
Radiate it
Think night and day about it
And you will see a miracle happen:
the greatness of your own life.
In a world of big powers, media, and monopolies
But of four and a half billion individuals
Networking is the new freedom
the new democracy
a new form of happiness.

• Advertising •

Advertising is gaining public notice for your business through means that require direct payment. Some forms of advertising are: display ads in publications; radio and television commercials; classified ads; billboards; phone books; and bus stop benches. Until recently, mass media advertising has typically been avoided by health care providers, mainly due to the impersonal nature and the presumed cost. It's becoming more commonplace to hear ads on the radio, see billboards on the roads and even encounter television ads promoting complementary health care. Still, most of these advertising techniques are usually employed by larger clinics rather than individual practitioners, or are announcing a specific event. Classified ads tend to be the most productive form of advertising for practitioners. Your advertising venues contribute to your overall image, so choose them carefully.

Advertising is best used when your target market is a mass market, your product or service is purchased frequently, the competition is high or your goal is to quickly create awareness of a new service or product.

The two essential elements for successful advertising are consistency and quality. Quality relates to the ad's style, wording and visual impact. Statistics reveal that an ad needs to be seen at least three times before it's noticed and seven times before it inspires the reader to take action. It works better to place a smaller (or shorter) ad on a regular basis than to do a big splashy ad one time only.

The steps in designing effective advertising are: Identify your target market, grab the reader's attention, highlight your differential advantage, list the benefits, state your offer, highlight the ad feature, request a response and provide a means of contact.

Print Advertising

Of all the advertising venues available print advertising (e.g., newspapers, magazines, trade journals and specialty publications) is the most preferred by health care providers.

Contact those publications and request an advertiser's media kit. These kits contain rates for display and classified ads, demographic statistics and a sample of the publication.

It can be difficult to sit down and create ad copy. Most people think they should start with the headline. Unless you are struck by a bolt of advertising genius (hey, it could happen!), begin by making a list of your benefits and determine the offer you want to make. Then write the body copy. Save the headline composition for last.

In many ways the headline is the most critical element of an ad. People's choice of whether to read or ignore your ad is often based on the headline's impact. Personalize the ad to an individual reader (use embedded commands).

You can have brilliant ideas, but if you can't get them across, your ideas won't get you anywhere.
— Lee Iacocca

Photographs are more convincing than drwan illustrations. They can increase response by 50%. Before and after pictures are also quite persuasive.

Exciting Headline Styles

News: Use words such as "New," "Presenting" or "Announcing."

Instruction/Advice: Use words such as "How to," "Why," "Which," "You," "This" and "Discover."

Testimonial: Utilize strong quotes from satisfied clients.

Compelling Offer: Use words such as "Free" and "Limited Offer."

Curiosity: Ask questions to inspire readers to want to know more. Use phrases such as "Do you feel (want, need, desire)."

Claim: Relay a success story.

Display Ad Tips

- Include an attention-grabbing, benefits-oriented headline.
- Have the subhead elaborate the headline benefit.
- Incorporate a strong visual image.
- Identify your target markets.
- Keep the body text paragraphs short and visually attractive. Don't skimp on information—studies show ads with more copy draw better than those with less. Then again, don't pack so much in that it requires a microscope to decipher the text.
- Use language that's geared toward your target market.
- Include powerful words such as "new," "free," "save" and "now."
- Use embedded commands.
- Provide a guarantee.
- Offer incentives.
- Broadcast on station WIIFM (What's In It For Me).
- Back up benefits with key features.
- Demonstrate credibility and reliability.
- Include testimonials.
- State your offer in clear, simple terms.
- Compel readers to take action.
- If you are selling a product, make it easy to respond: include a toll-free number, fax number and other ways to contact you such as e-mail or website; provide an order form; and offer to take credit cards.
- Include your logo, location and phone number.
- Border your ad—it makes small ads look bigger. Don't limit yourself to plain, straight-lined boxes, nor use overly baroque designs.
- Make the layout attractive and inviting.
- Use color whenever possible. A second color (in addition to the black ink) can increase the ad's effectiveness by 25 percent. The most eye-catching and frequently used color is red.

Busy layouts often pull better responses than neat ones. Vary shapes, sizes and colors. Keep in mind that too many extraneous props divert attention.

See pages 290-295 for additional design ideas.

According to Cahners Advertising Research Report, ads with benefits in the headlines and copy are 2-3 times more likely to be remembered than ads that don't stress benefits.

Figure 9.10   Sample Salon and Minispa Display Ad

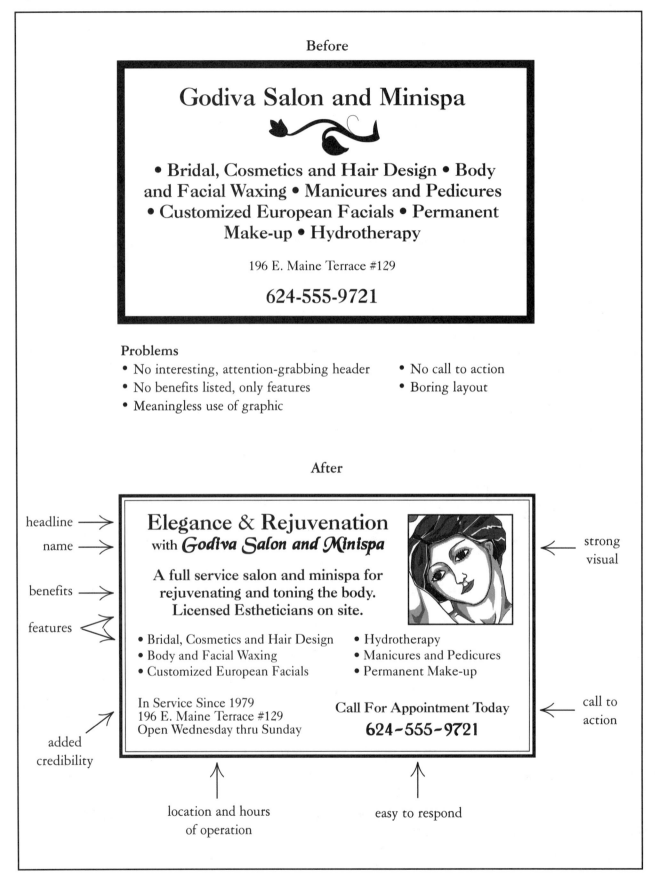

Figure 9.11   Sample Chiropractic Display Ad

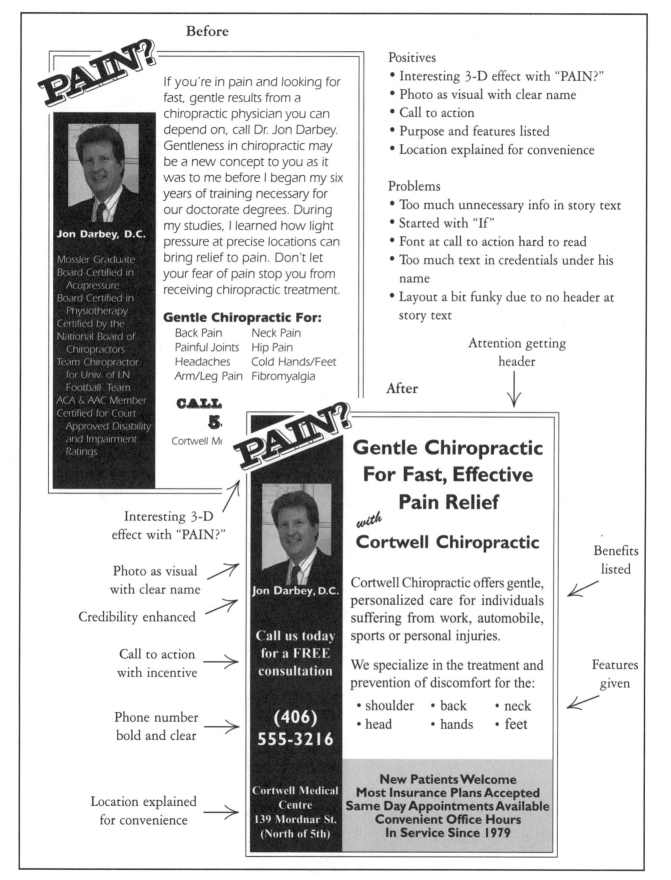

Before

PAIN?

If you're in pain and looking for fast, gentle results from a chiropractic physician you can depend on, call Dr. Jon Darbey. Gentleness in chiropractic may be a new concept to you as it was to me before I began my six years of training necessary for our doctorate degrees. During my studies, I learned how light pressure at precise locations can bring relief to pain. Don't let your fear of pain stop you from receiving chiropractic treatment.

Jon Darbey, D.C.

Mossler Graduate
Board Certified in Acupressure
Board Certified in Physiotherapy
Certified by the National Board of Chiropractors
Team Chiropractor for Univ. of LN Football Team
ACA & AAC Member
Certified for Court Approved Disability and Impairment Ratings

Gentle Chiropractic For:

Back Pain	Neck Pain
Painful Joints	Hip Pain
Headaches	Cold Hands/Feet
Arm/Leg Pain	Fibromyalgia

CALL
5
Cortwell Me

Positives
• Interesting 3-D effect with "PAIN?"
• Photo as visual with clear name
• Call to action
• Purpose and features listed
• Location explained for convenience

Problems
• Too much unnecessary info in story text
• Started with "If"
• Font at call to action hard to read
• Too much text in credentials under his name
• Layout a bit funky due to no header at story text

Attention getting header

After

Interesting 3-D effect with "PAIN?"

Photo as visual with clear name

Credibility enhanced

Call to action with incentive

Phone number bold and clear

Location explained for convenience

PAIN?

Jon Darbey, D.C.

Call us today for a FREE consultation

(406) 555-3216

Cortwell Medical Centre
139 Mordnar St.
(North of 5th)

Gentle Chiropractic For Fast, Effective Pain Relief
with
Cortwell Chiropractic

Cortwell Chiropractic offers gentle, personalized care for individuals suffering from work, automobile, sports or personal injuries.

We specialize in the treatment and prevention of discomfort for the:

• shoulder	• back	• neck
• head	• hands	• feet

New Patients Welcome
Most Insurance Plans Accepted
Same Day Appointments Available
Convenient Office Hours
In Service Since 1979

Benefits listed

Features given

Figure 9.12 Sample Counseling Display Ad

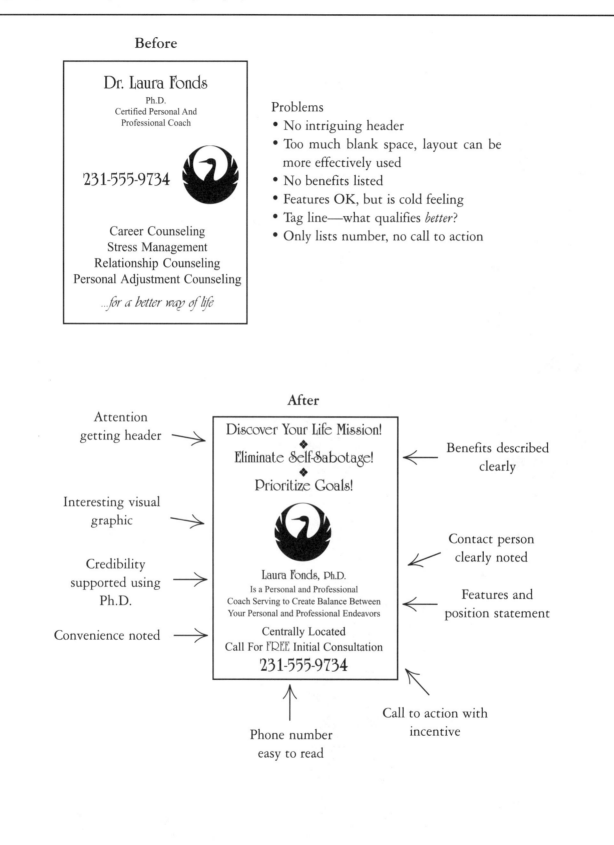

Before

Dr. Laura Fonds
Ph.D.
Certified Personal And
Professional Coach

231-555-9734

Career Counseling
Stress Management
Relationship Counseling
Personal Adjustment Counseling

...for a better way of life

Problems
- No intriguing header
- Too much blank space, layout can be more effectively used
- No benefits listed
- Features OK, but is cold feeling
- Tag line—what qualifies *better*?
- Only lists number, no call to action

After

Attention getting header →

Interesting visual graphic →

Credibility supported using Ph.D. →

Convenience noted →

Discover Your Life Mission!
❖
Eliminate Self-Sabotage!
❖
Prioritize Goals!

Laura Fonds, Ph.D.
Is a Personal and Professional
Coach Serving to Create Balance Between
Your Personal and Professional Endeavors

Centrally Located
Call For FREE Initial Consultation
231-555-9734

← Benefits described clearly

← Contact person clearly noted

← Features and position statement

Call to action with incentive

Phone number easy to read

Figure 9.13   Sample Acupuncture Display Ad

Both have:
- Attention-getting header
- Interesting graphic
- Benefits described
- Credibility enhanced
- Features added
- Call to action
- Easy-to-read phone number

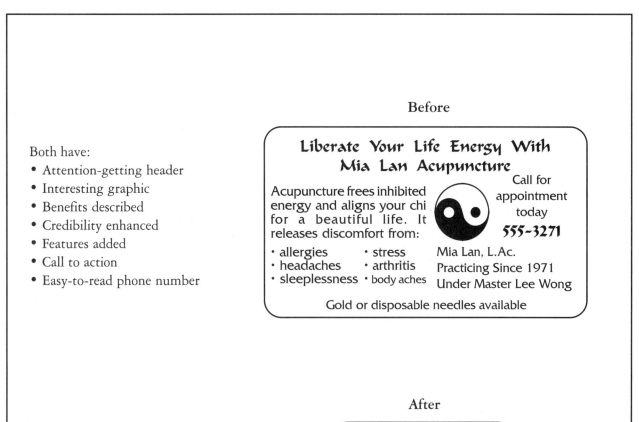

Before

Liberate Your Life Energy With Mia Lan Acupuncture

Acupuncture frees inhibited energy and aligns your chi for a beautiful life. It releases discomfort from:

· allergies   · stress
· headaches   · arthritis
· sleeplessness · body aches

Call for appointment today
555-3271

Mia Lan, L.Ac.
Practicing Since 1971
Under Master Lee Wong

Gold or disposable needles available

After

Layout flows better →

Liberate Your Life Energy With Mia Lan Acupuncture

Gold Needles Available

Acupuncture frees inhibited energy (chi) and releases discomfort from:

· allergies   · stress
· headaches   · arthritis
· sleeplessness · body aches

Call for appointment today

207-555-3271

Mia Lan, L.Ac.
Practicing Since 1971
Under Master Lee Wong

Figure 9.14   Sample Massage Display Ad

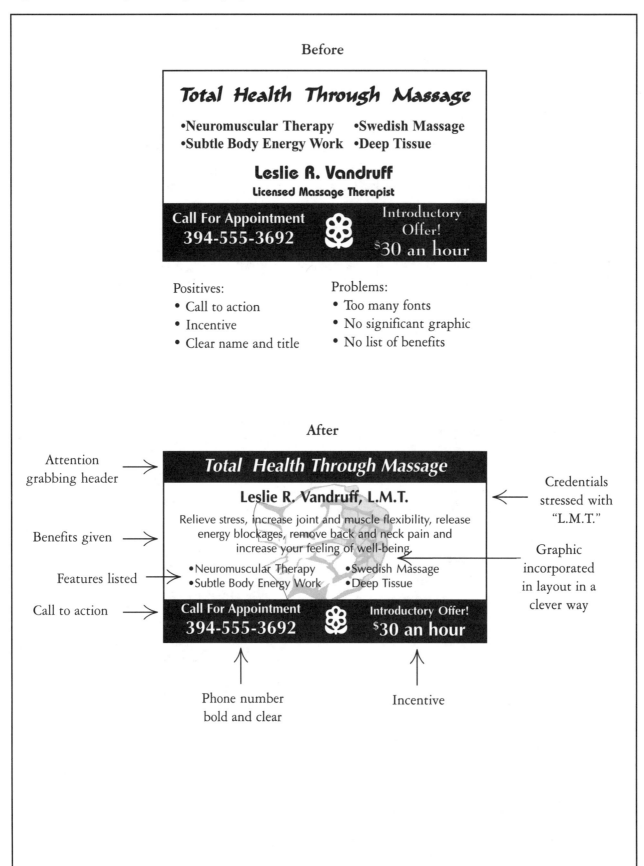

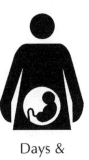
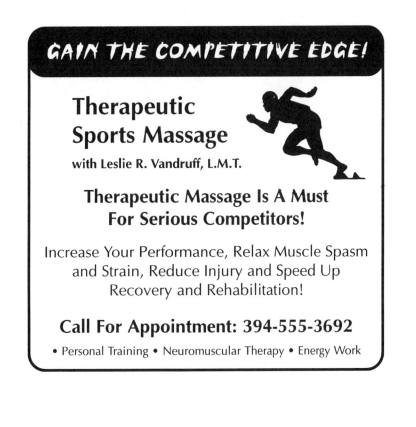

Classified Ads

Places to put listings include the telephone Yellow Pages, business directories, trade journals, local publications, magazines, newsletters and special interest books.

Listings (often referred to as classified ads) tend to be the most productive form of advertising for health care providers. A listing is a concise, engaging description of your practice or announcement that is placed in a specific section of a publication. Classified ads are generally much less expensive than display ads—and you don't need to employ a commercial artist.

The major advantage of a listing is inherent in its definition. People look at listings because they are interested in what's being offered. Contrast this with display advertising in which you have to grab the reader's attention.

You must have a catchy headline to make sure your listing stands out. Other ways to increase the visibility of your listing are to put the headline in bold capital letters, bold the whole ad, include some type of graphic design, ad color or box the ad. Follow the same general design tips for display advertising.

Figure 9.16   Sample Classified Ads

CLASSIFIEDS

To Gain Leads

Massage Therapy—General:
FREE stress/pain relief booklet. Call Leslie Vandruff, LMT for FREE booklet or info about therapeutic massage services. (394) 555-3692.

Massage Therapy—Sports:
SPORTS CHAMPIONS! Keep your competitive edge! Therapeutic sports massage. Call for FREE *Health Tips for Athletes* pamphlet. 394-555-3692.

Massage Therapy—Pre-Natal:
EXPECTANT MOTHERS! Nurture your wellness. Pre-natal massage eases the stresses of pregnancy. Call for FREE Healthy Pregnancy Tips brochure! 394-555-3692.

To Gain Clients

Massage Therapy—General:
STRESS RELIEF/PAIN RELIEF! Relaxing therapeutic massage releases tension and restriction from sports injuries, household accidents, repetitive movement and everyday stress. Neuromuscular Therapy, Subtle Body Energy Work, Swedish & Deep Tissue Massage available. Centrally located. For appointment or FREE stress/pain relief booklet, call Leslie Vandruff, L.M.T. 394-555-3692.

Massage Therapy—Sports:
SPORTS CHAMPIONS! Keep your competitive edge! Therapeutic sports massage increases your performance, relaxes muscle spasm/strain, reduces injury and speeds up rehabilitation! Equipment travels to you! Call for FREE *Health Tips for Athletes* pamphlet or for appointment. 394-555-3692.

Massage Therapy—Pre-Natal:
EXPECTANT MOTHERS! Nurture your wellness. Pre-natal massage eases the stresses of pregnancy, reduces edema, increases flexibility, boosts energy and enhances your sense of well-being for both you and your baby! Call for appointment or for FREE Healthy Pregnancy Tips brochure! 394-555-3692.

CLASSIFIEDS

To Gain Leads

Chiropractic:
BACK & NECK PAIN? **FREE** consultation. Call Cortwell Chiropractic Center for gentle, personalized chiropractic care. 555-3216, 139 Mordnar St. Ask for our **FREE** pamphlet on Tips for a Supple Spine.

Esthetics:
ELEGANCE & REJUVENATION. Weddings, proms, special occasions & gifts. Call Godiva Salon and Mini-spa for FREE brochure of services. 624-555-9721.

Counseling:
FEELING OUT OF SYNC? Create balance between your personal and professional endeavors. Call Dr. Laura Fonds for FREE initial consultation. 231-555-9734.

Acupuncture:
FREE Acupuncture information pack. Release discomfort from allergies, headaches, stress, sleeplessness, arthritis, body aches and more. 555-3271.

Nutrition:
FREE information! Learn how to achieve optimal health. Call for your free copy of our *Healthy Living Guide*. 555-9643

To Gain Clients

Chiropractic:
BACK & NECK PAIN? Do you suffer from work, auto, sports or personal injury? Call Cortwell Chiropractic Center for a **FREE** consultation. Gentle, personalized chiropractic care releases pain from your shoulder, back, neck, head, hands and feet. Guaranteed results. Most insurance accepted. Convenient office hours. 555-3216, 139 Mordnar St., Big Sky.

Esthetics:
ELEGANCE & REJUVENATION. Revitalize and tone your body. Weddings, proms, special occasions. Gift certificates available. Treat yourself to Godiva Salon and Min-ispa. Licensed estheticians on site. In service since 1979. 196 E. Maine Terrace #129. Open Wed-Sun. Call for appointment today. 624-555-9721.

Counseling:
FEELING OUT OF SYNC? Create balance between your personal and professional endeavors! Discover your life mission! Eliminate self-sabotage! Prioritize goals! Call Laura Fonds, Ph.D. for **FREE** initial consultation. Centrally located. 231-555-9734.

Acupuncture
ACUPUNCTURE FREES inhibited energy and aligns your chi for a beautiful life. Release discomfort from allergies, stress, headaches, sleeplessness, arthritis, body aches and more. Call Mia Lan Acupuncture for more info or for **FREE** consultation. Downtown location. 555-3271.

Nutrition:
Do you want to achieve **OPTIMAL HEALTH**? We can assist you in feeling strong, energetic and enlivened. Call Tracy Smith, N.D. for an appointment or to receive a **FREE** copy of our *Healthy Living Guide*. 555-9643.

Yellow Pages

The Yellow Pages provide year-round visibility to every person in your community (actually it's worldwide now that there's an Internet Yellow Pages). They are extensively utilized by the public for locating services.

Look to see how other health care providers list their practices. You needn't be overly concerned about an enhanced listing (additional lines of information) or display ad if you live in a city where there are only a few people who provide your specific services. Then again, it could be a great opportunity for you to stand out.

If you decide to not place a display ad, consider purchasing an enhanced listing, using a second color or placing a border around it.

Put your listing under the most logical category if you can only afford one listing, otherwise list under each applicable category.

Broadcast Advertising

The broadcast media (namely radio and television) reaches a wider audience than print advertising and has immediate impact. Unfortunately, you need to repeat the ad frequently because of the likelihood listeners or viewers won't be paying attention when your ad plays.

Radio Advertising

Health care providers are utilizing radio advertising more and more each day. Radio is still a personal medium and people respond well to it. It's also relatively inexpensive. You can dramatically increase the effectiveness by using it in combination with another type of marketing activity. The most common reasons to advertise on the radio are to: herald the opening of a new business; introduce new staff members; announce new services or products; and invite the public to attend special events such as workshops and open houses.

An option to traditional advertising is to sponsor a radio show or public service announcement. In return for sponsorship (which could be in dollars or services), your name gets mentioned during the show. For example: "The Monday Morning Alternative Music Hour brought to you by Cortwell Chiropractic Center."

Many radio stations offer prize packages to their listeners. Donate your services as part of a prize package and you receive a lot of free air play. For example, a massage therapist here in Tucson offered one massage for the Mother's Day Package the station was giving away. Her name (which is unusual—so it's easy to remember) was mentioned several times an hour for two weeks! This is an example of a shrewd investment: minimal cost—extremely high return.

Figure 9.17   Tips for Radio Advertising

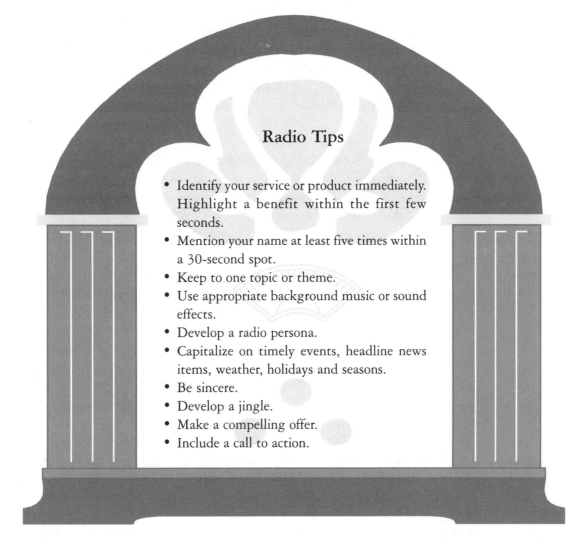

Radio Tips

- Identify your service or product immediately. Highlight a benefit within the first few seconds.
- Mention your name at least five times within a 30-second spot.
- Keep to one topic or theme.
- Use appropriate background music or sound effects.
- Develop a radio persona.
- Capitalize on timely events, headline news items, weather, holidays and seasons.
- Be sincere.
- Develop a jingle.
- Make a compelling offer.
- Include a call to action.

Television Advertising

Television is a powerful advertising vehicle. It reaches more people than any other single medium (the average household watches seven hours of television every day). While nationwide coverage is extremely expensive, local advertising is more affordable due to the abundance of cable networks and non-affiliated stations.

The two keys to successful television advertising are placement and quality. In terms of placement, if one of your target markets is stockbrokers, running your ad on *any* station in the morning isn't going to net you high results (their attention is on Wall Street). Regarding quality, consumers rate the value of your services and products on the production quality of your commercial. You can do damage to your reputation if your commercial looks cheap or hokey in any way.

Although most local television ads are designed to encourage the public to visit a location (e.g., a restaurant or a store), it's becoming more commonplace to see ads for health care providers.

Computer Advertising

Millions of people use the Internet daily to search for information, read news or to kick back and "surf." Having a "home page" with your services and products opens the "world" to you and you to the world. Take advantage of the technology available to expand your visibility and your network; positioning your business on the Internet enables prospective clients to easily and quickly find out about your services.

Initially, most commercial websites were created for product sales; now, with the relative ease and low cost involved to design and maintain a site, more service companies are setting up websites.

For those of you who aren't familiar with cyberspace terminology, here are a few basic definitions:

- Home page: The first page of your website.
- Website: A collection of web pages.
- Internet Service Provider (ISP): A private or public entity that provides dial-up access to the Internet.

For under $1,000 you can set up a multimedia "storefront" on the Internet's World Wide Web. The cost can be even less if you design and maintain your own website (although I highly recommend otherwise). The monthly rental cost for the space to host your site runs between $20-$40 for five megabytes of information (which is more than enough for most companies).

In addition to increasing your visibility you save money (printing and postage) and time (labor involved in assembling and mailing packets) by giving your clients and prospects the option of getting your information via the Internet.

Websites are extremely beneficial to practitioners who have aspects of their businesses that change frequently (e.g., classes, open houses, discounts, promotions and product specials). Changes can be updated in minutes at little or no cost—in comparison to the expense of reprinting brochures.

The two most common methods for health care providers to develop a web presence are to create their own website or rent a home page on another site (usually a professional association or a "health mall").

Regardless of where your site is technically located, you must let people know how to find you. Notify the Internet search engines (four of the most popular being Alta Vista, Lycos, Infoseek and Yahoo!) as well as other sites related to your specific field and your target market's interests. Many cities have websites that list local businesses and even provide direct links. Also advise people on your mailing list by sending them an announcement or publishing the address in your newsletter. Print your website address on all your marketing materials (e.g., business cards, brochures and letterhead).

Customer Service on the Internet: Building Relationships, Increasing Loyalty, and Staying Competitive
by Jim Sterne
John Wiley & Sons

Cyberwriting: How to Promote Your Product or Service Online
by Joe Vitale
AMACOM

The Internet Marketing Plan: A Practical Handbook for Creating, Implementing and Assessing Your Online Presence
by Kim M. Bayne
John Wiley & Sons

Laura Lemany's Web Workshop
by Laura Lemany
SAMS.NET

Marketing on the Internet
by J. Ellsworth & M. Ellsworth
John Wiley & Sons

The Web Page Design Cookbook
by William Horton
John Wiley & Sons

Web Publishing Unleashed
by William R. Stanek
SAMS.NET

To get repeat business you must keep your site current. Make it easy to use; if it takes too long to load because of the number or complexity of the graphic images, or if the site is difficult to navigate (not easy to directly move to where you want to go), people may leave your site before viewing everything and not return.

Pique viewers' interest by sponsoring contests, displaying valuable information, offering electronic coupons, giving online demos, posting surveys and including a "Tips of the Day" column.

Since there is virtually no space limitation, you can include photographs, animation and even audio and video clips. Before investing in a home page, check out similar sites. Note what appeals to you and incorporate those elements into your design.

Design Tips

- Compose a clear Table of Contents that takes up less than one screen.
- Include exciting headlines.
- Utilize simple graphics and plenty of "white space."
- Use a lightly shaded (and possibly textured) background.
- Employ animation sparingly.
- Concentrate on the message: Content, not looks, is what counts.

• Publicity •

Publicity is free media exposure for your practice. It's a powerful tool for any business—yet people rarely take the time to work the system. Some examples of publicity are news releases, announcements, feature stories, interviews and press conferences. Publicity differs from advertising in that you don't pay for the exposure (although some media outlets do give news exposure preference to advertisers).

The advantage of publicity over advertising is that this type of exposure lends an air of credibility to a business that advertising cannot. People are more likely to utilize your services if they read an article about you, listen to an interview with you on the radio or watch you on television than if they see an advertisement about your business. When a respected journalist or reporter makes a positive statement about you, it has much greater impact than if you said the same thing about yourself.

Take a moment to reflect upon an interview you've read about a local business person. What were your impressions? Did you feel a connection with the person? Would you experience the same things by seeing that person's advertisement? Many people I know have increased their businesses significantly through their publicity efforts. Also, most health care providers can't afford to place an advertisement that covers the same page space or air time as an interview.

Developing Media Relationships

Publicity is a powerful marketing tool; to get it you must supply interesting, factual and newsworthy information to media outlets such as radio, television, newspapers, magazines, newsletters and specialty publications. While it's the media's job to inform the public about interesting people and events, they are flooded with press releases and press kits. You need to capture their attention: to get free publicity you need to *market* yourself to the media. You must provide evidence that coverage of you or your business will benefit their readers, listeners or viewers. Media representatives tend to take interest in things that are new, have magnitude, contain an element of human interest or are beneficial to the community.

Press releases play an integral part in effective public relations. To generate ideas for press releases, think about what makes you unique—this is your "hook." In addition to your actual work, consider other aspects such as how long you have been in practice, your location, your training, the equipment and products you use, the types of clients you work with and any new changes you've made to your practice. Familiarize the media with your business. Send out press releases on any major business changes and events. The more often they see your name, the more recognizable you become. Your investment of a little time and postage can reap great rewards.

Become the Expert

Another idea for developing relationships with the media is to become the "expert in the field" who they reference as an information source. It's gratifying when someone from the media calls you for information or your opinion, even when the article isn't directly about you. To facilitate this, mail Rolodex-sized cards (with your name, business name, phone numbers and areas of expertise) to the editors and reporters of local publications, and to producers and hosts of radio and television shows. Put your major category of expertise on the protruding edge of the card.

Be Newsworthy

You increase your odds of being interviewed if you offer something newsworthy. But what makes an event newsworthy? That all depends upon the specific media. This is why it's important to research the different media outlets in terms of *their* target markets and to list the types of articles they write or shows they produce that relate to you. For example, does the newspaper often run interviews of local businesspeople? If so, what types of business owners have been featured? Is there a segment on a television news program that highlights healthy things to do? Are there any specialty publications or shows aimed at people who would be interested in your services?

Some ideas for creating a newsworthy image include staging events, such as free demonstrations or "massage-a-thons;" disseminating information that is unique or useful to the general public, such as announcing a new health care product or describing techniques to alleviate headache pain; forming a wellness group to study specific health-related topics; sponsoring a sports team by donating your services for

Media Hooks:

* You are unique
* You can prove you do it better than competition
* Your credentials
* Your cost is lower
* Process you use to get results
* Result is better, faster, cheaper etc.
* Length of time in business
* Experience in this field
* New to this field
* First company in the field
* Testimonials from satisfied customers/clients
* Your mission
* Your market(s)
* Your image
* Obstacles you have overcome
* Tie into something that has status
* Tie into something that is already happening
* Consistent image
* You are the expert

pre- and post-events and offering reduced rates for regular sessions; adopting a charitable cause; connecting with a celebrity; and giving an annual award or scholarship.

It's easier to get publicity if it's in an area that the media already covers. Ride on the coattails of a national trend. Also note upcoming events that will most likely generate publicity, such as charity events, tournaments and expositions. Find a way to connect with these activities either by volunteering, becoming a sponsor or donating your services. Then send press kits to the media. Check the newspaper for headlines that can be related to your services. Once you have developed an interesting angle, call the newspaper and offer your comments. Let them know you are available as a source for future related articles. Follow up this phone call with a letter, including your business card, the Rolodex-sized card and a brochure.

My philosophy is that not only are you responsible for your life, but doing the best at this moment puts you in the best place for the next moment.
— Oprah Winfrey

To get a mention in the media such as a listing in the calendar of events, a press release will suffice. If you want to announce a new location, additional staff, or an award, keep it simple and short. Some publications have a special section that highlights individuals and businesses in terms of being new, a change in status, relocation, staff additions, employee promotions and awards. These are usually 20 words or less. So, if you know what you want it to say, don't make it too wordy, lest you run the risk of the editor omitting crucial data. Send a black and white, head and shoulders photo along with the press release.

Press Releases

Your chances of capturing a media representative's interest in what you're doing are greatly increased if the press release can be quickly assessed. Presentation is crucial with press releases—so make certain yours are typed (double-spaced) on high quality paper, preferably letterhead; and that they conform to the preferred format standards of source information, the release date, a headline, the body and the conclusion. Keep your wording clear and conversational. Avoid using jargon.

See pages 337-338
Figures 9.18 and 9.19
for Sample Press Releases.

One page press releases work best. If it's more than one page, follow these guidelines: type "(more)" at the bottom of each page—except on the last page: type "End" or "30" or "###" after the final paragraph on the last page; and staple the pages together. After you have typed your press release, double check to make sure that you have included important dates, times, locations and contact numbers. Then proofread, proofread and proofread again.

Press Release Components

Source Information: Name, company, address and phone number. Put this in the top left-hand corner of the page.

Release Date: If the story or announcement can be printed as soon as it's received, type "For Immediate Release." If you want it posted on a specific date, type "For Release, Monday, October 7." In general it's best to have press releases that state

The influence on others must proceed from one's own person. In order to be capable of producing such an influence, one's words must have power, and this they can only have if they are based on something real, just as the flame depends on its fuel.
— The I Ching

"For Immediate Release." Otherwise you take the chance of the media representative putting it aside and forgetting about it. Place the release date below the source information and to the right side of the page.

Headline: This is a succinct summary of the content of the release. Word it in such a way that you put the information that would capture your reader's attention first, without making it sound like hype. Always type the headline in bold capital letters. Two examples of headlines are: "**FREE WORKSHOP ON INFANT MASSAGE**" and "**MELISSA BLUMENTHAL, NATIONALLY RENOWNED SPORTS PSYCHOLOGIST, HAS JOINED TOUCH, INC.**" Place the headline below the release date and center it between margins.

Body: This contains the details about the release. The first paragraph should be a concise statement, expressing the most important features first. Cover who, what, where, when, why and how. Use separate paragraphs for additional information or supplemental material. Write it in the "inverted pyramid style," as newspapers refer to it. That means placing the most important information at the top, as they cut from the bottom up. It's wise to use a multiple paragraph composition for the body because the space allotted for news stories and press releases constantly varies. This way, if they have extra space and you've provided them ample material, they will use it. Conversely, if their space is limited, it's easy for them to locate and use the vital information.

Conclusion: A separate paragraph indicating the action you want the reader, listener or viewer to take as a result of reading or hearing your story or announcement. You might type, "Call 555-5555 for more information" or "Stop by our Grand Opening on Saturday, October 12 from 10 a.m. to 2 p.m."

Figure 9.18   Sample Massage Press Release

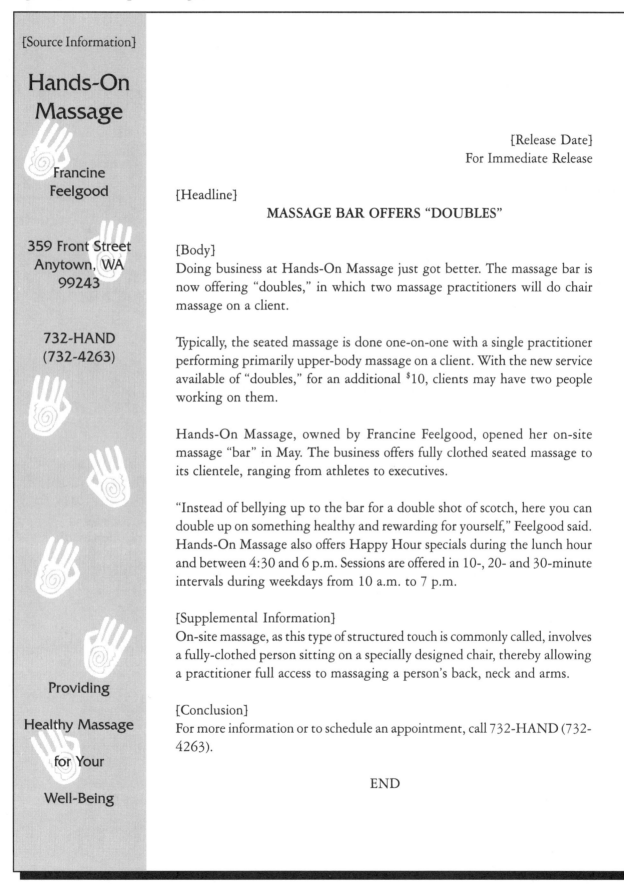

Hands-On Massage

Francine Feelgood

359 Front Street
Anytown, WA
99243

732-HAND
(732-4263)

Providing

Healthy Massage

for Your

Well-Being

[Release Date]
For Immediate Release

[Headline]

MASSAGE BAR OFFERS "DOUBLES"

[Body]
Doing business at Hands-On Massage just got better. The massage bar is now offering "doubles," in which two massage practitioners will do chair massage on a client.

Typically, the seated massage is done one-on-one with a single practitioner performing primarily upper-body massage on a client. With the new service available of "doubles," for an additional $10, clients may have two people working on them.

Hands-On Massage, owned by Francine Feelgood, opened her on-site massage "bar" in May. The business offers fully clothed seated massage to its clientele, ranging from athletes to executives.

"Instead of bellying up to the bar for a double shot of scotch, here you can double up on something healthy and rewarding for yourself," Feelgood said. Hands-On Massage also offers Happy Hour specials during the lunch hour and between 4:30 and 6 p.m. Sessions are offered in 10-, 20- and 30-minute intervals during weekdays from 10 a.m. to 7 p.m.

[Supplemental Information]
On-site massage, as this type of structured touch is commonly called, involves a fully-clothed person sitting on a specially designed chair, thereby allowing a practitioner full access to massaging a person's back, neck and arms.

[Conclusion]
For more information or to schedule an appointment, call 732-HAND (732-4263).

END

Figure 9.19   Sample Press Release for a Laughter Workshop

[Source Information]

Hands-On Massage

Francine
Feelgood

359 Front Street
Anytown, WA
99243

732-HAND
(732-4263)

Providing

Healthy Massage

for Your

Well-Being

[Release Date]
June 9, 2001

[Headline]

FREE LAUGHTER WORKSHOP

[Body]

A free workshop focusing on the benefits of laughter as an effective stress-reduction tool will be held Thursday, June 26 at 3 p.m. at Hands-On Massage, located at 359 Front St.

"People don't often take time out for themselves, a primary reason so many of us are stressed out," said Francine Feelgood, who is sponsoring the event. "Taking a break helps us do everything better. I really believe laughter is a tonic of life, so I want people to have a good laugh on us."

[Supplemental Information]

Hands-On Massage, with two "bars" in town, offers chair massage, involving a fully-clothed person sitting on a specially designed chair and being massaged on the back, neck and arms. Sessions are offered in 10-, 20- and 30-minute intervals during weekdays from 10 a.m. to 7 p.m. at its 359 Front St. and 62 Prescott Way locations. Along with happy hour specials, the business also offers "doubles," in which two practitioners work on a client, and recently began offering free 15-minute sessions to people celebrating their birthday.

[Conclusion]

To register for the workshop, to receive more information or to schedule an appointment, call 732-HAND (732-4263).

###

The Press Kit ~~~

If you want to be interviewed in print or on the air, send a press kit. Most health care providers get interviewed as a feature segment, but if you are requesting an interview in connection with an event, it can become news coverage. Press kit components include: a cover letter or press release; fact sheet; photograph; biography; brochure; business card; and supplemental information such as articles written about you or similar businesses, pamphlets stating the benefits of your services and a listing of previous media coverage. If your hook entails involvement with another event, include a stat sheet on the event. Papers can easily get misfiled, so it's wise to include identification such as company name, subject matter, contact person and telephone number on each piece of material. Ideally, put the information in a folder and enclose it in a 9"x12" envelope. Label the envelope "Press Kit" or "Media Kit" and then have it mailed or hand delivered.

The unwritten rule is: always put photographs on the left side of the press kit.

Cover Letters

The purpose of a cover letter is to grab the media representative's attention so he will read the rest of the material in your press kit. State who you are, your hook, what you are sending and ask for action. Ideally, this letter contains 100 words, but never more than 200 words.

Press Releases

(Please see previous section.)

Fact Sheets

Ensure accuracy by always including a one-page fact sheet that includes important, concise information. I use the following four categories: history, founder, awards and today.

History encompasses the technical information about the company, such as what the practitioner does, a mission statement and length of time in business.

Founder contains information on the health care provider's professional background. Some practitioners may wish to combine the history and founder categories.

Under the **Awards** category, list honors received.

The **Today** category gives a bit more information on the practice and lists statistics such as the number of current clients, type of work she has done recently, hours and any new announcements.

Biographies

This is a short biography of you and your practice. It's more conversational in tone than the fact sheet and includes the following: your philosophy; a description of the types of people you work with; the modalities you use; and special equipment and products you incorporate. Keep the length to two double-spaced pages. Some people omit the biography if their brochures contain this information.

Photographs

Put a caption describing the photograph and identifying all parties. This can be placed on the back or the front border.

Photographs convey a visual representation of who you are. Get professional publicity photos taken by a photographer. Most publications prefer black and white prints; it's also wise to keep a stock of color photos. Always put your name and phone number on the back of the photograph. If you are being profiled or listed under announcements, the publications often use the photo you send. When a reporter is doing an in-depth interview, they usually bring along a photographer.

Stat Sheets

Whenever your hook involves another event or includes a connection with a newsworthy company, provide the media with a stat sheet. Stat sheets are one-page summaries. They outline the event/company background (e.g., mission statement, inception date), highlight activities and list important dates, names and phone numbers.

Getting Interviewed ~~~
Print Coverage

Never underestimate the power of the written word. Many businesses have blossomed as a direct result of print publicity. Print media ranges from large daily newspapers to neighborhood weeklies, magazines, newsletters and specialty publications. Each publication has several departments, often with different editors. Some of the most common departments of interest for health care providers are: business, education, events calendar, features, health, community outlook, news and sports.

Research all the local publications. Familiarize yourself with their styles, the types of articles they run, and the people profiled. Find out the names of editors and reporters for each department so you can send your publicity materials to the appropriate people. Plan your publicity campaign well in advance. Some publications, particularly magazines, have a long lead time between getting material and having it printed.

Call the person in charge of the department where you would like coverage. Find out about their deadlines and preferred submission format. Be prepared to convey the essence of your story in 30 seconds. Then make certain that your press kit or press release is in the reporter's hands within 24 hours of your call. Call to confirm the material was received, and ask if the reporter needs any other information from you.

If the publication is unable or unwilling to write an article about you, then find out what the article submission guidelines for the publication are, and write the article yourself.

Guest editorials are spots for either individuals or representatives from a group to offer their opinions on major controversial issues. This is a good forum to educate the public about health care concerns—particularly if something has occurred within your community that doesn't support alternative care.

Most reporters do their interviews on location (e.g., your office or home). Occasionally they will meet you in a public place. At the end of the interview, give the reporter a copy of your fact sheet to ensure that the vital information (e.g., names, numbers and statistics) gets correctly conveyed.

There's no such thing as "off the record."

After you've been interviewed, send a short thank-you note to the reporter, stating how much you enjoyed the experience. Once the interview is published, send another follow-up. This time go into a bit more detail about one or two specific things (e.g., "I really appreciate the way you captured my philosophy by..."). Close the note by inviting the reporter to feel free to contact you in the future on this subject or similar topics.

Air Time

Radio and television interviews are great fun and can significantly enhance your public image. At the very least you'll be more recognizable to the general public after a television appearance. News programs, short features, talk shows, special programs and public service announcements are types of available air time.

Observe various programs to determine which ones would be the most suitable for your message. Cable television offers more opportunities than commercial stations. You can also produce or host your own show. Ascertain the following information for each show: program title, focus, day and time aired, producer's and host's name. Call the station to find out who would be the appropriate recipient of your proposal. As with print coverage, when talking with the producer/host, ask about preferences for being approached, how much time you should allow to elapse before doing follow-up and deadlines. Give a 30-second highlight of your story and make certain that all follow-up materials are received within 24 hours.

Once you are slotted to appear on a TV or radio program, watch or listen to the show at least once beforehand. This is imperative for television shows so you can see what the set looks like from the audience's perspective. It also affords you the opportunity to notice the style of clothing the host wears, the positioning of the chairs and whether the cameras tend to do full-length body shots or mainly head and shoulder shots. Note the backdrop color so you don't wear similar-colored clothing—or else you will literally fade into the background. Watch the host's interviewing style: Is there active participation in the discussions? Do questions encourage lengthy responses or does the host tend to dominate the show?

Many talk-show hosts ask the guest to submit a list of suggested questions. While this may seem intimidating, it's a great opportunity for you to shape the program. It gives you the power to ensure coverage of the most salient points about yourself, your business and your profession. It also solidifies the message you wish to convey.

Have a friend or colleague coach you by asking the questions you submitted. This helps you clarify your responses so you won't fumble for words during the interview. Also have your coach toss in a few questions of her own, just to help prepare you for responding to unexpected or ignorant inquiries (particularly if it's a call-in show).

Find out well in advance the directions to the studio, determine how long it takes to get there and verify the time you need to arrive (which is earlier than the actual taping time). If it's a television show, find out if the studio plans to provide you with a hair and make-up artist. Ask when the show will be aired, if they provide a copy of the program and when it will be available for you to pick up.

Bring an extra shirt just in case you spill something or the pattern clashes with the host's attire.

When you go to the interview, bring a copy of the suggested questions, a fact sheet and any other supporting materials. When appearing on television wear rich, dark colors. Avoid all white or "busy" patterns like checks, intricate, small designs or broad stripes. Jewelry should be simple and not flashy or dangling. Women: Apply makeup a bit heavier than normal and make sure your lipstick has a matte finish.

After you've been interviewed, send a short thank-you note to both the host and producer. Once the interview is aired, send another follow-up note. This time when you close the note suggest additional topic and areas of your expertise that could be explored on future shows.

Watch the video and listen to the tape for evaluation purposes. Assess your strengths and challenges. Note how well and thoroughly you responded to the questions, your demeanor and any changes you want to make for future appearances.

Programs to Target

News Programs: Getting coverage on your local news program may be the most difficult because reporters tend to cover hard news. The most likely angle to demonstrate newsworthiness is related to emergency situations, such as volunteering your services at an event that's already scheduled to be covered (e.g., providing free biofeedback sessions to firefighters during a record-breaking fire season).

Short Features: These segments last less than 10 minutes and are often included within a news program. Increase your odds of coverage by tying in your business with another soft news event, such as a health awareness week, the Great American Smoke-Out or sporting events.

Talk Shows: Talk shows and live interview shows are excellent forums for introducing the public to your business and the benefits of your services. It's usually much easier to get coverage on a talk show than to arrange for a taped feature interview. Hosts are always looking for interesting guests. Some shows include audience interaction. As a health care provider, you have an abundance of information to share with the public. Plus, if the show is on television, you can give a demonstration. I know of a massage therapist who managed to give a demonstration on the radio. He brought in a massage chair to the station and worked on the deejays while they were on the air. They relayed their experiences (along with their oohs and aahs of relaxation) to the audience while the therapist described what he was doing and the benefits of massage. The station's phone lines were ringing off the hook.

Special Programs: These programs are devoted to your specific business, your profession or your area of expertise. They last from 15 to 60 minutes. Usually you are the sole guest but occasionally a producer will chooses a program topic and slates several interviewees. Panels are another option for theme-centered shows.

Public Service Announcements: Although these announcements are usually reserved for non-profit organizations, you can get your public service announcement broadcast if it provides information that benefits the community.

Calendar Announcements: These announcements are often handled by the person in charge of public service announcements. The event must be free for a business owner to get it announced.

Planning Your Publicity Campaign

Research media outlets and design your public relations plan at least six months in advance to get the best results. Timing is critical. Sometimes publications have deadlines months before the distribution date. In some instances it may take you months or even years to get coverage.

In the spring of 1994 I decided to test myself and see if what I've been telling people about getting coverage still held true. In the first three months following my initial contacts I was interviewed by one newspaper, appeared on two television shows, interviewed on one television news program and was a guest on one radio program. The next five months generated another newspaper interview, three more television shows and four radio programs. In January 1996, 20 months after the original contact, I was profiled in a magazine.

Publicity coverage can dramatically increase your success. The disadvantage of utilizing publicity to build your practice is the lack of control. You can never be certain if or when you will get coverage or if the coverage will portray you the way you desire.

Be sure to coordinate activities to follow up your media coverage. Arrange workshops, introductory seminars and open houses to take place within three weeks and then two months after a scheduled publicity coverage.

How to Contact the Media

The mail, telephone, fax machines, e-mail and personal delivery are all useful means to approach the media. The method chosen depends on the newsworthiness of your materials and the media representative's interest in them. Some will prefer to talk with you first and others defer until they've seen your press kit. When you are confirming the media contact's name and address, you can ask the receptionist if she knows how the contact prefers to receive information.

Don't alienate the media by not playing according to their rules. Also don't hesitate to ask them what their rules are—although most of them follow certain guidelines, everyone has their own peculiarities and preferences. The most important thing to remember is to be patient, polite and courteous.

See pages 346-347 **Figures 9.20 and 9.21** for Sample Media Pitch Letters.

Mail

Mailing materials is the most common and generally preferred method to approaching the media. The major problem is the plethora of mail they receive. Call to confirm receipt of your press release or kit within two days after it should have arrived. Send the materials to a specific person. If you are unable to get the name, address it to the relevant department (e.g., city desk editor, calendar editor or evening news producer).

Time the mailing of your releases so they are appropriately received. Some publications have a deadline date of several months before printing. Daily newspapers prefer lead time of least one week in advance of the date you want the announcement to appear.

Another suggestion to get feedback is including a stamped, self-addressed reply postcard. List the following questions: Are you planning to use this information? If so, when? Do you want more information? If so, what? Would you be interested in receiving materials of a similar nature in the future? Comments?

Telephone

At some point the media has to be contacted by telephone, either to make an initial contact or a follow-up call. Always find out first if the journalist/producer/host is free to talk. Then be brief and straight to the point. Find out which is preferred: talking about the story over the phone or sending (or resubmitting) written materials first. When making an initial contact, you are more likely to generate interest if you have several potential angles to your story.

Persistence Pays!

Your Initial Phone Call Might Go Something Like This:

"Good morning, I'm Liza Montoya from Healing Touch Massage. Is this a good time to talk? I'm participating in a fund raiser for Health Awareness Week. I'm offering free demonstrations on self-massage techniques as well as donating five gift certificates for massages. Stress is the leading cause of illness, and massage is one of the best methods for reducing stress. I think your readers/listeners/viewers could greatly benefit by becoming more aware of the steps they can take to reduce stress and learning some simple self-massage techniques."

Sample Follow-up Script to Media Pitch Letter:

"Good afternoon, this is Liza Montoya from Healing Touch Massage. Is this a good time to talk? I'm calling about the press kit I sent, highlighting the Health Awareness Week fund raiser in which I'm participating. Health Awareness Week is approaching quickly and I was just wondering if there is any other information I can send you about myself or the fund raiser?"

> **Sample Follow-up Script to Media Pitch Letter**
>
> **(3rd or 4th Follow-up Call):**
>
> *"Good afternoon, this is Liza Montoya from Healing Touch Massage. Is this a good time to talk? We spoke several weeks ago about you interviewing me. You seemed very interested, particularly after you received my materials. We were going to discuss Oriental therapies, including techniques to relieve pain, such as headaches. Since we last talked, an article about ways to de-stress your life appeared in* Prevention *magazine. Taking personal responsibility for your well-being is a hot topic and the information I can provide fits in well."*
>
> **If Contacting the Print Media Say:**
>
> *"If you are unable to do a feature, I would be willing to submit a written article."*

For events that you would like covered remind the newspapers, radio and TV stations the day before or the morning of the event.

Faxes

While faxed materials are acceptable many people do not like to receive uninvited faxes. Plus, they never look as nice as materials printed on your letterhead. Use faxes for press releases but not press kits. When you call to confirm the name of a specific recipient, ask if that person likes to receive faxed press releases or prefers them mailed. Fax machines are more commonly used for sending follow-up materials and press releases that only request an announcement be made.

e-mail

Like faxes, e-mail is becoming more commonplace but you can lose a lot of the emphasis of design layout (e.g., paper texture and color), and text italics and bolding if it isn't sent as an attachment. The positive aspect is that your release won't need to be retyped, so a harried reporter with space to fill might choose to publish your release out of convenience.

In Person

Deliver your publicity materials in person to the media outlets that are the most important to you. The receptionist usually takes the materials; occasionally you will be able to talk with the reporter/editor/host. If you are able to talk with the right person, be brief and to the point. Do not expect the person to be able to conduct the interview right then.

Post Coverage Follow-up

Whenever you get press coverage, send a thank-you note to the reporter who covered the story. Send thank-you notes to the host and producer whenever you appear on a show. It also never hurts to send a quick thank-you to the appropriate editors when your press releases get published. Acknowledgment is a vital element in building rapport. The greater your level of rapport, the more likely your next story will get the attention it deserves.

Figure 9.20   Sample Print Media Pitch Letter

Healing Touch Massage
321 W. Prickly Pear Way
Needles, CA 92363
619-555-1212

April 4, 2001

Alice Adams
The Desert Daily
111 Arid Lane
Needles, CA 92364

Dear Ms. Adams,

Americans are constantly looking for new ways to feel and look better. This search has contributed to a multi-billion dollar health-food/vitamin industry. Instead of focusing on the newest, flashiest product to emerge in the marketplace, I'd like to propose an alternative viewpoint.

Massage is one of the best methods for reducing stress and increasing circulation, providing the recipients with an easy, affordable manner in which to feel good. Touch has been around since the beginning of time; therapeutic touch has been in practice for thousands of years.

My name is Liza Montoya. I am a licensed massage therapist, in practice for six years. I specialize in Oriental therapies such as acupressure and shiatsu. I find that many people are fascinated by this approach to well-being. I believe your readers would benefit by increasing their awareness of wellness alternatives. I could also provide them with information on specific pressure points they can work themselves to relieve pain, such as headaches. If we do this as an interview, I could also arrange for you to watch a session and/or receive a treatment. This would provide you with a more direct experience of the work.

I've enclosed my brochure, some information on shiatsu, a fact sheet, a copy of an interview in which I was featured and a photograph.

I will call you next week to see if you are interested. I look forward to talking with you soon.

Sincerely,

Liza Montoya

Liza Montoya
enclosures

Figure 9.21   Sample Television Pitch Letter

Healing Touch Massage
321 W. Prickly Pear Way
Needles, CA 92363
619-555-1212

September 11, 2001

Chad Evans
KTXZ
123 Broadcast Avenue
Needles, CA 92361

Dear Mr. Evans,

Hello! This is Liza Montoya. I am writing to follow up on our conversation this morning. I think I would make a great guest for your HealthBeat program. Americans are constantly looking for new ways to improve their well-being—contributing to a multi-billion dollar health-food/vitamin industry. Massage is one of the best methods for reducing stress and increasing circulation, thus providing the recipients with an easy, affordable manner to feel good and lead a happier, more productive life.

I am a licensed massage therapist, in practice for six years. I specialize in Oriental therapies such as acupressure and shiatsu. I find that many people are fascinated by this approach to wellness and I believe your viewers would enjoy learning about this modality. I could also provide them with information on specific pressure points they can work themselves to relieve pain, such as headaches.

I've enclosed my brochure, some information on shiatsu, a fact sheet, a copy of an interview and a photograph.

I will call you next week to see if you are interested in booking me for your show. I look forward to talking with you soon.

Sincerely,

Liza Montoya

Liza Montoya
enclosures

• Community Relations •

Refer to Chapter Four, page 56

for more ideas on goodwill and community relations.

Community relations increase your visibility and enhance your image, but only if it's clear you are doing the activities to serve the community and not just to build your business. You can cultivate these relations by: devoting your time and services to a charity or community organization; assembling a disaster relief team; giving presentations in public schools (career day, health education week); sponsoring an activity such as "adopt a highway" or a "massage-a-thon" for a special cause; developing a newsworthy persona outside of being a health care provider; hosting your own radio show or public access cable show; giving free demonstrations; sponsoring a public interest program; and becoming a spokesperson for your profession (or even other activities you are involved in such as hobbies, sports or civic organizations).

Fund Raisers

One of the easiest ways to gain visibility and promote your practice while doing good is to donate your services for fund-raising events. Target the appropriate groups according to your purpose (be it for professional advancement or personal gratification).

There are two ways of spreading light: to be the candle or the mirror that reflects it.
— Edith Wharton

One idea is to choose a charity that has special meaning to you and donate a day's revenues. Send announcements to your colleagues, clients and the media informing them of the designated day and date. Depending on the type of service you provide, you could hold this "event" in a public place (check with your local zoning and licensing board first). You can make it a regular event such as once a quarter or even once a month.

Another option is to announce to your clients that for every specified dollar amount (say $50) they donate to your favorite charity, they get a free treatment (such as a half-hour session or an adjunct service). Caution: Communicate up front the exact services you are offering. You may qualify recipients by requiring a copy of the check *and* a receipt for proof. It's a good idea to notify the charity and even the media.

If one of your major goals is to increase your visibility in the community, donate your services to events that are attended by people in your target market or those that are highly publicized. For major fund raising events, make certain your donation is substantial enough to be considered one of the top prizes: this increases the likelihood of you being included in all the various types of promotions, advertising and media coverage.

• Cooperative Marketing •

Cooperative marketing is a great solution to overcoming marketing reluctance. By combining some of your marketing tasks with others, you not only save time and money, you also generate a powerful synergy; the creative process is significantly enhanced by additional input. Also by pooling your resources, you may be able to afford more imaginative, elaborate, expensive and long-term marketing projects—there's strength in numbers.

The three most common types of cooperative marketing alliance are: practitioners who offer the same service to different markets; the same service to the same market; and different services to the same market.

Cooperative marketing doesn't just make better use of your promotional budget. Some of the most dreaded aspects of marketing become less of a chore when you don't have to do them alone. For instance, even though public speaking is one of the most effective means of promotion, many people are so uncomfortable being in front of a group, they don't schedule any speaking engagements. Presentations, seminars and demonstrations are much less intimidating and make a greater impact when done by two people. It isn't necessary to do everything by yourself!

As much as most practitioners claim they do not believe in "competition," I find that very few actively share in marketing their practices. Many are unwilling to even brainstorm ideas with their colleagues for fear of someone else successfully implementing their plans. We need to alter this scarcity consciousness.

A great way to ease into working with other practitioners is to do a small-scale promotional activity. You can increase the magnitude of your co-ventures as you build confidence in yourself, your co-marketers and the process.

Costly promotions such as mass mailings, booths at conventions and display advertising become affordable when shared by several people.

See Chapter Three, pages 41-43 for tips on risk taking.

Same Service—Different Markets

The following are hypothetical samples of triads of health care providers that specialize in the same modality but work with diverse target markets:

Acupuncturists: one mainly works with people in recovery programs, another targets the geriatric population, the third works with people with disabilities.

Rolfing® practitioners: one targets construction workers, another works with physical therapy clients, the other works mainly with athletes.

On-site seated chair massage therapists: one works on hair stylists, one targets attorneys, the other works with car salespeople.

Hypnotherapists: one targets other health care professionals, another works with abuse survivors, the third works with corporate executives.

Marketing Ideas

In developing a marketing plan with other practitioners that provide the same service to a different market, concentrate on broad-based promotions. Some avenues to consider are:

Any activity becomes creative when the doer cares about doing it right, or better.
— John Updike

- Share a booth at conferences, health fairs and expositions. Don't limit your exposure to just the traditional venues; consider participating in home shows, business expos, state and county fairs, and community art festivals.
- Advertise in local publications and perhaps even on the radio or television.
- Co-write an article and submit it to your local publications.
- Contact the media to do interviews.
- Give presentations to the general public.

Same Service—Same Markets

The best time to join forces with others who provide the same service to the same target market is when the market is too big for you to handle yourself. A common instance is when you contract to provide services for a large corporation. Depending on the size of the company, you may even need numerous practitioners. Another similar situation arises when you are working with a specialty group such as an athletic team.

Marketing Ideas

The joint promotions to consider are niche-oriented and include activities such as:

- Submit proposals to corporations for your services.
- Send direct mailings to specific groups of people.
- Give in-person or video presentations.
- Volunteer at athletic events.
- Sponsor an athletic or charitable group (e.g., underprivileged children).

Different Service—Same Markets

One of the most effective means of cooperative marketing is between providers of different services (and products) to the same market. In this case let your market determine the people to gather in your joint ventures. Review your target market profiles to assist you in compiling this list. The following examples give you an idea of the possible ways to match specific markets with the appropriate service providers:

- Most athletes could use the services of a massage therapist, sports physician, personal trainer and hypnotherapist.
- People active in personal growth might be interested in seeing a massage practitioner, Rolfing® practitioner, hypnotherapist, counselor and aromatherapist.
- Pregnant women might assemble a health care team consisting of a massage therapist, midwife, gynecologist, Lamaze instructor and nutritionist.

Unique pairings can generate a lot of attention, so extend your combined promotional efforts to include other businesses—not just adjunct health care providers—who share the same markets. Some examples are: health food stores, restaurants, educational organizations, hair salons that use natural products, bookstores, specialty clothing shops and cultural groups. You can let your imagination run free in creating promotions to reach the same target market. The following examples demonstrate the scope of possibilities.

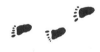

A candle loses nothing of its light by lighting another candle.
— James Keller

Marketing Ideas

- Design health-care/well-being packages for businesses and special interest groups. In addition to the standard health care providers such as massage therapists, counselors, chiropractors, and physicians, consider including a vendor of ergonomic devices like chairs or pillows, a new age bookstore for relaxation tapes and self-improvement products, a health food restaurant to supply healthy snacks and a biofeedback specialist for stress management.

- Place cooperative advertisements in local publications. If you are in a professional building or shopping complex, get together with the business owners to do joint advertising for bringing people to your location. You can also sponsor an open house for the public, advertising free demonstrations, music, munchies and door prizes.

- For those who are not conveniently located next to one another, consider sharing advertising to promote the benefits of each other's services. This might include health care providers and related businesses. A recent advertisement in my community paper displayed a chiropractic service, a massage therapist and a bookstore.

See Chapter Six, pages 157-162 for "Partnership" guidelines.

- Sponsor an event such as a fund raiser for a local charity or a health awareness day. If possible, participate in events such as major races by providing a booth for refreshments or your services.

- Design a special flier that describes the services, products and benefits of the people involved in the cooperative venture. Another possibility is to combine your separate promotional materials into one packet and send a direct mailing to potential clients.

- Co-sponsor seminars on health-related topics. For example, develop a stress management workshop with a counselor, aromatherapist and a new age bookstore.

- Create packages for celebrations: holidays, birthdays, "thank-goodness-tax-season-is-over" and anniversaries. For example, you could put together a Valentine's Day special that includes dinner, flowers, music and massage for two.

Cooperative marketing provides you with the means to expand the scope of your promotional ventures. Also, your marketing endeavors will be more successful, fun, and less risky if you participate with others in joint activities.

Begin now to develop a working relationship with at least three other people—one person from each category. Start out with small projects—until you feel confident about your ability to work well together. Create an alliance proposal that includes the purpose, priorities, goals, financial outlays and interaction expectations.

Cooperative Marketing Exercise

- List at least two people who do similar work as you but target different markets.
- List at least two people in allied fields who share your market.
- List at least two people in totally different businesses who also share your target market.
- List at least three marketing projects that would be a lot more fun to do with others.

• Companies that Market for You •

Almost every person I know in a service business—health care providers, artists, restauranteurs and consultants—wish that someone could handle their marketing. This reluctance to market oneself can be a major block to success—but it doesn't have to be. Many companies offer products, workshops and services to teach health care providers how to better market themselves and to assist them in achieving their goals.

In addition to assistance some companies provide marketing services for health care providers. These services range from obtaining client referrals to job placements to coordinating cooperative marketing ventures to supplying clients.

Evaluating Marketing Services

Over the next few years there will be a dramatic rise in the number of services and products made available to assist health care providers in their marketing. Besides the nationally-oriented service companies, there is tremendous growth potential for companies specializing in marketing on a statewide, regional or even citywide basis.

Assessing the relative value of any given company involves researching the company, evaluating the cost for services provided and determining if the presentation and activities of the company complement your image.

The initial research is important to make companies accountable for what they claim. Request copies of the following materials: health care provider recruitment brochures;

marketing materials given to prospective clients; and a list of marketing ventures (including the actual dates) with samples of ads. If the company offers a published directory, get a copy of it. If they don't want to just give it to you, offer them a fee which can be deducted from the service contract if you decide to sign up. After you've collected the materials, contact at least three other members for their feedback about the organization.

Evaluate the fit. Ask questions to determine their experience, philosophy and knowledge of your industry. It's imperative that you trust them and are able to communicate well. Find out if their marketing efforts tend to target a specific type of client, type of health care service or geographic area. Check to see if the promotions and advertising done by the company address your specific target markets. If not, determine if they are at least compatible.

While reviewing their marketing materials, ask yourself the following questions: Do you like the types of marketing the company does? Does it match your image? Does this fit in with your current marketing plan?

Consider the activities for which you might be responsible. For instance, will your contract require you to make presentations, volunteer at events or post fliers around town? Are you comfortable with the other members?

If you've decided that the marketing company is compatible with your values and goals, evaluate the cost. Unfortunately, this is not a very straightforward task, particularly if the company is new and has not collected success statistics.

If you think you can, you can. And if you think you can't, you're right.
Mary Kay Ash

Questions to Consider

- Does the company's marketing endeavors adequately cover your geographical area? For instance, even if a company takes out advertisements in national publications, what are they doing on a local level?
- Can you afford to do this?
- Can you afford not do to this?
- How much would it cost to do similar marketing yourself?
- Can you more effectively organize local practitioners into cooperative ventures?
- Does this complement your marketing plan?
- Would it be a better use of your time and money investing in other marketing activities?

In deciding upon whether to invest in any particular marketing company, calculate the number of sessions or new clients it would take to pay for this service. Nothing is risk-free, so I suggest that if you feel the potential reward is worth the risk, do it. Successful marketing involves a myriad of activities; don't tie up a significant portion of your marketing budget in any one method.

These types of marketing companies can be of great support in supplementing your current marketing endeavors and in essence become part of your marketing team. Keep in mind that if you hire the services of marketing companies, they are only one venue. It's not wise to rely upon services like these to totally fill your practice.

Also realize that just because a company is young and might not have a substantial track record yet, it still can be a good choice. All companies have to be a "start-up" at some point.

The potential down side to utilizing the services of a marketing company is that they might not do what they claim and they usually aren't personal. People tend to choose health care providers (particularly for long-term work) out of an experience of the practitioner either directly or through a personal recommendation. While these types of services can be extremely helpful in augmenting your practice, ultimately *you* are the best person to market yourself.

•Choosing a Graphic Artist•

The major promotional expense most health care providers incur is the design and production of business cards, brochures and other visual promotional materials. Rarely is this process an easy one; most of us "non-artists" don't know how to communicate well with people in the graphics or printing industry.

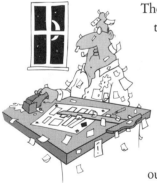

The first step is finding a good graphic artist who can take your ideas and transform them into exquisite printed materials. With the advent of desktop publishing, many people are calling themselves graphic artists when in reality they are adept word processors—they can make type look good on a page and even insert your artwork in an attractive manner; a true artist can turn your basic concept into a magnificent finished product.

To select an appropriate graphic artist get recommendations from your colleagues. Interview prospective artists. Look at their portfolios. Find out the types of clients they have. Ask if they have ever worked with any health care providers in general and your field specifically.

After choosing an artist, give the artist a sample session. One of the best brochures I had was designed by a graphic artist who was also a client. Since he had a direct experience of me and my work, he was better able to translate that into a brochure.

Some people are clear about what they want in their promotional pieces (particularly brochures), while others don't even know where to start. You save yourself considerable time and money if you are able to give your artist all (or most of) the written material. (Graphic artists are not necessarily advertising copy geniuses.) Be certain that the design and content of your promotional pieces are appropriate for your target markets, establish your credibility and focus on the benefits you provide.

Occasionally, things just don't work out and you need to cut your losses and find another artist. Personalities and communication styles don't always mesh.

Anecdote

For example, when I returned to Tucson in the mid-1980s, I realized it was time to redo my brochures for my coaching and training practice but I wasn't exactly sure what I wanted. I decided to go to a highly acclaimed public relations and advertising company. I met with the director, shared with him the "feel" that I wanted and submitted the basic copy (which needed significant editing—it was four pages long). I also gave him a description of my current clientele and target market: small business owners, mostly women between ages 25 and 55, with busy lifestyles, working in health care, retail, restaurant and other service industries. Well, when I received the first draft of my brochure, the cover had a caricature of a male golfer hitting a hole-in-one. They obviously did not understand my market or what would appeal to them. It was at this point that I should have found another design firm. But, I thought that if we communicated more, they would understand what I wanted and do a great job (after all, they were an award-winning company). Alas, that didn't occur. Even though they technically fulfilled their agreement and produced a brochure template, I never used it—the brochure just wasn't right.

Contracts ⚘

Most of the dissatisfaction involved in designing promotional materials stems from three areas: the final product not matching your expectations, the project taking longer than anticipated and being charged more than you budgeted. The one step you can take to avoid misunderstandings is to create a written contract that clearly delineates the job and the responsibilities of both you and the artist. Include these details:

- A precise description of the project (e.g., design a two-color brochure with at least two photos and one graphic image; create gift certificates; design layout for office sign; and alter current letterhead, envelopes and business cards to match new brochure).
- A listing of the major steps involved and the person responsible.
- A timeline of target dates for all of the major phases and the final date of completion.
- A description of what exactly you are to furnish.
- A detailed estimate of the cost (including what constitutes possible additional charges—for instance, how many alterations are included in the base price).
- Clarification of who actually "owns" the artwork. If you do not put this into your agreement, you may discover (to your dismay) that you are only able to use items such as a logo on the specific materials designed by the artist.

- An explanation of how the final work will be done: Will you be given the final printed product, a computer disk or camera-ready art? If you are given art, will you be provided with color separations, and will the work be typeset or computer generated?

If the artwork is from a computer, define the image resolution you desire. Most laser printers output at 600 dpi (dots per inch). Graphic artists usually have printers with 1200 dpi resolution (the higher the number of dots, the sharper the image). For example, most artwork that is printed directly to film uses 1200 to 2400 dpi. This industry is changing so rapidly—you can even take your final copy on computer disk to a service bureau and they can output the information at 1200 dpi (the cost per page ranges from around $2 to $15—depending on whether you want the artwork printed on paper or film).

- A recourse policy if either party fails to meet stated responsibilities (e.g., the artist is three weeks late or you dislike the final product).

If you have concerns or ideas, don't wait to express them until you receive the final proof. Keep in mind that you can renegotiate along the way. If you or the artist decide to alter something, make sure you are advised of the possible repercussions in terms of time and cost. If a lot is involved, put it in writing so both parties continue to have a clear idea of each other's expectations. You may decide the proposed change is not worth the cost.

Your printed marketing materials are your major promotional tools. They should be attractive, and effectively communicate who you are and the benefits of your service. When you find an artist who is in sync with you and able to convert your ideas into graphic images, invest the time in developing and nurturing that relationship—it can be invaluable to your career.

• Marketing Ideas from A to Z •

A

- Acknowledgments: Always thank the person, company or organization that refers a client to you. Make sure to acknowledge others when they have been a help—either in writing or with a small token of appreciation.

- Adopt-a-Highway: This is an excellent tool to increase visibility, but it can backfire if you don't keep the area clean. If you are a one-person business, consider joining with others. The highway sign could say "This road sponsored by the Associated Reflexologists of Santa Cruz." Make a banner (with your company name and number) that you can affix to the reflective garments you wear while cleaning the road. Post a sign in your office that says, "Proud sponsors of Highway 101."

- Advice Column: Write an advice column regarding your field for a local publication. Not only is this educational, it builds your credibility by demonstrating your degree of expertise.

- Announcements: Inexpensive promotional tools to enhance your visibility and keep you connected. Send out postcards to your current clients and choice prospective clients to announce special offers, speaking engagements and changes that occur in your practice (e.g., the addition of new staff, a change in status, the incorporation of innovative techniques or equipment).

- Answering Machines/Voice Mail: Necessary for communication with clients when you are busy. Keep your message welcoming and short; they are a good method of keeping clients informed of your status (as long as the message is current).

- Answering or Appointment Services: Some people appreciate human contact more than a machine. Be sure the service is reliable and accurate. Appointment services can be a boon to your practice; they must have up-to-date status of appointment times.

- Articles: Write articles for magazines, newspapers, trade journals, in-house publications and newsletters published by other organizations.

- Assumptions: Don't assume anything when it comes to your clients; find out by asking them. Making assumptions is one of the most detrimental actions taken in business as well as in personal affairs.

- Attire: You and your staff represent your business. Clients develop an attitude about your business based upon the way you look at work (e.g., slovenly appearance equals slovenly service).

- Auctions: Donating services/products for silent and not-so-silent auctions provides you with free advertising and support for your community.

- Audio Cassettes: Can be used effectively and inexpensively as talking brochures or as a means of instructing clients on how to do homework (e.g., visualizations, affirmations, exercises and stretches). As something unique you can also reply to correspondence or inquiries by audio tape.

B

- Bags: Imprint bags with your company name, logo and position statement. Many people reuse bags, so your information gets seen repeatedly.

- Bake Sales: Sponsoring or participating in local fund raising events, such as bake sales, helps promote you as an active member of your community and gets your name out to the public. You can even sell healthy baked goods at your office and donate the proceeds to charity. Be creative! Make cookies, cakes and cupcakes in the shapes of hand, feet or a full body.

- Banners: Not only can these have your name, but your slogan and/or logo to be used at a booth or special event.

- Benefits: Donating services/products as door prizes gives you free publicity and says you are interested in helping in your community.

- Billboard Advertising: Seen by many people and is a good way of informing the public about you and your services. Look for high traffic locations such as well traveled main streets and intersections. Keep your copy short and to the point.

- Birthday Cards: These cards demonstrate your concern and thoughtfulness. You can really make a client's day by enclosing a coupon for a free treatment or product.

- Board Meetings: If you sit on the board of any organization, regular attendance and participation can lead to opportunities for marketing your services and products.

- Book Signings: Co-sponsor a book signing at a local bookstore by a respected author in your field. Meeting the buying public and establishing rapport with the bookstores' sales staff is crucial for authors.

- Booths: Many companies design booths that are inexpensive and portable. Booths accord you a quick and easy-to-find location for malls, health expos and local events.

- Breakfasts: Volunteering to speak at local business "breakfast" clubs is a "free" marketing tool. Having breakfast with potential networking associates is a great way to start your day.

- Brochures: Provides overall information about your business. Include logo, slogan, mission statement, methodology, expertise, *benefits* and a photo of you.

- Business Cards: More than just your name, address and phone, it's a visual representation of you and your business. It can become a mini-brochure describing some of the benefits of your services/ products. Set a number of cards to distribute in a certain period of time (e.g., 250 cards in one week) and go into stores, professional offices and just pass them out to people you meet on the street). Give a magnetized business card to each new client and every guest at your open houses and public speaking events. Most people put them on refrigerator doors where they are regularly seen, which makes them much more effective than a business card that gets relegated to a drawer.

- Business Plan: Your business plan is the road map to your success. A thorough business plan has a marketing plan built into it.

C

- Catalogs: For those who sell products or offer training programs, catalogs are excellent marketing tools. Feature each item and its benefits. Look into bulk mailing rates for cost savings.

- Celebrations: Celebrate milestones (e.g., opening, moving, anniversary, 100th client) and invite your clients, colleagues and prospective clients to celebrate with you. Provide refreshments, music and fun.

- Canvassing: Take brochures, cards, fliers or circulars around to area businesses letting them know you are there, who you are and what you can do for them. Distribute information to your target markets.

- Circulars: Make circulars informative, short and easy to distribute on car windshields, to use as bag stuffers, post on bulletin boards and place on counters.

- Classified Ads: There are many possible places to place ads such as newspapers, trade journals, magazines, local business and health papers and event programs (e.g., tournaments, concerts, fund raisers).

- Cleanliness/Neatness: A messy or dirty environment spills over in concept for clients to the way you conduct business and provide services. Fortunately, so does being clean and neat.

- Client Calls: Clients like to know they're appreciated and cared about. Follow-up calls are essential.

- Client Contact: Each minute spent with a client is a marketing minute. To make those minutes work for you provide excellent service, improve your relationship and offer helpful products.

- Client Names: We all know how good it feels when people we work with remember our name and use it. This demonstrates that they are important, cared about and acknowledged.

- Clinics: Offer clinics (hands-on, educational workshops) on your specific service or general wellness. In addition to clinics you host offer them in conjunction with other activities such as sporting events, tournaments, health fairs and store celebrations.

- Columnists: Some write stories or series of articles on health related issues; find out about the columnists in your area and propose an interview or provide information to them.

- Comment Cards: Give your clients the opportunity to voice their opinions about you and your company. Include one in your Welcome Kit, stack them in the waiting area and mail them to all your clients at least once a year.

- Community Calendars: Various organizations, radio stations, and Public TV provide calendars of events for the community. If you are sponsoring or participating in a public event or conducting a seminar, have it posted on the various community calendars available in your area.

- Competition: If you cannot fulfill a client's request (other than ones that may be illegal or unethical), or feel that another service/practitioner would best suit a client's needs, refer them to your "competition" so they can be served. They will remember you had their best interests in mind and not just your pocketbook.

- Computer Bulletin Boards: Local computer groups have bulletin boards where members can post information about themselves and their services. Membership is usually free.

- Computerized Telemarketing: This is the age of "surfing the net." Having a "home page" with your services and products opens the "world" to you and you to the world. Take advantage of the technology available to expand your visibility and your network.

- Conferences: Attending or participating in service/product related conferences is another form of marketing and public exposure. Again, use that booth you designed to your best advantage.

- Connections With Others: Let other related businesses know you will display signs and have information available in your office if they will do the same for you.

- Consultations: A free consultation gives you the opportunity to demonstrate your expertise, answer questions and hand out information. Also, offer free services for local special events.

- Contests: People love to play games! Contests bring attention to your business and add names to your mailing list. It's best to get people to come to your business to enter.

- Convenience/Speed: Make it easy and fast for clients to do business with you. Time is valuable to both you and those you serve.

- Coupons: Terrific for marketing to prospective clients (e.g., 50% off the first visit) and rewarding loyal ones (one free session after each 10 visits). Coupons do not cheapen your practice if they are tastefully done. Many health care providers (e.g., dentists, optometrists, chiropractors and touch therapists) offer introductory specials.

- Create Heros: Whenever an employee does something exceptional or a client reaches a particular milestone in treatment, celebrate their accomplishment and give them something tangible such as a certificate.

- Credit Cards: Making it easier for people to pay, makes it easier for them to buy.

D

- Days/Hours of Operation: Keep them consistent as much as possible for optimum dependability. You increase your chances for success if your hours and days of operation are more convenient for clients than your competitors' schedules.

- Decor: First impressions are important. Your office should reflect your identity and create an atmosphere where clients feel comfortable, safe and relaxed. Add a festive touch by coordinating flowers, signs and holiday displays.

- Demonstrations: Allow prospective clients to see/experience first hand what your services and products are all about first hand.

- Dinners/Lunches: After letting people know who you are through introductory letters, postcards and other marketing tools, follow-up with a call, an appointment or get together for dinner/lunch. Don't just "do" dinner/lunch; get to know each other, explore common goals in your fields and determine how you can assist each other.

- Direct Calling: Speaking directly with potential clients, other professionals, networking associates and your clients adds the personal touch to your marketing strategy.

- Direct Mail: Postcards, fliers, catalogs, notices and announcements are inexpensive methods of staying in communication with your clients.

- Direct Mail Coupons/Card Packs: Coupons are given to and compiled by companies and mailed to target markets; participants share in the mailing costs.

- Direct Referrals: Referring clients directly to other professionals is one of the strongest threads in networking and is usually reciprocal. Setting up a network of related services and products is one of the best tools for effective business growth.

- Directories: Take out listings in appropriate directories. Publish a directory of local allied health care providers to be given away at major events, mailed out in promotional campaigns and distributed to other health care providers.

- Discount Sales: Giving a discount can help a prospective client decide to try your services and products. Used for rewards, introductions and referrals.

- Display Kudos: Frame and display any press, complimentary letters and awards where they can be seen. This allows others to see your dedication and service to your profession. If you have too many to display at once, rotate them regularly.

- Distribution: Given the products you sell, utilize as many methods of distribution for sale as possible to gain the widest spectrum. The same applies to distributing information about services and products.

- Donate Services to Charities: Even donating an hour a week to a charity or community cause creates goodwill and word-of-mouth marketing.

- Door Hangers: Effective tool for reaching potential clients when your target market is geographically based. It must convey immediate action (e.g., "Get rid of that nagging backache today!"). Inspire the recipient to give you a call by offering a discount, invitation to a seminar or free educational literature.

E

- Emergencies: Coordinate an emergency response team of health care providers to be ready during tough times like floods, hurricanes, fires or blizzards.

- Expos & Health Fairs: Participating in these events is an excellent venue for networking: gives you exposure to other professionals in your field as well as their products and services; provides an opportunity to meet potential clients; and makes use of that booth you created.

F

- Fax Machines: Another piece of equipment that optimizes your ability to communicate and disseminate information in a timely manner. You can fax appointment reminders, announcements and press releases.

- Flea Markets: This is a place where you can reach large numbers of people while demonstrating your products and services (and utilizing that booth).

- Fliers: Used for short announcements about upcoming events, sales and changes in service; whatever is happening with your business that the public needs to know about. In addition to posting them around town mail at least 25 per week to prospective clients.

- Free of Charge: Once in awhile, do something free of charge for your clients; perhaps a modality such as a hot pak or upon seeing they are enjoying having their feet rubbed, let them know and give them an extra five minutes.

- Frequent Buyer Cards: Offer an exclusive discount on products or services) to frequent clients. Give a free session or product after a set number (e.g., "Your 11th session is free!") or dollar amount of purchases.

G

- Gifts: Instead of always giving candy or food as gifts, help enrich someone's mind with a book, inspirational bookmark or a mug with a meaningful message. Establish goodwill and loyalty by giving small gifts to employees for work well done or that extra mile they go for you.

- Gift Certificates: Wonderful way for clients to share their experience with others and a great marketing tool for you (e.g., a gift certificate for a session on a client's birthday!). Keep in mind that the profit isn't generated from the sale of the certificate, but from the subsequent sessions.

- Golf Resorts: Post a sign offering a free session to members who have made a verifiable hole-in-one.

- Grand Openings: This is a "grand" way of letting people know who you are, where you are and what you are all about.

- Greeting Cards: These are a good method of connecting with clients, networking associates and referring professionals just to wish them good tidings.

H

- Health Clubs: Submit a proposal for the health club to purchase gift certificates to give as an incentive to new members who pay in full upon initiation or when members reach a milestone goal.

- Holidays: Decorate your office to match the holiday, offer special discounts for holidays and give specialty gifts (e.g., cinnamon-scented oil for Thanksgiving, sports bottles for the Summer Solstice).

I

- Introductory Letters: Send letters to allied health care providers to develop mutual referrals. Send at least two letters each week until you have amassed your desired network.

- Introductory Seminars: The focus is introducing your services/products to prospective clients. Having introductory prices available helps fence sitters make a move in your direction.

- Invitations: Can be verbal, hand-delivered or mailed. Invite people to see your facilities, come to a free demonstration or call for information. Warmly given or nicely printed on paper, make sure your offer is inviting.

J

- Jargon: Avoid using jargon unless you are certain your market/clients know the terminology.

- Jingle: Create a catchy tune and phrase that easily identifies your company (particularly for radio and television advertising).

K

- Keynote Speeches: Advise your professional associations and community organizations that you are available as a keynote speaker.

- Kiosk: Post promotional materials on kiosks at malls, colleges and pavilions. Check for regulations first.

- Kites: Design a kite with your logo and fly it prominently.

- Knowledge is Power: Ascertain your current and potential clients' needs, desires and goals.

L

- Lectures: Giving lectures on your service/products provides credibility to you as a professional, educates the public and becomes a vehicle for sales.

- Little Things: Make doing little things for clients a matter of business policy. These little things help establish client loyalty.

- Location: This is an important component to the success of a business. A poor location can break a business even if your service and products are good. If you are in an area that is inconvenient or unsafe, people will seek out other providers.

- Logo: A graphic representation of your business that helps people quickly recognize your company.

M

- Mailing Lists: Keep accurate and up to date. Include clients, prospects, practitioners, networking associates and companies/individuals in related fields. Trade lists with others who provide services or products to your target markets.

- Memberships: Join professional associations, business groups and service organizations.

- Mistakes: We all make them and the best way to handle them is with no excuses—just plain honesty. Create a "goof gift" to give to clients when you or a staff member makes a mistake.

N

- Networking: A very important part of marketing; join networking organizations, community service organizations, clubs; and participate in community special events. Networking is a great way to establish trust and build professional relationships.

- Newcomers Welcome Kit: Include several business cards, brochure, pertinent information, product samples and educational/promotional materials on the benefits of your services/products.

- Newsletters: Used as a consistent marketing tool, they establish your expertise and educate the public. Newsletters can also be sent to other health professionals and potential clients for marketing purposes. Another idea is to write articles or place ads in other's newsletters.

- Newspaper: Submit opinion pieces, articles, letters to the editor, press releases and calendar listings. Get a newspaper reporter to interview you. Also place display and classsified ads.

O

- Open Houses: Hold quarterly and special holiday open houses for colleagues, businesses in your community, prospects and clients.

- Order Forms for Product Sales: Have these available for quick, impulse sales as well as for those who like to ponder. The elements to successful product sales are quality, availability and convenience.

P

- Painted Cars/Car Signs: Provides great coverage as you go through your day; draws attention as it's unusual to see unique, eye-catching things on cars.

- Package Deals: Putting together packages for services and products that save clients money can improve sales without increasing marketing costs.

- Pamphlets: Detailed information about you, your services, philosophy, mission statement, benefits, specific techniques and health tips.

- Park or Street Bench Advertising: Another underutilized method of reaching the general public. Place ads on benches that are seen by your target markets (e.g., in front of stores they patronize).

- Parties: Plan theme parties such as "Fluid Motion" and decorate the place with pictures of sea creatures (or stuffed toys), play ocean music and show videos of underwater life moving gently, easily and fluidly. You can also have clients sponsor parties where you demonstrate your services to their friends.

- Pens: Pass out imprinted pens to clients, colleagues and people involved with your target markets.

- Personalized gift items: Also known as premiums and specialty advertising. Keep an assortment of inexpensive, fun, useful items to give away.

- Phone Attitude: How the phone is answered can either foster or damage a relationship. Remember warmth, enthusiasm and helpfulness are key marketing tools. "Yeah, what do you want? I'm tired and you're bothering me" attitude doesn't work!

- Postcards: Fast, easy and inexpensive method of reminding clients of follow-ups, appointments, announcements or just saying hello. Also a good technique for generating new clients.

- Posters: Have posters made to put in windows or on bulletin boards at related businesses (e.g., health food stores, sports facilities and fitness clubs).

- Press Conferences: Generally used by large companies and firms in order to relate information affecting the general public.

- Press Releases: Short statements for publication (in magazines, newspapers, newsletters and journals) or broadcast (radio and television) regarding your services, products and publications. Advise your "net" of exciting events such as hiring someone, forming an association, expanding your services, adding new equipment, hosting an open house or facilitating a workshop. Also send press releases to clients and colleagues.

- Pricing: One of the main factors clients use in choosing services/products. Find out what the going rates are in your area and set your prices accordingly.

- Professional Journals: Not only a good place to advertise, but also to write articles and make yourself known. Writing adds to your credibility as a professional.

- Public Awareness Campaign: Join with other people in your specific field and create a public awareness campaign through advertisements, articles, interviews and public speaking.

- Publicity: Inform the media about anything newsworthy concerning your business.

- Public Service Tie-In: Sponsor events such as the blood donor mobile unit, police fingerprint unit for children or fire department home safety seminars.

- Public Speaking: Give talks at business associations, clubs and public service organizations. Join an organization like Toastmasters to learn platform speaking techniques and gain confidence.

Q

- Qualify: Design your marketing materials so that they actually pre-screen clients.

- Quotes: Use quotes from people who are prominent within your target market.

R

- Radio: An advertising medium that reaches large numbers of people. Take an ad, sponsor a program, become a guest speaker on local talk shows or host a health care talk show.

- Raffles and Prizes: Providing services/products for special events for raffles and prizes helps in getting your name out to the public.

- Receptions: Often given to welcome and introduce new employees, associates and mergers.

- Referral Networks: Essential as a marketing tool; not only benefits you but provides the opportunity for you to assist others with their growth and prosperity.

- Referral Cards: These cards encourage clients to promote your practice. Traditional referral cards offer the recipient a discount (e.g., $10 off the initial session). If you really want to inspire enthusiasm from your clients, offer them the same discount whenever a card is redeemed.

- Refreshments: Offering healthy tidbits (e.g., bottled water, juice, tea, fruit) to clients creates an atmosphere of warmth and caring. A small gesture as this can produce a dramatic effect.

- Reprints: Advertising is costly and articles appear in print only once. You can inexpensively reprint them so they're available for mailings, handouts and signs.

- Restaurants: Place a display with your cards and brochures next to the cash register (and put coupons from the restaurant in your waiting area).

- Retreats: Either sponsor a retreat or provide your services at retreats held by local companies and associations.

- Reunions: Attend class reunions and let people know what you are doing. Host a reunion for all your clients who have completed a treatment course.

- Rewards/Incentives/Gifts: Submit proposals for companies to offer your services for customer or employee rewards. They could offer certificates for sales incentives, to honor employees of the month, to use as premiums with their customers and to give as holiday gifts for employees (it's certainly classier than a gift certificate for a frozen turkey).

S

- Sandwich Boards: Directs the public to your products and services at your location. Make sure they are colorful and easy to read from a distance.

- Satisfied Customers: One of the most valuable marketing tools is a customer who is satisfied with your quality of service and its value. They are your greatest ally and the impetus for your word-of-mouth campaign.

- Scholarships: Sponsor an academic or sports scholarship for children, young adults or members of your target markets.

- Scripts: Providing your employees with scripts for various circumstances helps guide them in representing your business to its optimum and aids in deterring the disasters "winging it" can create.

- Searchlights: A flashy, unique way to direct people to your location and draw attention to a special event.

- Seminars: Establishes you as an authority in your field, lends credibility, provides a catalyst for your services and products, and educates the public.

- Service: One of the main reasons clients select and stay with a business. Good or poor service means client retention or loss and ties directly into marketing through word-of-mouth.

- Shopping Cart Signs: Many people are in a hurry and stressed when shopping—especially after work. Create a sign that makes them think about how good they would feel after utilizing your service/products.

- Sign Language: Learn to communicate in sign language so you can offer services to the hearing impaired.

- Signs (Inside): Hang signs and posters announcing specials. Also emphasize services such as "Gift Certificates Available."

- Signs (Outdoors): Your sign should be clear and large enough to be easily seen. Include your logo if economically feasible. Your location sign needs to be easily and quickly identifiable.

- Skywriting: How often do you see writing in the sky? Gets your attention, huh?

- Smiles/Greetings/Goodbyes: Rarely thought of as a marketing tool, yet reflect on how often you go back to a business where no one smiles, greets you warmly or says, "Good-bye, I hope we helped you and look forward to seeing you again."

- Solicitation Letters: Sent to prospective clients asking them to try your services/products or to professionals seeking mutual referrals.

- Special Events: Encourage publicity by being a sponsor of (or participating in) local events or holding unusual events at your place of business.

- Special Promos & Displays: Boost marketing efforts with "in-store" displays featuring your products, cards, brochures and fliers that explain your services and benefits. Attract business by providing discount fliers that can be redeemed at the time of the appointment.

- Sponsor an Event or Community Activity: Involves your business in the community and helps you meet potential clients.

- Sponsor an Athletic Team: Print T-shirts with your name and logo for the team to wear; show up at the games to support your team; and display a sign in your office that says, "Proud sponsor of the ABC Cycling Team!"

- Sporting Events: Volunteer your services at local sporting events, senior and special Olympics.

- Statement Stuffers: Include information about specific products or services whenever you send out statements to clients. You can also place your brochure in other people's billing statements (just make sure they go to your target markets).

- Stationery: A visual representation of your business; make sure it conveys your desired image.

- Surveys/Questionnaires: Great way to get the "pulse" of your clients and discover what you are doing right and what needs to be changed: find out what clients want, like, dislike and their opinion of your services.

- Sweepstakes: Another interactive method of calling attention to your business and getting additional names for your mailing list.

T

- Television: Become a guest on local television shows. Place commercials which demonstrate your services and/or products and their benefits—fully utilize the dynamics of music, words and pictures.

- Testimonials: Nothing hits home like personal accounts of the success of your products and services; use in marketing tools, advertising and seminars. Always use full names and if possible the title, company and city.

- Theme Festival: Band together with nearby businesses and hold a gala event such as "Spring Festival" or "Winter Warm-Ups."

- Theme Week: Devote a week to a particular activity (e.g., Mobility Week) and set up activities centering on mobility issues. Coordinate with your local government to sponsor city-wide events.

- Toll-Free (800/888) Numbers: For those marketing products, giving seminars or conducting lectures, having a toll-free number gives prospective clients an additional reason to call, even if it's just for information. That information call can turn into a sales call.

- Tournaments: Volunteer short treatment sessions for participants. You can also sponsor a refreshment stand—just be sure you have a large display sign or banner. Offer free sessions to the winners or even propose that the tournament coordinators purchase a number of certificates to be given as prizes.

- Trade Directory: Advertise in local trade directories. They are usually the first place people look when they want your specific service and/or products.

- Trainings: Training other professionals establishes your credibility and expertise. They range from an evening class to a weeklong intensive training.

- Transit Advertising (buses, taxis, depots): Directs the public to your services and products as your image is driven all over town and seen by those who have to wait for their rides.

U

- Umbrellas: If you live in a rainy city, purchase a stock of umbrellas with your logo imprinted on them and loan/give them to clients who forget their own.

- Uniforms: Create a unique, professional image by putting your logo, position statement or favorite design on clothing.

V

- Vacation Nights: Sponsor a "health" vacation with guest speakers, activities, drawings and show slides (e.g., spa destinations, great places to hike and boat).

- Videotapes: A unique method of presenting and demonstrating your services and products which can be left with other professionals for marketing; have clients view them while waiting to see you; use as part of a proposal for a corporate contract; and show as an educational tool for the public.

- VIPs: Turn your customers into VIPs. Give them the opportunity to avail themselves of special sales and promotions.

- Voice Mail Services: Can be used as a primary message service or to back up an answering machine in case of mechanical failure.

W

- Welcome to My Office Kit: Send a welcome kit to all new clients as soon as they book their first appointment.

- Window/Store Front Displays: Create an inviting display showing your services or products; make it colorful and catchy to grab the public's attention and change it frequently. These can also be created at related businesses, not just your own. Some malls even rent "Window Display" areas in front of vacant stores or have special display alcoves.

- Word-of-Mouth: One of the most powerful resources for business; satisfied and dissatisfied clients talk and talk and talk....

- Workshops: Conduct workshops/classes in your area. Advertise in newspapers and local magazines, mail fliers and hang posters. Do free lectures which you can advertise at no cost by sending out Public Service Announcements (PSAs) to print media and radio stations.

- Writing Articles: Good method of demonstrating knowledge in your field, educating the public and making yourself known.

X

- X-Rays: If you are a chiropractor or dentist, offer free x-rays upon initial visit.

Y

- Yellow Pages: Used extensively by the public for locating services. Place your listing under the most logical category if you can only afford one listing, otherwise list under each applicable category.

Z

- Zoological society: Sponsor an animal or event at your local zoo. Sponsorships are often published in the society's newsletters and if the contribution is significant, the zoo might even place a plaque (with your name) on its premises.

• Marketing Schedule •

Invest at least 15 percent of your time in marketing activities to maintain your practice. To successfully grow your practice, you may need to spend two to three times this amount of time. The following sample marketing schedule is based on eight hours per week.

Marketing Schedule

Daily

- Give clients samples, premiums, educational materials and discount coupons for friends.
- Confirm the next day's appointments.
- Place three phone calls to prospective clients and follow-up calls to current clients.
- Demonstrate/incorporate at least one product per session.
- Review client files prior to each session.

Weekly

- Distribute 75 business cards, 50 brochures and 25 fliers.
- Call one allied health care provider to initiate an affiliation or to follow up.
- Attend one networking function.
- Spend at least one hour working on a long-term project.
- Contact one group regarding a future speaking engagement.
- Send birthday cards and notes to clients.

Monthly

- Spend at least two hours reviewing your marketing plan and doing research.
- Meet with a business support group twice.
- Send two letters of introduction to allied health care providers.
- Meet with two allied health care providers.
- Give two presentations.
- Send out press releases about your public speaking engagements.
- Donate services to your favorite charity.
- Tabulate information from Client Comment Cards and make necessary changes.
- Work with the media: send press releases and kits, do appropriate follow-up.

Quarterly

- Hold one open house, do a "party" and sponsor an event.
- Update client educational materials and rearrange the product display area.
- Send a newsletter to clients, colleagues and prospects.
- Offer some type of special promotion and do a cooperative marketing project.
- Read at least one practice-building book.
- Get interviewed by the paper, radio, television or specialty publication.

Annually

- Take part in at least two trade shows, fairs or expos.
- Send out a client survey.
- Attend at least one practice-building workshop.

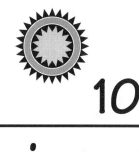

10

The Business Plan

• Introduction •

A business plan serves many functions and it can dramatically increase your chances of success. It's a powerful declaration of your goals and intentions, a written summary of what you aim to accomplish and an overview of how you intend to organize your resources to attain those goals.

Developing an effective business plan generally requires a considerable amount of time. You have to do a lot of honest thinking in addition to some technical research. If you have completed the exercises throughout *Business Mastery*, most of the groundwork is done!

If you are starting a practice, a business plan assists you in clarifying your vision, evaluating the marketplace, calculating your costs, forecasting your growth and determining your risks. For those of you who have been in business for a while, a new or updated plan can rejuvenate your practice.

A business plan addresses these issues: What are you offering? Who will your clients be? What needs do your services satisfy? How will your potential clients find you? How much money do you plan on making? What actions do you intend on taking to ensure success?

The odds of getting a loan from a bank are greatly increased if you submit a typed business plan. You will be perceived as a lower risk because it demonstrates your business savvy.

The major components of a business plan are a description of the business, the long-range and short-term goals, a financial forecast and a marketing plan. A business plan is a motivational tool for keeping you on track. It can be so easy to get caught up in day-to-day working and not take the time to plan the strategies to ensure future success, or become overwhelmed and miss opportunities.

Using a business plan as a reference keeps you focused. Inscribing how and what you want encourages you to be more realistic. It also assists you in anticipating and avoiding problems, or at least be prepared so that you can overcome them—thus minimizing your risks. Transcribing clearly stated goals gives you a basis for evaluating progress. In creating a business plan you become aware of the finances that are really required to start and maintain a thriving business.

Finally, by developing a business plan you may discover steps vital to your success and happiness that you may have otherwise been unaware of or overlooked.

The majority of work you have been doing thus far has set the stage for your business plan. The rest of this chapter is a business plan outline. Before you go to your journal or computer, scan through the chapter; this provides a sense of the direction and scope of the plan. Use this outline to refine what you have already written (by completing the exercises from the other chapters) and to clarify the other details that are requisites for your success.

When your business plan is complete, type it (or print it from a computer) and put it in a three-ring binder. This type of binder allows you to easily update your plan and add information (e.g., copies of reports and sample promotional materials). Plus this keeps all the major business documents in one place. If you are submitting the business plan for a loan, consider taking your documents to a print shop and having them copied and bound.

Outline Summary

• Business Plan Outline •

Cover Page ❦

The cover page is simply the first page of the business plan. Include a title (e.g., "Business Plan for The Healthy Alternative"), and below it put your name, address and telephone numbers.

Table of Contents ❦

The table of contents lists all of the business plan sections with corresponding page numbers. Title each document you include in the Appendix.

Owner's Statement ～

A one page description of the business and the owner. Include the following: the business name, address, phone numbers, fax number, e-mail address and website address; your name, home address, home phone number; a summary of your business experience and philosophy; and a brief business description (the year the business was established and current financial status).

Efforts and courage are not enough without purpose and direction.
— John F. Kennedy

Executive Summary ～

The executive summary consists of business plan highlights. This section is of critical importance if you are applying for financial backing; it must convince lenders and investors that your business will succeed. Although the summary appears at the beginning of the business plan, it's best to write it last (and keep it to three pages or less).

Purpose, Priorities and Goals ～

This section is a detailed description of your career plan. State your overall career purpose and at least six priorities; your long range (3-5 year) purpose, at least six priorities and at least two goals per priority; and your short term (1-2 year) purpose, at least six priorities and at least three goals per priority. Note: Many of these declarations assist you in being clear and motivated—and can be quite personal. You may want to censor some of these statements if you are submitting this plan for a loan.

The SMA Resource Directory contains hundreds of listings from product vendors to equipment manufacturers to business services to Internet contacts www.sohnen-moe.com

Business Description ～

This section provides background about your practice. Begin by writing a brief history of your company and your basic purpose/mission statement. Describe the following: the services you offer and products you sell; special product used; equipment; the physical location; and the unique features that distinguish your practice from others (e.g., experience, variety of services and techniques, pricing, location, outcalls, product sales, equipment, supplies, credit terms, management abilities and financial standing). If you sell products, include a product register with the suppliers' names, define your position in the chain of distribution and specify the types of clients who purchase products.

Include photographs of your office in your business plan portfolio.

Marketing ～

Marketing is the pivotal component of a business plan. Begin by depicting the image you wish to convey. Next describe your target markets and clarify your differential advantage. Follow with a competition analysis—including steps you'll take to meet any challenges.

The major section is the strategic action plan. Outline your marketing goals for all four areas (promotion, advertising, publicity and community relations). Delineate a timeline, budget and rationale for each strategy. If you sell products include a description and cost for the following: inside displays; additional sales staff (include training); equipment; and special promotions, discounts and sales.

Set a marketing budget per year. Tabulate the cost to market your services and the cost to market your products. Determine the total marketing costs and calculate the actual cost per potential client.

Close this section with a summary of how your marketing strategies will enable you to succeed.

Risk Assessment

Risk assessment is a demonstration of your ability to anticipate and manage risks. Detail the effects your competition has on all phases of your business. List possible external events that might occur to hamper your success: a recession, new competition, shifts in client demand, unfavorable industry trends, problems with suppliers and changes in legislation. Identify potential internal problems such as income projections not realized, long-term illness or serious injury. Then generate a contingency plan to counteract the most significant risks.

Financial Analysis

This section consists of statements about your income potential, fees, current financial status and financial forecast.

Determining income potential can be tricky. Contact your professional society or several of the major teaching institutions (for your specific field) to get this information. You may have to do some informal research because this data has not been compiled for every profession. Describe the existing business conditions. Where do you stand in the current "state of the art"? Describe the projections and trends for your specific profession (nationally and locally). List the average income for practitioners in your specific field (both nationally and locally) for the first six months of practice, the first year, the second year, and the third year. If possible, include the average number of clients for those same times.

List your service fees; including introductory offers, pre-paid package discounts, professional courtesy discounts and sliding fee scales. Enumerate the amenities to be absorbed in pricing (e.g., credit offered, out-calls, parking, consultations, extended business hours, educational materials, samples and supplies). Describe your competition's effect on pricing.

Determine the equipment, supplies and inventory needed for next 12 months, clarify your acquisition plan (buy, consign or lease) and prioritize the purchases. Calculate

It's never too late—in fiction or in life—to revise.
— Nancy Thayer

Genius begins great works, labor alone finsihes them.
— Joseph Joubert

how much money you'll need to open your business and the annual operations budget for each of the next three to five years. Generate this information from a computerized accounting program or use the following forms found in Appendix A: Start-Up Costs Worksheet, Opening Balance Sheet, Business Income and Expense Forecast, Monthly Business Expense Worksheet, Monthly Personal Budget Worksheet, and Cash Flow Forecast. Put the actual worksheets in this section or the appendix.

Calculate a break-even analysis. Determine at what client (or sales) volume your business will break even. This is the point where total costs equal total income. You may need to update this every few months to accurately reflect your business growth.

List your potential funding sources, describe exactly how you anticipate spending the money received and note how any loans are to be secured.

When you get right down to the root of the meaning of the word "succeed," you find it simply means to follow through.
— F. W. Nichol

Operations ~~~

This section is an overview of your business organization, procedures and policies. Identify the management qualifications needed to run the "business" part of your practice and assess your strengths and challenges.

For businesses that have a staff, list the various functions and estimate the number of people needed for each function. Describe the training required and state your compensation plan.

If you have a group practice, describe the various functions and the person(s) responsible. Indicate the level of authority for each person (e.g., hiring, firing, scheduling and purchasing).

Specify the legal form of ownership you've chosen and the reasons why. Cite the requisite licenses, permits and insurance coverage.

Write a brief overview of your company policies and procedures. Also include details on safety precautions. Determine your security needs (consider client screening, location safety, ample lighting for the parking lot and night travel) and develop a plan to reduce these types of risks.

Close this section with an accounting and control summary. Clarify who does the bookkeeping (you or another). Set a production schedule (e.g., daily, weekly, monthly, quarterly, annually) for the following types of management reports: checking account balance; service reports such as the total number of return clients or the number of clients in relation to the time spent per client; product sales reports; balance sheets; profit and loss statements; condition of client accounts; expense reports; insurance reimbursement aging; forecasting; and inventory reports.

The Business Mastery Supplement Sohnen-Moe Associates, Inc. This text-based disk for PC and Macintosh computers contains a 58-page sample massage therapy business plan in addition to the client correspondence and marketing letters.

Success Strategies ᷈

List your goals for developing your success strategies. Specify your methods for implementing your business plan and having a prosperous practice. Include activities such as developing strategic plans, creating monthly flow charts, identifying decision points, reviewing and revising your plans, creating a business support system, networking and choosing appropriate advisors.

I've got to keep breathing. It'll be my worst business mistake if I don't.
— Sir Nathan Meyer Rothschild

Appendix ᷈

The types of additional information or documents (if any at all) to be included in this section depend upon the nature of your business plan. If your business plan is mainly for your personal use, you may not need to add anything else. But if you intend on using your business plan to obtain financial backing, consider including the following data. This list is only a guide. Check with the specific lending institutions or investors to find out their requirements.

- Personal net worth statement.
- Copies of last two year's income statements and balance sheets.
- List of client commitments.
- Copies of business legal agreements.
- Credit status reports.
- News articles about you or your business.
- Photographs of your location.
- Copies of promotional material.
- Letters of recommendation from your clients.
- Key employee resumés.
- Personal references.

• Supplement •

If your business plan is to be used in securing a loan, it's recommended to incorporate the following additional information into the previous sections of the business plan.

The Executive Summary

- State the type of business loan(s) you're seeking (e.g., term loan, line of credit or mortgage).
- Summarize the proposed use of the funds.
- Calculate the projected return on investment.
- Write a persuasive statement of why the venture is a good risk.

The Financial Analysis

- Describe the loan requirements: the amount needed, the terms and the date by which it's required.
- State the purpose of the loan, detailing the facets of the business to be financed.
- Provide a statement of the owner's equity.
- List any outstanding debts. Include the balance due, repayment terms, purpose of the loan and status.
- Document your current operating line of credit—the amount and security held.

Add a Section Titled "References"

- List all pertinent information regarding your current lending institution: branch, address, types of accounts and contact person(s).
- List the names, addresses and phone numbers of your attorney, accountant and business consultant.

Appendix A

Wheel of Life

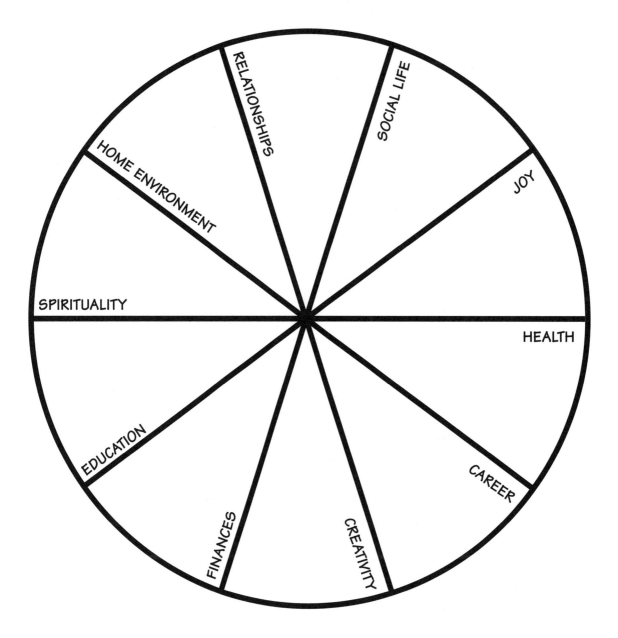

High Priority Activities

High priority activities are the "20 percent" ones that produce 80 percent of your results. Before you can begin to increase the time spent in those important activities, you must identify them.

Think about the various activities involved in your business. List at least ten of the most important things you do in the center column on the form below. Then in the left hand column rate them in the order you think is most important to your success. In the right hand column rate them in the order of how much time you spend in each activity.

Importance	Activity	Time Spent
_____	_____	_____
_____	_____	_____
_____	_____	_____
_____	_____	_____
_____	_____	_____
_____	_____	_____
_____	_____	_____
_____	_____	_____
_____	_____	_____
_____	_____	_____
_____	_____	_____
_____	_____	_____
_____	_____	_____
_____	_____	_____
_____	_____	_____
_____	_____	_____

The more you focus on your high priority activities, the more productive you will be. You may also discover some conflicts. If this happens, refer to your purpose, priorities and goals. They usually will provide direction. Sometimes you have to make difficult decisions and then either delegate the other activities, simplify them or eliminate them. It's also recommended that you show your list to a colleague. It's possible that you overlooked something or you may need to switch some of your priorities—and it's usually easier for someone else to be objective.

Daily Plan

Day/Date: _____

Purpose: _____

Priorities: _____

_____

_____

_____

_____

Goals: _____

_____

_____

_____

_____

Thought for the day: _____

_____

What supplies/information do I need? _____

_____

_____

_____

To Do List

Imperative:

_____

_____

_____

_____

_____

_____

_____

_____

Important:

_____

_____

_____

Desirable:

_____

_____

_____

What did I accomplish today? _____

_____

_____

Time Tracking Sheet

	Mon	Tue	Wed	Thu	Fri	Sat	Sun	Goal	Actual
Health/Exercise									
Play									
Reading									
Planning									
Phone									
Appointments									
Driving									
Promo/Networking									
Seminars									
Bookkeeping									
Proposals									
Client Files									
Repair/Maintenance									
Letters									
Follow-up									
Operations									
Meetings									
Volunteer									
Miscellaneous									
TOTAL									

Strategic Planning

Today's Date: _____ Target Date: _____ Date Achieved: _____

Purpose: _____

_____

_____

Priority: _____

_____

_____

Situation Description: _____

_____

_____

_____

Objective: _____

❑ Capitalize on this strength ❑ Change this condition ❑ Other: _____

Goal: _____

_____

_____

Benefits of Achieving This Goal: _____

_____

_____

Possible Courses of Action:

1. _____

_____

2. _____

_____

3. _____

_____

4. _____

_____

Best Course of Action: _____

_____

_____

_____

Proposal Outline:

1. _____
_____
2. _____
_____
3. _____
_____
4. _____
_____

Advantages:

_____
_____
_____
_____

Potential Conflicts/Disadvantages:	Solutions:
1. _____	1. _____
2. _____	2. _____
3. _____	3. _____
4. _____	4. _____
5. _____	5. _____
6. _____	6. _____

Action Required To Begin:

_____
_____
_____
_____
_____

Resources Needed:

_____
_____
_____
_____
_____

Specific Steps To Achieve This Goal	Target Date	Person Responsible
1. _____	_____	_____
2. _____	_____	_____
3. _____	_____	_____
4. _____	_____	_____
5. _____	_____	_____
6. _____	_____	_____
7. _____	_____	_____
8. _____	_____	_____
9. _____	_____	_____
10. _____	_____	_____
11. _____	_____	_____
12. _____	_____	_____
13. _____	_____	_____
14. _____	_____	_____
15. _____	_____	_____
16. _____	_____	_____
17. _____	_____	_____
18. _____	_____	_____
19. _____	_____	_____
20. _____	_____	_____
21. _____	_____	_____
22. _____	_____	_____
23. _____	_____	_____
24. _____	_____	_____
25. _____	_____	_____

Contact/Referral Records

Name: _____

Company: _____

Title: _____

Address: _____

Phone: (work) _____ (home) _____

Referred by: _____

Follow-up: _____

_____

_____

Notes: _____

_____

_____

_____

_____

Date	Time	Action/Outcome

Business Mileage Sheet

Date	Beginning Mileage	Ending Mileage	Total Mileage	Destination	Purpose

Bank Reconciliation Form

Balance   __/__/__
month   day   year   _____

Plus Receipts   _____

Less Disbursements   _____

Balance   __/__/__
month   day   year   _____

Balance Statement   __/__/__
month   day   year   _____

Deposits In Transit   _____

                                     _____

                                     _____

                                     _____

Plus Total Deposits In Transit   _____

Outstanding Checks   _____

                                     _____

                                     _____

                                     _____

                                     _____

                                     _____

                                     _____

                                     _____

                                     _____

                                     _____

                                     _____

                                     _____

Less Total Outstanding Checks   _____

Bank Balance   __/__/__
month   day   year   _____

Opening Balance Sheet

Date: _____

— ASSETS —

Current Assets

Cash and bank accounts		$ _____
Accounts receivable		$ _____
Inventory		$ _____
Other current assets		$ _____
TOTAL CURRENT ASSETS	(A)	$ _____

Fixed Assets

Property owned		$ _____
Furniture and equipment		$ _____
Business automobile		$ _____
Leasehold improvements		$ _____
Other fixed assets		$ _____
TOTAL FIXED ASSETS	(B)	$ _____
TOTAL ASSETS	(A+B=X)	$ _____

— LIABILITIES —

Current Liabilities (due within next 12 months)

Bank loans		$ _____
Other loans		$ _____
Accounts payable		$ _____
Other current liabilities		$ _____
TOTAL CURRENT LIABILITIES	(C)	$ _____

Long-term Liabilities

Mortgages		$ _____
Long-term loans		$ _____
Other long-term liabilities		$ _____
TOTAL LONG-TERM LIABILITIES	(D)	$ _____
TOTAL LIABILITIES	(C + D = Y)	$ _____
NET WORTH	(X - Y = Z)	$ _____
TOTAL NET WORTH AND LIABILITIES	(Y + Z)	$ _____

Start-Up Costs Worksheet

Item	Estimated Expense
Open Checking Account	$ _____
Telephone Installation	$ _____
Equipment	$ _____
Office (e.g, first & last month's rent, security deposit)	$ _____
Supplies (e.g, linens, books, folders, pens, stamps)	$ _____
Stationery & Business Cards	$ _____
Marketing	$ _____
Decorating & Remodeling	$ _____
Furniture & Fixtures	$ _____
Legal & Professional Fees	$ _____
Insurance (e.g., property, auto, liability, malpractice)	$ _____
Utility Deposits	$ _____
Beginning Inventory	$ _____
Installation of Fixtures & Equipment	$ _____
Licenses & Permits	$ _____
Professional Society Membership	$ _____
Other	$ _____
TOTAL	$ _____

Business Income and Expense Forecast

One Year Estimate Ending   month / day / year

— PROJECTED NUMBER OF CLIENTS —

For Your Services   _____

For Your Products   _____

     TOTAL NUMBER OF CLIENTS   _____

— PROJECTED INCOME —

Sessions $ _____

Product Sales $ _____

Other $ _____

     TOTAL INCOME   (A) $ _____

— PROJECTED EXPENSES —

Start-up Costs $ _____

Monthly Expenses (x 12) $ _____

Annual Expenses $ _____

     TOTAL EXPENSES   (B) $ _____

     TOTAL OPERATING PROFIT (OR LOSS)   (A - B) $ _____

     CAPITAL REQUIRED FOR THE NEXT 12 MONTHS $ _____

Monthly Business Expense Worksheet

Expense	Estimated Monthly Cost	x 12
Rent	$	$
Utilities	$	$
Telephone	$	$
Bank Fees	$	$
Supplies	$	$
Stationery and Business Cards	$	$
Insurance	$	$
Networking Club and Professional Society Dues	$	$
Education (e.g., seminars, books, professional journals)	$	$
Business Car (e.g., payments, gas, repairs, insurance)	$	$
Marketing	$	$
Postage	$	$
Entertainment	$	$
Repair, Cleaning, Maintenance and Laundry	$	$
Travel	$	$
Business Loan Payments	$	$
Licenses and Permits	$	$
Salary/Draw*	$	$
Staff Salaries/Payroll Expenses	$	$
Taxes	$	$
Professional Fees	$	$
Decorations	$	$
Furniture and Fixtures	$	$
Equipment	$	$
Inventory	$	$
Other	$	$
TOTAL MONTHLY	$	
TOTAL YEARLY		$

In most instances it's not wise or appropriate to take draw for the first 6-12 months.

Monthly Personal Budget Worksheet

	Estimated Monthly Cost	x 12
INCOME		
Income (Draw) From Business	$ _____	$ _____
Income From Other Sources	$ _____	$ _____
TOTAL INCOME	$ _____	$ _____
EXPENSES		
Rent/Mortgage	$ _____	$ _____
Home Insurance	$ _____	$ _____
Health Insurance	$ _____	$ _____
Utilities	$ _____	$ _____
Telephone	$ _____	$ _____
Auto: (payments, gas, repairs)	$ _____	$ _____
Food	$ _____	$ _____
Household Supplies	$ _____	$ _____
Clothing	$ _____	$ _____
Laundry/Dry Cleaning	$ _____	$ _____
Education	$ _____	$ _____
Entertainment	$ _____	$ _____
Travel	$ _____	$ _____
Contributions	$ _____	$ _____
Health	$ _____	$ _____
Home Repair and Maintenance	$ _____	$ _____
Self-Development	$ _____	$ _____
Outstanding Loans and Credit Card Payments	$ _____	$ _____
Miscellaneous Expenses	$ _____	$ _____
TOTAL EXPENSES	$ _____	$ _____
BALANCE (+/-)	$ _____	$ _____

Cash Flow Forecast

Month: _____ _____ _____

	Estimate	Actual	Estimate	Actual	Estimate	Actual
BEGINNING CASH $						
Plus Monthly Income From:						
Fees $						
Sales $						
Loans $						
Other $						
TOTAL CASH AND INCOME $						
Expenses:						
Rent $						
Utilities $						
Telephone $						
Bank Fees $						
Supplies $						
Stationery and Business Cards $						
Insurance $						
Dues $						
Education $						
Auto $						
Marketing $						
Postage $						
Entertainment $						
Repair, Maintenance and Laundry $						
Travel $						
Business Loan Payments $						
Licenses and Permits $						
Salary/Draw $						
Staff Salaries/Payroll Expenses $						
Taxes $						
Professional Fees $						
Decorations $						
Furniture and Fixtures $						
Equipment $						
Inventory $						
Other Expenses $						
TOTAL EXPENSES $						
ENDING CASH (+/-) $						

Weekly Income Ledger Sheet

Month _____ Day _____ Year _____ Page _____

Date	Client Name	Amt Paid	Ck #	Services	Products	Type	Location	Company	Notes

Service Income: $_____ Product Income: $_____ Total Income: $_____ # Sessions: _____ New Clients: _____ Ongoing: _____

Monthly Disbursement Ledger Sheet

Month _____ Day _____ Year _____ Page _____

Date	Description	Ck #	Amt Pd	Rent / Utilities	Maintenance / Telephone	Supplies / Postage	Marketing / Advertising	Travel / Auto	Furniture / Equipment	License / Dues	Education / Insurance	Books / Inventory	Bank Fees / Entertainment	Misc. / Draw
TOTAL														

Business Expenses Summary Sheet

EXPENSE	Jan	Feb	Mar	Apr	May	Jun	Jul	Aug	Sep	Oct	Nov	Dec	Total
Advertising													
Auto													
Bad Debts													
Bank Fees													
Depreciation													
Draw													
Dues and Fees													
Education													
Entertainment													
Equipment													
Furniture													
Insurance													
Interest													
Inventory													
Licenses													
Loan Payments													
Maintenance													
Parking													
Permits													
Postage													
P.O. Box Rental													
Printing													
Professional Fees													
Promotion													
Rent													
Repairs													
Staff Salaries													
Supplies													
Taxes													
Telephone													
Travel													
Utilities													
Other													
Other													
Other													
Other													
TOTAL													

Client Status Report

Name: _____ Date: _____

Please identify current problem areas in your body by drawing the appropriate symbols on the diagrams below.

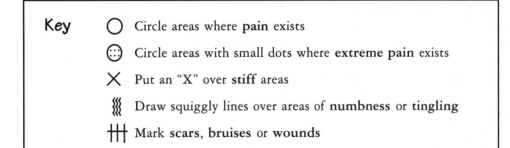

Key

○   Circle areas where **pain** exists

⊙   Circle areas with small dots where **extreme pain** exists

✕   Put an "X" over **stiff** areas

〰   Draw squiggly lines over areas of **numbness** or **tingling**

卌   Mark **scars, bruises** or **wounds**

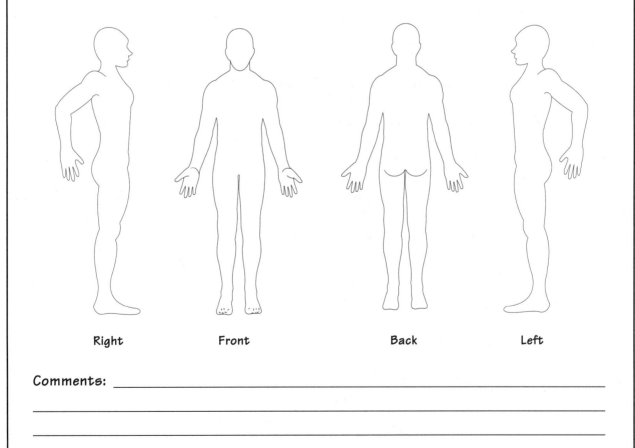

     Right   **Front**   **Back**   **Left**

Comments: _____

_____

_____

_____

_____

Client Health Information Sheet

Name:_____ Date:_____

Who referred you to this office? Name:_____

    ❏ Yellow Pages   ❏ Advertisement   ❏ Sign   ❏ Other: _____

Present symptoms: What is your major complaint or condition you want to improve?_____

_____

When did you first notice major complaints?_____

What brought it on?_____

_____

What activities aggravate the condition? _____

_____

Is this condition getting progressively worse?   ❏ Yes   ❏ No

    Please Explain:_____

_____

Does this condition interfere with work? ❏ Y ❏ N   Sleep? ❏ Y ❏ N   Daily Routine? ❏ Y ❏ N

    Please Explain: _____

_____

What have you done to get relief?_____

_____

Has there been a medical diagnosis?   ❏ Yes   ❏ No

    If so, by whom? _____

    Please Explain: _____

_____

Have you had X-rays taken? ❑ Yes ❑ No

If yes, by whom? _____

What are your intentions or expectations for this visit? _____

_____

_____

Are you now under medical/therapeutic treatment? ❑ Yes ❑ No

If yes, for what condition? _____

_____

_____

Please list your care provider's name and phone number: _____

_____

List any medications (including aspirin) and nutritional supplements you are taking: _____

_____

Describe the exercise activities you do (include frequency): _____

_____

List other therapies you receive: _____

_____

Please list (date and description) any accidents or operations: _____

_____

Please list any additional comments regarding your health and well-being: _____

_____

_____

_____

_____

Client Intake Form

Date: _____

Name: _____ Sex: ❑ Male ❑ Female

Address: _____

City: _____ State: _____ Zip: _____

Daytime Phone #: _____ Evening Phone #: _____

Social Security #: _____ Driver's License #: _____

Date of Birth: _____ Occupation: _____

Employer: _____

Employer's Address: _____

Marital status: ❑ Single ❑ Married

Children's Names and Ages: _____

Name of Spouse/Significant Other: _____

Preferred Appointment Day and Time: _____

Insurance Carrier: _____ Policy #: _____

ID #: _____ Group #: _____ Claim #: _____

Adjuster's Name: _____

Adjuster's Address: _____

City: _____ State: _____ Zip: _____

Telephone #: _____ Extension: _____

Time and Date of Insurance Verification: _____

Primary Health Care Provider: _____

Provider's Address: _____

City: _____ State: _____ Zip: _____

Telephone #: _____ Extension: _____

Permission to Consult with Primary Provider? ❑ No ❑ Yes _____ (please initial if yes)

In Case of Emergency, Please Notify:

Name: _____ Telephone #: _____

Relationship: _____

*Please note that if you are billing insurance companies, your clients will have to
fill out a claim form (most likely a HCFA-1500) that duplicates most of this information.

Client Intake Form

Date: _____

Name: _____

Address: _____

City: _____ State: _____ Zip: _____

Home Phone: _____ Work Phone: _____

Occupation: _____ Employer: _____

Date of Birth: _____ Marital Status: ❑ Single ❑ Married

Children's Names and Ages: _____

Name of Spouse/Significant Other: _____

Preferred Appointment Day and Time: _____

Referred By: Name: _____

     ❑ Yellow Pages ❑ Ad ❑ Sign ❑ Other: _____

What are your long-term skin care goals? _____

_____

What are your goals for this treatment? _____

_____

Present Symptoms: What is your major complaint or condition you want to improve? _____

_____

What activities and products have you used to address this condition? _____

_____

What activities or products aggravate the condition? _____

_____

What activities or products improve the condition? _____

_____

Are you under medical/therapeutic treatment? ❑ Yes ❑ No

    If yes, for what condition? _____

_____

Please list your care provider's name and phone number: _____

List any medications (including aspirin) and nutritional supplements you are taking: _____

_____

Specify any known allergies: _____

_____

Please list any additional comments regarding your skin care or general well-being: _____

_____

_____

Health History

Check the following conditions that apply to you, past and present. Please add your comments to clarify the condition.

Musculo-Skeletal
- ❏ Headaches
- ❏ Joint stiffness/swelling
- ❏ Spasms/cramps
- ❏ Broken/fractured bones
- ❏ Strains/sprains
- ❏ Back, hip pain
- ❏ Shoulder, neck, arm, hand pain
- ❏ Leg, foot pain
- ❏ Chest, ribs, abdominal pain
- ❏ Problems walking
- ❏ Jaw pain/TMJ
- ❏ Tendonitis
- ❏ Bursitis
- ❏ Arthritis
- ❏ Osteoporosis
- ❏ Scoliosis
- ❏ Bone or joint disease
- ❏ Other: _____

Circulatory and Respiratory
- ❏ Dizziness
- ❏ Shortness of breath
- ❏ Fainting
- ❏ Cold feet or hands
- ❏ Cold sweats
- ❏ Swollen ankles
- ❏ Pressure sores
- ❏ Varicose veins
- ❏ Blood clots
- ❏ Stroke
- ❏ Heart condition
- ❏ Allergies
- ❏ Sinus problems
- ❏ Asthma
- ❏ High blood pressure
- ❏ Low blood pressure
- ❏ Lymphedema
- ❏ Other: _____

Skin
- ❏ Rashes
- ❏ Allergies
- ❏ Athlete's Foot
- ❏ Warts
- ❏ Moles
- ❏ Acne
- ❏ Cosmetic surgery
- ❏ Other: _____

Digestive
- ❏ Nervous stomach
- ❏ Indigestion
- ❏ Constipation
- ❏ Intestinal gas/bloating
- ❏ Diarrhea
- ❏ Diverticulitis
- ❏ Irritable bowel syndrome
- ❏ Crohn's Disease
- ❏ Colitis
- ❏ Adaptive aids
- ❏ Other: _____

Nervous System
- ❏ Numbness/tingling
- ❏ Twitching of face
- ❏ Fatigue
- ❏ Chronic pain
- ❏ Sleep disorders
- ❏ Ulcers
- ❏ Paralysis
- ❏ Herpes/shingles
- ❏ Cerebral Palsy
- ❏ Epilepsy
- ❏ Chronic Fatigue Syndrome
- ❏ Multiple Sclerosis
- ❏ Muscular Dystrophy
- ❏ Parkinson's disease
- ❏ Spinal cord injury
- ❏ Other: _____

Reproductive System
- ❏ Pregnancy:
  - ❏ Current ❏ Previous
- ❏ PMS
- ❏ Menopause
- ❏ Pelvic Inflammatory Disease
- ❏ Endometriosis
- ❏ Hysterectomy
- ❏ Fertility concerns
- ❏ Prostrate problems

Other
- ❏ Loss of appetite
- ❏ Forgetfulness
- ❏ Confusion
- ❏ Depression
- ❏ Difficulty concentrating
- ❏ Drug use _____
- ❏ Alcohol use _____
- ❏ Nicotine use _____
- ❏ Caffeine use _____
- ❏ Hearing impaired
- ❏ Visually impaired
- ❏ Burning upon urination
- ❏ Bladder infection
- ❏ Eating disorder
- ❏ Diabetes
- ❏ Fibromyalgia
- ❏ Post/Polio Syndrome
- ❏ Cancer
- ❏ Infectious disease (please list)
  _____
- ❏ Other congential or acquired
  disabilities (please list)_____
  _____
- ❏ Surgeries _____
- ❏ Other: _____

For clients who need mobility assistance, please give your height: _____ weight: _____

Please list any additional comments regarding your health and well-being: _____

_____

I have stated all conditions that I am aware of and this information is true and accurate. I will inform the health care provider of any changes in my status.

Client's Signature: _____ Date: _____

Client Treatment Plan

Date: _____

Client: _____

Assessment: _____

_____

_____

_____

Goals: _____

_____

_____

_____

Client Preferences: _____

_____

_____

_____

Treatment Plan: _____

_____

_____

_____

Notes: _____

_____

_____

_____

_____

_____

Client Session Notes

Date: _____

Client: _____

Current Session Number: _____ Date of First Session: _____

Observations: _____

_____

_____

Goals for Current Session: _____

_____

_____

Description of Specific Techniques Used: _____

_____

_____

Were the Goals Achieved? _____

_____

_____

Goals and Notes for Further Sessions: _____

_____

_____

Other Recommendations to Client: _____

_____

_____

Comments: _____

_____

_____

Client Session Notes

Client Name: _____

Skin Analysis: Texture: ❑ Fine ❑ Medium ❑ Coarse   Hydration: ❑ Good ❑ Poor
                  Elasticity: ❑ Good ❑ Poor

Condition	Location	Date Noticed	Changes
❑ Sensitivity	_____	_____	_____
❑ Suntan	_____	_____	_____
❑ Couperose	_____	_____	_____
❑ Pustules	_____	_____	_____
❑ Milia	_____	_____	_____
❑ Clogged Pores	_____	_____	_____
❑ Anomalies	_____	_____	_____
❑ Hyperpigmentation	_____	_____	_____
❑ Hypopigmentation	_____	_____	_____
❑ Warts	_____	_____	_____
❑ Secretions	_____	_____	_____

Initial Treatment: _____

Treatment Administered: _____

_____

Products Used: _____

_____

Additional Recommended Services: _____

_____

Recommended Treatment Frequency: _____

Recommended Products: _____

_____

Subsequent Visits:

Date	Treatment	Results/Notes	Products Used

Sign-In Sheet

Welcome! Please inform us if you have had any changes to your name or address, have a new insurance company/policy, or additional information that might help us serve you better. Thank you very much.

Date: _____   Time   Changes ✓

1. _____   _____   _____

2. _____   _____   _____

3. _____   _____   _____

4. _____   _____   _____

5. _____   _____   _____

6. _____   _____   _____

7. _____   _____   _____

8. _____   _____   _____

9. _____   _____   _____

10. _____   _____   _____

11. _____   _____   _____

12. _____   _____   _____

13. _____   _____   _____

14. _____   _____   _____

15. _____   _____   _____

16. _____   _____   _____

17. _____   _____   _____

18. _____   _____   _____

19. _____   _____   _____

20. _____   _____   _____

New Client Checklist

Initial Call

Date: _____

Staff Member Taking the Call: _____

Client Name: _____ Account Number: _____

Address: _____

_____

Phone Numbers: (Home) _____ (Work) _____

Who Referred the Client: _____

Reason for the Appointment: _____

Insurance Information (if applicable): _____

Client Informed of Major Policies: ❏ Yes   ❏ No

Determine if Client Has Special Needs: _____

_____

Prior to Appointment	Date:	Staff Initials:
Welcome Packet mailed:	_____	_____
Insurance Verified:	_____	_____
Confirmation Call Placed:	_____	_____
Previous Records Received:	_____	_____

First Appointment

Intake Forms Completed:	_____	_____
Financial Arrangements Settled:	_____	_____

Client Check-Out

Fee Received:	_____	_____
Samples and Educational Material Dispensed:	_____	_____
Prescriptions Written:	_____	_____
Products Sold:	_____	_____
Next Appointment Scheduled:	_____	_____

Follow-Up

Client Check-in Call:	_____	_____
Referral Letter Sent:	_____	_____
Progress Notes Sent:	_____	_____

Insurance Pre-Approval Form

Entry Date: _____

Patient's Name: _____ Phone: _____

Social Security No.: _____ Date of Birth: _____

Employer: _____ Phone: _____

Referring Physician: _____ Phone: _____

Date of Injury: _____

Insured's Name: _____ Phone: _____

Social Security No.: _____ Date of Birth: _____

Insurance Company: _____ Phone: _____

Street Address: _____

City: _____ State: _____ Zip: _____

Policy #: _____ Plan #: _____

Claim #: _____ Member #: _____

Group #: _____ I.D. #: _____

Type of Insurance: ❏ Group   ❏ PIP/Auto   ❏ Workers' Compensation

Effective Date of Policy: _____

Is There A Deductible? ❏ Yes ❏ No   Amount: _____

Is The Deductible Met? ❏ Yes ❏ No   Amount Remaining: _____

Co-Pay Amount: _____ Maximum # of Visits: _____

Maximum Dollar Amount: _____

Percentage Policy Pays for the Following Services:

Office Visit _____ Acupuncture _____ Massage _____ Physiotherapy _____ Counseling _____

Chiropractic _____ Supports _____ X-Rays _____ Physical Therapy ___ Vitamins _____

Adjuster's Full Name: _____

Phone #: _____ Extension #: _____

Time and Date of Call: _____

Approved For: _____

Send: ❏ Notes: _____   ❏ Rx: _____   ❏ Interim Report: _____

     ❏ Initial Report: _____   ❏ Progress Report: _____

Financial Agreement

Please read this agreement carefully.
We will be happy to answer any questions you may have.

I, _____ (client), understand that my insurance is an agreement between the insurance company and myself.

I understand that _____ (health care provider), will assist me in billing my insurance carrier. However, I am fully responsible for any payments due that are denied by my insurance company.

I assign payments to be made on my behalf to this provider for any services furnished to me. I authorize any holder of information about me to release such information needed to determine these benefits or to assist in the collection of payment for services.

If the bills for services are not paid within sixty (60) days by my insurance carrier, I am responsible for the balance on the sixty-first (61st) day.

In the event my insurance company does not pay in full for services provided, I hereby authorize the health care provider to charge all past due payments to my credit card listed below.

In the event fees are not paid as requested, a collection agency and possibly legal action may follow. If so, I _____ (client), will be responsible for all reasonable costs associated with the collection of such fees, including attorney and court costs.

I have read and understand this financial agreement.

Signature: _____ Date: _____

Credit Card Number: _____ Expiration Date: _____

Name of Cardholder as it Appears on Credit Card: _____

Massage Therapy Informed Consent

I, _____ , (client) understand that massage therapy provided by, _____ , (massage therapist) is intended to enhance relaxation, reduce pain caused by muscle tension, increase range of motion, improve circulation and offer a positive experience of touch. Any other intended purposes for massage therapy are specified below:

_____

_____

The general benefits of massage, possible massage contraindications and the treatment procedure have been explained to me. I understand that massage therapy is not a substitute for medical treatment or medications, and that it is recommended that I concurrently work with my Primary Caregiver for any condition I may have. I am aware that the massage therapist does not diagnose illness or disease, does not prescribe medications, and that spinal manipulations are not part of massage therapy.

I have informed the massage therapist of all my known physical conditions, medical conditions and medications, and I will keep the massage therapist updated on any changes.

I have received a copy of the therapist's policies, I understand them and agree to abide by them.

_____   _____
Client Signature   Date

Appendix B

• A Barrier-Free Practice •

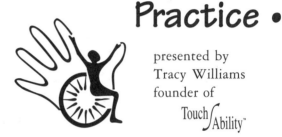

presented by
Tracy Williams
founder of
Touch∫Ability™

Health care providers help clients recognize and release barriers that block spiritual, emotional, mental and physical growth. Their services are especially beneficial for people with physical disabilities and special needs. This segment of the population represents a vital and largely untapped market. Alternative health care represents a service they genuinely value and appreciate. Personally, professionally and even financially there are numerous benefits to working with these populations.

Benefits ～

Referrals

There is a tight network of people with special needs—a tremendous potential source of referrals. Few people have training and experience with such clients, so those who do are widely sought out.

Marketing Advantages

There are unique marketing possibilities for practitioners. Contact rehabilitation centers, hospital wellness clinics, social services agencies, summer camps and support groups to promote your services and create new programs. Educate doctors and medical personnel about the benefits of alternative therapies to people with special needs.

Personal Gowth

Working with a physically challenged population allows practitioners to confront their own fears and weaknesses, usually an empowering experience. Practitioners who work with clients with special needs report enormous personal and spiritual growth.

Professional Growth

Practitioners who create an accessible practice serve all people better. Through working with clients with extreme conditions, you'll gain new understanding of the body's potential, enriching your service to everyone.

Who are People with Special Needs? ᜪᜪ

People with special needs are those who have a physical or mental impairment that substantially limits one or more major life activities. Their conditions range from arthritis to quadriplegia, from blindness to epilepsy. In addition to being limited in their physical capacities, many are dealing with chronic pain, depression and secondary complications resulting from their conditions. Ostracism and discrimination are also a common experience.

As you might expect, people with disabilities are interested in anything that might improve the quality of their lives. Alternative therapies have much to offer physically challenged individuals, both mentally and physically. People with congenital conditions like cerebral palsy and spina bifida experience relief from chronic pain. Permanently impaired war veterans with missing limbs have discovered that touch therapy, acupuncture and hypnotherapy relieve accumulated stress. People with degenerative diseases such as multiple sclerosis or muscular dystrophy find that bodywork improves flexibility and range of motion. Aquatherapy, acupuncture and shiatsu have helped seniors with arthritis and other conditions.

Like many other minorities, individuals with disabilities began organizing and campaigning in the 1960s for better access and other civil rights and protections. This activism ultimately led to the passage of the Americans with Disabilities Act (ADA) in 1991, which guarantees people with disabilites the right to participate equally in mainstream society. The ADA has boosted the determination of people with disabilities to fully participate in life.

Practitioner Accommodations ~~~

Safe Body Mechanics

There are a number of techniques that health care providers must learn to ensure safe and comfortable handling of physically challenged clients. Many people with disabilities need complete or partial assistance simply to be put in position for treatment. Competence in body mechanics skills comes from practice; hands-on practical training is essential to learn these sensitive skills. Some practitioners are taught these skills in school (e.g., nurses, physical therapists, and personal care attendants) and are valuable resources to call upon for guidance. Many community colleges and professional organizations offer courses for caregivers.

Of course, your most important teacher is the client. Communicate with your clients and encourage them to communicate with you. Ask questions, outline procedures, listen and follow instructions. People with disabilities know what works for them.

Some clients may be accompanied by a caregiver, who may be able to provide demonstrations and coaching on how best to work with the client.

Communication

An authentic therapeutic relationship with a client who has special needs depends on clear, honest, mature and good-humored communication. People with disabilities often have poor self-esteem and are accustomed to being ignored and treated rudely. Even many medical professionals rarely take the time to understand their situation.

Practitioners need to listen carefully to their clients' instructions and reactions, and be able to maintain an approach that is natural and matter-of-fact. There is an etiquette for working with people with disabilities; for example, help should be offered only when asked for. It's a good idea to incorporate mobility assistance into the flow of the session, so that activities of dressing and undressing, turning, positioning, and propping become stretching and range-of-motion exercises.

See Appendix A, pages 398-402 for sample Health Intake Forms.

In working with people with disabilities, it's extremely important to gather information before beginning treatment. A thorough initial interview takes at least 30 minutes and should establish rapport as well as elicit vital information.

During the session, observe and make note of outstanding qualities about the client's posture, breathing patterns, facial expressions, gait and limb mobility. Pay special attention to personal needs and requests, anatomical changes and vulnerable mental/emotional conditions. Keeping a record of anatomical features from session to session enables you to track progress.

Practitioners gain their clients' respect if they're sensitive to issues people with disabilities face daily and are open to learning about their life experiences. Be aware that your work may trigger emotional reactions for both yourself and your clients. Deep fears about body disassociation, helplessness and isolation may come up. Pay attention to your own reactions—maybe even record your thoughts and feelings in a journal. As you review your notes, you will see your own emotional/spiritual progress.

Medical Issues

When working with people with disabilities, be aware that medical problems sometimes arise. At the beginning of your relationship with a physically challenged client, ask your client to have their physician complete a release form covering medically relevant information. During the intake interview, be sure to review the client's health history. It's also important to discuss such personal care issues as bowel and bladder management, skin care and mobility assistance. At all times, respect the clients' feedback as they discover new ways to reach their fullest potential. The client controls the session while you supply the energy and techniques to address their priorities. The team approach keeps everyone safe and satisfied.

Accessibility

If you want to accommodate people with special needs, the inside and outside of your business must be accessible. In selecting a business location, check whether architectural and communication accommodations exist or could be made.

The following guidelines summarize accessibility considerations suggested by the ADA. The Internal Revenue Service allows a deduction of up to $15,000 per year for expenses associated with improving access. Small businesses may also qualify for tax credits. For a free code of Federal Regulations (ADA), contact the Department of Justice.

See Chapter 7, page 182 for tax information on form 8826 Disabled Access Credit.

- **Parking and passenger loading zones** must be available as close as possible to the entrance, with ramps and curb cuts to enable easy access. Reserved spaces should have a sign posted showing the symbol of accessibility.

- **Ramps** should be built with the least possible slope (1:12, or one inch height for every foot in length). Recommended width is 36 inches (915 mm) with level landings at the bottom and top.

- **Floor surfaces** should be smooth and slip-resistant. Unpaved exterior ground surfaces (as well as deep pile carpeting) can be unsafe for people who use wheelchairs and other mobility aides. Walks, ramps, stairs and curb ramps must be stable and firm. Carpet should be no thicker than ½ inch (13 mm) and securely attached with a firm backing.

- **Doorways** must be 32 inches (815 mm) wide with the door able to open 90 degrees. Thresholds at doorways must not exceed ¾ inch (19 mm) in height. Ideally, the doors would be automatic or power-assisted. Door hardware (handles, pulls, latches, locks and other operating devices) must be easy to operate for someone with arthritis who has a limited ability to grasp, pinch or twist their wrist. Hardware should be mounted no higher than 48 inches (1220 mm) above the floor.

- **Restrooms** must have enough maneuvering space for a person using a wheelchair to get in and out. A standard accessible toilet stall (five-by-five feet) has a minimum depth of 56 inches (1420 mm). Install a raised toilet seat, grab bars, and a full-length mirror. To make sinks accessible to people who use wheelchairs, leave an open space under the basin. Be sure to remember that their legs may touch the plumbing, so insulate the hot water pipe to prevent burns.

- **Clear passage** for a wheelchair is 32 inches (815 mm). Rearrange tables, chairs, vending machines, display racks and other furniture to ensure clearance. A person in a wheelchair needs a clear space of 60 inches (1525 mm) diameter to make a 180-degree turn.

- **Miscellaneous:** The telephone should be easy to reach and the water fountain should have a paper cup dispenser. Also keep on hand a package of disposable pads, a box of rubber gloves, a urinal and a physical therapy transfer belt. These items can be purchased at a medical supply or drug store. Even though you may never need these health care tools, they should be available for exceptional circumstances.

Resources ~~~

Special populations are a marketing dream come true. People with disabilities have a close network of associates and therefore generate valuable word-of-mouth promotion. As noted earlier, they also tend to be repeat customers. The main challenge is establishing yourself as a credible, empathetic and respectful practitioner. Understanding their situation and using the right language with an appropriate attitude is critical to establishing credibility.

Independent Living is a worldwide political action movement driven by the spirit of the disability-rights movement. Throughout the country, Independent Living Centers (ILCs) offer public education and awareness programs to inform the public about the choices, achievements and lifestyles of people with disabilities. These organizations offer a way for practitioners to approach people with disabilities as well as a source of information and educational material.

See page 417
for a listing of
Independent Living
Resources.

Touch/Ability™ was established by Tracy Williams, M.S., a rehabilitation counselor, to bring together healing arts practitioners and people with special needs. Touch/Ability offers workshops and learning programs that prepare healing arts practitioners to practice with exceptional clients. For more information write Touch/Ability at P.O. Box 30987, Tucson, AZ 85751-0987 or call 520-743-7566.

• Business Organizations •

This directory lists general national and international organizations whose purpose is to support people in small business. Some of these organizations offer education information, contacts and resources. Others provide benefits such as group insurance rates and discounts on products. Many of these orgnizations offer information free of charge—but be sure to check. For specialized business support organizations, please refer to the Encyclopedia of Associations.

American Assn of Home Based Business
P.O. Box 10023
Rockville, MD 20849
301-310-3130; 301-963-9153
www.aahbb.org

American Business Women's Assn
9100 Ward Parkway, Box 8728
Kansas City, MO 64114 0728
816-361-6621; 800-228-0007
www.abwa.org

American Entrepreneurs Assn
2392 Morse Ave
Irvine, CA 92714
800-482-0973

American Federation of Small Business
407 S. Dearborn Street
Chicago, IL 60605-1111
312-427-0207

American Home Business Assn
4505 S Wasatch Blvd, Suite 140
Salt Lake City, UT 84124
800-664-2422; 801-273-2399
www.homebusinessworks.com

American Management Assn
1601 Broadway
New York, NY 10019-1201
212-586-8100
www.amanet.org

Assn of Small Business Development Centers
3108 Columbia Pike, Suite 300
Arlington, VA 22204
703-271-8700
www.asbdc-us.org

Best Employers Association
2515 McCabe Way
Irvine, CA 92614-6243
949-756-6100; 800-854-7417

Council of Better Business Bureaus
4200 Wilson Boulevard Ste. 800
Arlington, VA 22203
703-276-0100
www.bbb.org

Entrepreneurship Institute
3592 Corporate Dr, Suite 101
Columbus, OH 43231
614-895-1153; 800-736-3592
www.tei.net

Health Insurance Assn of America
555 13th St NW, Suite 600 E
Washington, DC 20004
202-824-1600
www.hiaa.org

Home Office Assn of America
133 E 58th St., Suite 711
New York, NY 10022
800-809-4622; 212-588-9097
www.hoaa.com

Independent Business Alliance
1 Ramada Plaza
New Rochelle, NY 10801
800-559-2580
www.ibaonline.com

Insurance Information Institute
110 Williams St, 24th floor
New York, NY 10038-1008
800-331-9146; 212-669-9200
www.iii.org

Int'l Council for Small Business
3674 Lindell Blvd
St. Louis, MO 63108-3302
314-977-3628
www.icsb.org

Nat'l Assn of Home Based Businesses
10451 Mill Run Circle, Suite 400
Owings Mills, MD 21117
410-363-3698
www.usahomebusiness.com

Nat'l Assn for Female Executives
PO Box 469031
Escondido, CA 92046-9925
800-634-6233
www.nafe.com

Nat'l Assn for the Cottage Industry
PO Box 14850
Chicago, IL 60614
773-472-8116

Nat'l Assn for the Self-Employed
PO Box 612067
Dallas, TX 75261-2067
800-232-6273; 800-551-4446
www.nase.org

Nat'l Assn of Women Business Owners
1411 K St NW, Suite 1300
Washington, DC 20005-3404
800-556-2926; 202-347-8686
www.nawbo.org

Nat'l Business Association
5151 Beltline Road, Suite 1150
Dallas, TX 75240
972-991-5381
www.nationalbusiness.org

Nat'l Federation of Independent Business
53 Century Blvd., Suite 300
Nashville, TN 37214-1341
800-634-2669; 615-872-5300
www.nfib.com

Nat'l Foundation of Women Business Owners
1411 K Street NW, Suite 1350
Washington, DC 20005-3407
202-638-3060; 202-638-3064
www.nfwbo.org

Nat'l Small Business United
1156 15th Street NW, Suite 1100
Washington, DC 20005
800-345-6728; 202-293-8830
www.nsbu.org

Quality Performance Network
201 E Dundee Rd
Palatine, IL 60074
800-429-7724; 800-776-0072
www.usccsbi.com

Service Corps of Retired Executives
409 3rd St. SW   4th Floor
Washington, DC 20024
800-634-0245; 800-205-6762
www.score.org

Small Business Legislative Council
1010 Massachusetts Ave NW, Suite 400
Washington, DC 20001
202-639-8500

Small Business Network
P.O. Box 30149
Baltimore, MD 21270-0149
410-581-1373
www.usahomebusiness.com

Small Business Service Bureau
554 Main Street, Box 15014
Worcester, MA 01615-0014
508-756-3513
www.sbsb.com

Support Services Alliance
PO Box 130
Schoharie, NY 12157-0130
800-322-3920; 518-295-7966
www.ssainfo.com

U.S. Chamber of Commerce
1615 H Street NW
Washington, DC 20062-0001
800-638-6582; 800-659-6000
www.uschamber.org

U.S. Dept of Commerce Business Assistance
14th St NW
Washington, DC 20230-0001
800-644-8818; 202-377-3176

U.S. Department of Labor
200 Constitution Avenue NW
Washington, DC 20210-0001
202-693-4650
www.dol.gov

U.S. Department of the Treasury (IRS)
1111 Constitution Ave NW
Washington, DC 20224
800-829-3676; 800-566-2041
www.irs.gov

U.S. Government Printing Office
732 N Capital St NW
Washington, DC 20401-0003
202-512-0000
www.access.gpo.gov

U.S. Small Business Administration
409 Third St SW
Washington, DC 20416
800-827-5722; 800-205-6600
www.sba.gov

• Independent Living Resources •

These organizations provide resource materials on issues related to independent living and disability rights. These cross-disability resources include rehabilitation equipment, workshops, technical assistance, database searches, referrals, newsletters, directories and conferences. Their advocacy efforts advance the full integration and participation of persons with disabilities.

ABLEDATA
8455 Colesville Rd, Suite 935
Silver Spring, MD 20910-3319
800-227-0216; 301-608-8998
TTY 301-608-8912
www.abledata.com

Disability & Business Tech Assistance Center
800-949-4232

Independent Living Research Utilization
  Program
2323 S Shepherd, Suite 1000
P.O. Box 20095
Houston, TX 77019
713-520-0232; 713-520-5136
Fax 713-520-5785

National Council on Independent Living
2111 Wilson Blvd, Suite 405
Arlington, VA 22201
703-525-3406; TTY 703-525-4153
Fax 703-525-3409   DIMENET.nicl

National Health Information Center
Department of Health & Human Services
P.O. Box 1133
Washington, DC 20013-1133
301-565-4167; 800-336-4797
Fax 301-984-4256

National Organization of Rare Disorders
100 Rt 37 / P.O. Box 8923
New Fairfield, CT 06812-1783
203-746-6518; 800-999-6673

National Rehabilitation Info Center
8455 Colesville Rd, Suite 935
Silver Springs, MD 20910-3319
800-346-2742; 301-588-9284
http://www.NARIC.com/NARIC

U.S. Department of Justice
(provides free ADA materials)
800-514-0301; TDD 800-514-0383

World Institute on Disability
510 16th St, Suite 100
Oakland, CA 94612-1500
510-763-4100 TTY 510-208-9493
Fax 510-763-4109

• Professional Associations •

This register contains the major health care professional associations (some provide malpractice insureance). The total list including the specialized, auxiliary and local branches numbers in the thousands. If you are interested in discovering the scope of this field or learning more about any particular association, look through the "Health and Medical" section of the Encyclopedia of Associations.

Aerobics & Fitness Assn of America
15250 Ventura Blvd, Suite 200
Sherman Oaks, CA 91403-3297
800-446-2322; 818-990-5468
www.afaa.com

Aesthetics' Int'l Assn
2611 N Beltline Rd #140
Sunnyvale, TX 75182
877-968-7539; 972-932-8380
www.dermascope.com

Alexander Technique Int'l
1692 Massachusetts Ave., 3rd Floor
Cambridge, MA 02138
888-668-8996; 617-497-2242
www.ATI-net.com

Alliance for Alternatives in Healthcare
PO Box 6279
Thousand Oaks, CA 91359 6279
805-374-6003; 805-379-1580
www.alternativeinsurance.com/html/
alliance_membership.html

Amer Foundation for Alternative Health
25 Landfield Ave
Monticello, NY 12701
914-794-8181; 914-794-5861

American Academy of Envir Medicine
7701 E Kellogg, Suite 625
Springfield, IL 62707-1705
316-684-5500; 316-684-5709
www.aaem.com

American Academy of Medical Acupuncture
5820 Wilshire Blvd., Suite 500
Los Angeles, CA 90036
323-937-5514
www.medicalacupuncture.org

American Acupuncture Assn
4262 Kissena Blvd
Flushing, NY 11355-3213
718-886-4431; 718-463-0808

American Alliance of Aromatherapy
PO Box 309
Depoe Bay, OR 97341
800-809-9850; 800-809-9808
www.healthy.net/pan/pa/aromatherapy/aaat/
aathm.htm

American Art Therapy Assn
1202 Allanson Road
Mundelein, IL 60060-3808
888-290-0878; 847-949-6064
www.arttherapy.org

Amer Assn for Teachers of Oriental Medicine
2700 W Anderson Lane #204
Austin, TX 78757
512-451-2866
www.aatom.org

Amer Assn of Acup & Bio-Energetic Medicine
2512 Manoa Rd
Honolulu, HI 96822
808-946-2069; 808-946-0378

American Assn of Alternative Healing
PO Box 10026
Sedona, AZ 86339-8026
www.cris.com/Aaah/toc.htl

American Assn of Anatomists
9650 Rockville Pike
Bethesda, MD 20814-3998
301-571-8314; 301-571-0619
www.faseb.org/anatomy

American Assn of Equine Practitioners
4075 Iron Works Pkwy
Lexington, KY 40511-8462
859-233-0147; 859-233-1968
www.aaep.org

American Assn of Oriental Medicine
433 Front St
Catasauqua, PA 18032-2526
800-500-7999; 610-266-1433
www.aaom.org

American Assn of Prof Hypnotherapists
4149-A El Camino Way
Palo Alto, CA 94306
650-323-3224
www.aaph.org

American Assn of Critical-Care Nurses
101 Columbia
Aliso Viejo, CA 92656-1491
800-839-2226; 949-362-2000
www.aacn.org

American Assn of Naturopathic Physicians
8201 Greensboro Dr, Suite 300
Mc Lean, VA 22102
703-610-9037; 703-610-9005
www.naturopathic.org

The American Assn of Orthopaedic Medicine
90 S Cascade Ave Ste 1230
Colorado Springs, CO 80903
800-992-2063; 719-475-0032

American Athletic Trainers Assn
660 W Duarte Rd
Arcadia, CA 91007
626-445-1978

American Board of Hypnotherapy
16842 Von Karman Ave #475
Irvine, CA 92606
800-634-9766; 949-261-6400
www.hypnosis.com/abh

American Board of Medical Specialties
1007 Church St #404
Evanston, IL 60201
800-776-2378; 847-491-9091
www.healthy.net/pan/cso/cioi/abms

American Botanical Council
P. O. Box 144345
Austin, TX 78714-4345
512-926-4900; 512-926-2345
www.herbalgram.org

American Chiropractic Assn
1701 Clarendon Blvd
Arlington, VA 22209-2700
800-986-4636; 703-276-8800
www.acatoday.com

American Chronic Pain Assn
P. O. Box 850
Rocklin, CA 95677
916-632-0922

American College of Nurse Midwives
818 Connecticut Ave NW, Suite 900
Washington, DC 20006
202-728-9860; 202-289-4395
www.acnm.org

American Counseling Assn
5999 Stevenson Ave
Alexandria, VA 22304-3300
800-347-6647; 703-823-9800
www.counseling.org

American Craniosacral Therapy Assn
11211 Prosperity Farms Rd, D-323
Palm Beach Gardens, FL 33410-3487
877-942-2782; 561-622-4334
www.acsta.com

American Dance Therapy Assn
2000 Century Plaza, Suite 108
Columbus, MO 21044
410-997-4040; 410-997-4048
www.adta.org

American Dental Assistants Assn
203 N. LaSalle St. Ste. 1320
Chicago, IL 60601-1225
800-733-2322; 312-541-1550
www.add1.com

American Dental Assn
211 E Chicago Ave
Chicago, IL 60611
312-440-2500; 312-440-2800
www.ada.org

American Dental Hygienists' Assn
444 Michigan Ave, Suite 3400
Chicago, IL 60611
312-440-8900; 312-440-8929
www.adha.org

American Dietetic Assn
216 W Jackson Blvd, Suite 800
Chicago, IL 60606
800-877-1600; 312-899-0040
www.eatright.org

American Electrology Assn
106 Oak Ridge Rd
Trumball, CT 06611-5213
203-374-6667; 203-372-7134
www.electrology.com

American Healing Arts Alliance, Int'l
803 N 9th St
Fort Smith, AR 72901
501-758-2422
www.ahaa.cjb.net

American Herb Assn
PO Box 1673
Nevada City, CA 95959
530-265-9552
www.jps.net/ahaherb

American Herbalists Guild
1931 Gaddis Rd
Canton, GA 30115
770-751-6021; 770-751-7472
www.healthy.net/herbalists

American Holistic Health Assn
PO Box 17400
Anaheim, CA 92817-7400
714-779-6152
ahha.org

American Holistic Medical Assn
6728 Old McLean Village Dr
Mc Lean, VA 22101-3906
703-556-9728; 703-556-9245
www.ahmaholistic.com

American Holistic Nurses Assn
P.O. Box 2130
Flagstaff, AZ 86003-2130
800-278-2462
www.ahna.org

American Holistic Veterinary Medical Assn
2214 Old Emmorton Rd
Bel Air, MD 21015-6106
410-569-0795; 410-569-2346
AHVMA@compuserve.com

American Horticultural Therapy Assn
909 York St
Denver, CO 80206
303-331-3862; 303-331-0095
www.ahta.org

American Institute of Homeopathy
801 N Fairfax St, Suite 306
Alexandria, VA 22314
703-246-9501
www.healthy.net/aih/

American Massage Therapy Assn
820 Davis Street, Suite 100
Evanston, IL 60201-4444
847-864-0123; 847-864-1178
www.amtamassage.org

American Medical Massage Assn
PO Box 272
Gainesville, VA 20156-0272
540-351-0807
www.americanmedicalmassage.com

American Medical Student Assn
1902 Assn Dr
Reston, VA 20191
800-767-2266; 703-620-6600
www.amsa.org

American Music Therapy Assn
8455 Colesville Rd, Suite 1000
Silver Spring, MD 20910
301-589-3300; 301-589-5175
www.musictherapy.org

American Natural Hygiene Society
11816 Racetrack Rd
Tampa, FL 33626-3105
813-855-6607
www.anhs.org

American Naturopathic Assn
1413 K St NW, Suite 852
Washington, DC 20005
202-682-7352; 202-909-7855
www.wnho.org.ana.htm

American Naturopathic Medical Assn
PO Box 96273
Las Vegas, NV 89193
702-897-7053; 702-897-7140
www.anma.com

American Nurses Assn
600 Maryland Ave SW, Suite 100 W
Washington, DC 20024
800-274-4262; 202-651-7000
www.ana.org

American Occupational Therapy Assn
4720 Montgomery Ln / PO Box 31220
Bethesda, MD 20824-1220
800-377-8555; 301-652-2682
www.aota.org

American Oriental Bodywork Therapy Assn
1010 Haddonfield-Berlin Rd, Suite 408
Voorhees, NJ 08043
856-782-1616; 856-782-1653
www.healthy.net/aobta

American Osteopathic Assn
142 E Ontario St
Chicago, IL 60611-2818
800-621-1773; 312-280-5800
www.aoa-net.org

American Pain Society
4700 W Lake Ave
Glenview, IL 60025
847-375-4715, 847-375-6315
www.ampainsoc.org

American Physical Therapy Assn
1111 N Fairfax Street
Alexandria, VA 22314-1488
800-999-2782; 703-683-6748
www.apta.org

American Polarity Therapy Assn
PO Box 19858
Boulder, CO 80308
303-545-2080; 303-545-2161
www.PolarityTherapy.org

American Preventive Medical Assn
9912 Georgetown Pike, Suite D-2
Great Falls, VA 22066
800-230-2762; 703-759-0662
www.apma.net

American Psychiatric Assn
1400 K Street, NW
Washington, DC 20005
888-357-7924; 202-682-6000
www.psych.org

American Psychological Assn
750 First St NE
Washington, DC 20002-4242
202-336-5500
www.apa.org

American Public Health Assn
800 I St NW
Washington, DC 20001-3710
202-789-5600; 202-789-5681
www.apha.org

American Reflexology Certification Board
P.O. Box 620607
Littleton, CO 80162
303-933-6921

American Reiki Masters Assn
PO Box 130
Lake City, FL 32056
904-755-9638

American Skin Assn
150 E 58th St 33rd Floor
New York, NY 10155-0002
800-499-7546; 212-753-8260
www.skinassn.org

American Soc for the Alexander Technique
PO Box 60008
Florence, MA 01062
800-473-0620; 413-584-2359
www.alexandertech.org

American Society of Alternative Therapists
P.O. Box 703
Rockport, MA 01966
978-281-4400
www.asat.org

American Society of Clinical Hypnosis
130 East Elm Court Suite 201
Roselle, IL 60172-2000
630-980-4740; 630 351 8490
www.asch.net

American Veterinary Chiropractic Assn
623 Main
Hillsdale, IL 61257
309-658-2620; 309-658-2622
www.healthy.net/pan/pa/vet/avca

American Veterinary Medical Assn
1931 N Meacham Rd Suite 100
Schaumburg, IL 60173-4360
800-248-2862; 847-925-8070
www.amva.org

American Yoga Assn
PO Box 19986
Sarasota, FL 34276
941-927-4977; 941-921-9844
www.americanyogaAssn.org

Aquatic Alliance Int'l
50 Prospect St #2
Lebanon, NH 03766
888-775-2744; 802-728-1390
www.mindspring.com/~aai_getwet/index.htm

Aquatic Exercise Assn
3439 Technology Dr, Unit 6
Nokomis, FL 34275-3627
800-232-9283; 941-486-8600
www.aeawave.com

Aquatic Therapy & Rehab Institute, Inc.
Rte 1 Box 218
Chassell, MI 49916-9710
906-482-9500; 906-482-4388
www.atri.org

Arthritis Foundation
1330 W Peachtree St
Atlanta, GA 30309
800-283-7800; 404-872-7100
www.arthritis.org

Assn for Applied Psycophysiology & Biofeedback
10200 W 44th Ave, Suite 304
Wheat Ridge, CO 80033-2840
303-422-8436; 303-422-8894
www.aapb.org

Assn for Holotropic Breathwork Int'l
P.O. Box 7169
Santa Cruz, CA 95061-7169
www.breathwork.com

Assn for Transpersonal Psychology
45 Franklin St, Suite 313
San Francisco, CA 94102
800-899-0573; 415-863-9941
www.atpweb.org

Assn for Worksite Health Promotion
60 Revere Dr #500
Northbrook, IL 60062
847-480-9574; 847-480-9282
www.awhp.org

Assn of Labor & Childbirth Educators
PO Box 382724
Cambridge, MA 02238-2724
888-222-5223; 617-441-2500
www.server4.hypermart.net/alacehq

Assn of Mass Therapists/Wholistic Practitioners
17878 106 Ave #207
Edmonton, AB T5S 1V4 Canada
403-484-2010
www.amtwp.org

Assn of Massage Therapists Australia
PO Box 627
South Yarra, VIC 3141 Australia
613-9-510-3930; 613-9-521-3209
www.amta.asn.au

Assn of Vegetarian Dietitians & Educators
3835 State Rte 414
Burdett, NY 14818
607-546-7171; 607-546-4091
www.vegedine.com

Associated Bodywork & Massage Professionals
1271 Sugarbush Dr
Evergreen, CO 80439-9766
800-458-2267; 303-674-8478
www.abmp.com

Assn for Humanistic Psychology
45 Franklin St #315
San Francisco, CA 94102-6017
415-864-8850; 415-864-8853
http://ahpweb.org

Assn for Play Therapy
2050 N Winery Ave, Suite 101
Fresno, CA 93703
559-252-2278; 559-252-2297
www.iapt.org

Assn for the Advancement of Sports Potential
PO Box 185
Unionville, PA 19375-0085
800-223-7014; 800-793-1881
www.eqbinc.com

Assn of American Physicians and Surgeons
1601 N Tucson Blvd, Suite 9
Tucson, AZ 85716
800-635-1196; 520-327-4885
www.aapsonline.org

Assn of Natural Medicine Pharmacists
PO Box 150727
San Rafael, CA 94915-0727
415-453-3534; 415-453-4963
www.anmp.org

Assn of Women's Health, Obstetric and
Neonatal Nurses
2000 L St, Suite 740
Washington, DC 20036
800-673-8499; 800-245-0231
www.awhonn.org

Australian Traditional Medicine Society
Suite 12/27 Bank St
Wiloughly, NSW 2068 Australia
www.atms.com.au

Biofeedback Certification Institute of America
10200 W 44th Ave #310
Wheat Ridge, CO 80033
303-420-2902; 303-422-8894
www.bcia.org

Bowen Technique Assn: UK
PO Box 4358
Dorchester, Dorset DT2 7XX England
44-0700-269-8324
www.bowen-technique.co.uk

BowTech Pty. Ltd.
PO Box 733
Hamilton, VIC 3300 Australia
610-3-5572-3000;   610-3-5572-3144
www.bowtech.com

British Columbia Acupressure Therapists' Assn
PO Box 8143
Camax, BC V8M 3R8 Canada
250-920-9986
www.islandnet.com

C.J. Jung Foundation
28 E 39th St
New York, NY 10016-2555
212-697-6430; 212-953-3989
www.cgjungpage.org/nyjung99.html

California Coalition on Somatic Practices
P.O. Box 5611
San Mateo, CA 94402-0611
650-574-5579; 909-659-9751
www.somatic.com/ccsp

Canadian Assn of Rubenfeld Synergists
112 Lund St
Richmond Hill, ON L4C 5V9 Canada
905-883-3158
www.rubenfeldsynergy.com

Canadian Federation of Aromatherapists
843479 Oxford Rd 84 RR #3
Lakeside, ON N0M 2G0 Canada
519-475-9038

Canadian Massage Therapist Alliance
365 Bloor St E, Suite 1807
Toronto, ON M4W 3L4 Canada
416-968-2149
www.collinscan.com/collins/clientspgs/cmta.html

Canadian Reiki Assn
PO Box 40026 RPO Marlee
Toronto, ON M6B 4K4 Canada
416-783-9904
http://ourworld.compuserve.com/home/pages/
canadian_reiki_assn

Canadian SportsMassage Therapists Assn
3444 78 St
Edmonton, AB T6K 0E9 Canada
780-461-7211
www.csmta.ca

College of Massage Therapists
427 Eglinton Ave W, Suite 2
Toronto, ON M5N 1A4 Canada
416-489-2626
www.cmto.com

College of Massage Therapists
103-1089 W Broadway
Vancouver, BC V6H 1E5 Canada
604-736-3404
www.cmtbc.bc.ca

Club Spa USA: The Day Spa Assn
PO Box 5232
West New York, NJ 07093
201-865-2065; 201-865-5361
www.clubspausa.com

Coalition for Natural Health
1220 L St, PMB 100-408
Washington, DC 20005
800-586-4264; 800-598-4264
www.naturalhealth.org

Compassionate Touch
20 Swan Ct
Walnut Creek, CA 94596
925-935-3906
www.journeyofhearts.org/compassionatetouch

Complementary Alternative Medical Assn
PO Box 373478
Decatur, GA 30037-3478
404-284-7592
www.camaweb.net

Complementary Medicine Assn
4649 E Malvern
Tucson, AZ 85711
520-323-6291

Council of Coll of Acup & Oriental Medicine
1010 Wayne Ave, Suite 1270
Silver Spring, MD 20910
301-608-9175
www.ccaom.org

Council on Chiropractic Education
8049 N 85th Way
Scottsdale, AZ 85258-4321
480-483-8877; 480-483-7333
www.cce-usa.org

Craniosacral Therapy Assn
North America:
1110 Birchmount Rd Unit 21
Scarborough, ON M1K 1S7 Canada
416-755-7734
www.crannnosacraltherapy.org
UK:
Monomark House, 27 Old Gloucester St
London, WC1N 3XX England
www.craniosacral.co.uk
U.S.:
4636 Gordon Dr
Boulder, CO 80303
303-499-4675
www.craniosacraltherapy.org

Dermatology Nurses Assn
East Holly Ave / Box 56
Pitman, NJ 08071
609-256-2330; 609-589-7463

Esalen Massage and Bodywork Assn
Highway 1
Big Sur, CA 93920-9616
831-667-3000; 831-927-5885
www.esalen.com

European Assn of Sports Massage
Postbus 302
Arhem, 6800 AH Holland
www.universal.nl/users/NGS/EAS/defeasen.html

Federation Quebecoise de Masseurs et
   Massotherapeutes
1265 Mont-Royal est, Bureau 204
Montreal, QC H2J 1Y4 Canada

The Feldenkrais Guild
3611 SW Hood Ave, Suite 100
Portland, OR 97201
800-775-2118; 503-221-6612
www.feldenkrais.com

Fibromyalgia Alliance of America
PO Box 21990
Columbus, OH 43221-0990
888-716-6711; 614-457-4222
www.fmaa.org

Fibromyalgia Network
PO Box 31750
Tucson, AZ 85751
800-853-2929
www.fmnetnews.com

Florida State Massage Therapy Assn
1089 W Morse Blvd, Suite C
Winter Park, FL 32789
877-376-8248; 407-628-2772
www.fsmta.org

Flower Essence Society
PO Box 459
Nevada City, CA 95959-0459
800-736-9222; 530-265-9163
www.flowersociety.org

Flying Doctors of America
4015 Holcomb Bridge Rd #350
Norcross, GA 30092
770-209-9277; 770-446-9634
www.fdoamerica.org

Foot Reflexology Awareness Assn
P.O. Box 7622
Mission Hills, CA 91346-7622
818-361-0528
www.foot-reflexologist.com

Foundation for the Advancement of
Chiropractic Tenets & Sciences
1110 N Glebe Rd, Suite 1000
Arlington, VA 22201
703-528-5000; 703-528-5023

Georgia State Massage Therapy Assn
P O Box 550915
Atlanta, GA 30305
770-869-7999; 770-841-0039

Gerson Institute
P.O. Box 430
Bonita, CA 91908-0430
619-585-7600; 619-585-7610
www.gerson.org

Hawaiian Lomilomi Assn
15-156 Puni Kahakai Loop
Pahoa, HI 96778
808-965-8917
www.lomolomi.org

Healing Touch Int'l
12477 W Cedar Dr, Suite 202
Lakewood, CO 80228
303-989-7982; 303-989-0581
www.healingtouch.net

Hellerwork Int'l
3435 M St
Eureka, CA 95503
800-392-3900; 707-441-4949
www.hellerwork.com

Herb Research Foundation
1007 Pearl St #200
Boulder, CO 80302
800-748-2617; 303-449-2265
www.herbs.org

Holistic Dental Assn
PO Box 5007
Durango, CO 81301
970-259-1091
www.holisticdental.org

Homeopathic Council for Research & Ed.
50 Park Ave
New York, NY 10016-3075
212-684-2290

Hospital-Based Massage Network
5 Old Town Square, Suite 205
Fort Collins, CO 80524
970-407-9232
www.hbmn.com

The Institute for Somatic Sciences
P.O. Box 265
Marne, MI 49435
616-837-7743

Institute of Noetic Sciences
475 Gate Five Rd, Suite 300
Sausalito, CA 94965
800-383-1394;   415-331-5650
www.noetic.org

Int'l Academy of Myodontics
7-6-7 Ohjima
Kohco-Ku, Japan 136
215-345-1149

Int'l Acad of Nutrition & Preventive Medicine
PO Box 926
Asheville, NC 28802-0926
704-252-1406
www.healthfinder.gov/text/orgs/HR0937.htm

Int'l Alliance of Healthcare Educators
11211 Prosperity Farms Road, D-325
West Palm Beach. FL 33410-3487
800-311-9204; 561-622-4334
www.iahe.com

Int'l American Colon Therapists Assn
11739 Washington Blvd
Los Angeles, CA 90066-5944
310-390-5424
www.allredtec.com

Int'l Assn for Colon Hydrotherapy
P O Box 461285
San Antonio, TX 78246-1285
210-366-2888; 210-366-2999
www.healthy.net/pan/pa/iact

Int'l Assn for Regression Research and Therapies
PO Box 20151
Riverside, CA 92516-0151
909-784-1570; 909-784-8440
www.aprt.org

Int'l Assn for the Study of Pain
909 NE 43rd St, Suite 306
Seattle, WA 98105-6020
206-547-6409; 206-547-1703
www.halcyon.com/iasp

Int'l Assn of Counseling Services
101 S.Whiting St, Suite 211
Alexandria, VA 22304
703-823-9840; 703-823-9843
www.iacsinc.org

Int'l Assn of Fitness Professionals
6190 Cornerstone Court E, Suite 204
San Diego, CA 92121-3773
800-999-4332; 858-535-8979
www.ideafit.com

Int'l Assn of Hygienic Physicians
4620 Euclid Blvd
Youngstown, OH 44512
330-788-0526; 330-788-0093
www.cisnet.com/iahp/

Int'l Assn of Infant Massage
1891 Goodyear Ave, Suite 622
Ventura, CA 93003
800-248-5432; 805-644-8524
www.iaim-us.com

Int'l Assn of Infant Massage
56 Sparsholt Rd
Barking, Essex 1G11 7YQ England
www.iaim.org.uk

Int'l Assn of NLP
342 Massachussetts Ave
Indianapolis, IN 46204
317-636-6059
www.nlp.org

Int'l Assn of Pfrimmer Deep Muscle Therapists
1105 S New St
Champaign, IL 61820
800-484-7773
www.pfrimmer.com

Int'l Assn of Yoga Therapists
PO Box 2418
Sebastopol, CA 95473
707-928-9898
www.yrec.org/iayt.htm

Int'l Breatherapy Assn
2973 21st Ave
San Francisco, CA 94132
415-681-3051
www.umissatsang.org/IBA.htm

Int'l Chiropractic Assn
1110 N Globe Rd Ste 1000
Arlington, VA 22201
800-423-4690; 703-528-5203
www.chiropractic.org

Int'l College of Applied Kinesiology
6405 Metcalf Ave, Suite 503
Overland Park, KS 66202-3929
913-384-5336; 913-384-5112
www.icak.com

Int'l Council of Reflexologists
PO Box 17356
San Diego, CA 92177-7356
905-884-0294
www.icr-reflexology.org

Int'l Council of Reflexologists
PO Box 30513
Richmond Hill, ON L4C 0C7 Canada
905-884-0294
www.icr-reflexology.org

Int'l Federation of Reflexologists
78 Edridge Rd
Croydon, Surrey CR0 1EF England
www.reflexology.ifr.com

Int'l Foundation of Bio-Magnetics
5447 E Fifth St, Suite 111
Tucson, AZ 85711
888-473-3812; 520-323-7951
www.planet-hawaii.com/bio-magnetics

Int'l Foundation of Oriental Medicine
P.O. Box 640625
Oakland Gardens, NY 11364-0625
718-886-4431; 718-463-0808

Int'l Guild of Prof. Electrologists
803 N Main St, Suite A
High Point, NC 27262
800-830-3247; 910-841-6631
www.igpe.org

Int'l Institute of Reflexology
5650 First Ave N
Saint Petersburg, FL 33733-2642
727-343-4811; 727-381-2807
www.reflexology-usa.net

Int'l Iridologists Assn
RR2, S18A, C4
Lumby, BC V0E 2G0 Canada
250-547-2281
www.Iridology.RDSweb.net

Int'l Loving Touch Foundation, Inc.
PO Box 16374
Midway, OR 97292
503-253-8482; 503-256-6753
www.lovingtouch.com

Int'l Massage Assn Group
92 Main St PO Drawer 21
Warrenton, VA 20188-0421
800-776-6268; 540-351-0800
www.imagroup.com

Int'l Medical & Dental Hypnotherapy Assn
4110 Edgeland, Ste.800
Royal Oak, MI 48073-2285
800-257-5467; 248-549-5594
www.infinityinst.com/imdha_about.htm

Int'l Myomassethics Federation
26 W Washington, Suite B
Howell, MI 48843
888-463-4454
imfhomeoffice@yahoo.com

Int'l Myotherapy Assn
PO Box 65240
Tucson, AZ 85728-5240
800-221-4634; 520-529-3979
www.bonnieprudden.com

Int'l New Thought Alliance
5003 E Broadway Rd
Mesa, AZ 85206-1301
480-830-2461; 480-830-2561
www.websyte.com/alan/inta.htm

Int'l NLP Trainers Assn
1201 Delta Glen Ct
Vienna, VA 22182-1320
703-757-7945; 703-757-7946
www.inlpta.com

Int'l Shen Therapy Assn
3213 W. Wheeler #202
Seattle, WA 98199
206-298-9468; 206-283-1256
www.shentherapy.org

Int'l Society for Med & Psychological Hypnosis
1991 Broadway #18-B
New York, NY 10023-5827
212-874-5290; 914-764-1445

Int'l Society for the Study of Subtle Energies &
   Energy Med.
11005 Ralston Rd #100D
Arvada, CO 80004
303-425-4625; 303-425-4685
www.issseem.org

Int'l Society of Naturopathy
1434 Fremont Ave
Los Altos, CA 94024-6159
650-967-1232

Int'l Somatic Movement Educ & Therapy Assn
148 W 23 St #1H
New York, NY 10011
718-229-7666; 718-242-1129

Int'l Spa Assn
2365 Harrodsburg Rd, Suite A32S
Lexington, KY 40504
888-651-4772; 606-226-4326
www.experienceispa.com

Int'l Sports Massage Federation
2!56 Newport Blvd
Costa Mesa, CA 92627
949-642-0735; 949-642-1729

The Int'l Thai Therapist Assn
47 W Polk St #100-329
Chicago, IL 60605
800-354-6303; 773-792-4121
www.thaimassage.com

Int'l Veterinary Acupuncture Society
PO Box 271395
Fort Collins, CO 80527-1395
970-266-0666; 970-266-0777
www.ivas.org

Irish Massage Therapist Assn
Kemple's Annex
Menlo, Galway Ireland
011-353-01-760-211

Israel Assn for Massage and Bodywork
Rehov Eshel #10
Tel Aviv, Israel
972-8-931-8247

Israel Reflexology Assn
Sholomo Ha Melech #37
Tel Aviv, Israel

Japan Holistic Medical Society
Sun Palace 612 8-12-1 Nishi-Shinjuku
Shinjuku-ku
Tokyo, 16 Japan
03-3-366-1380

Jin Shin Do Foundation
1084 G San Miguel Canyon Rd
Royal Oaks, CA 95076
831-763-7702; 831-763-1551
www.jinshindo.org

London & Counties Society of Physiologists
PO Box 1611
Fort Qu'Appelle, SK S0G 1S0 Canada
306-332-3873
lcsp.cdn.br@sk.sympatico.ca

Massage Australia
PO Box 13
Windang, NSW 2528 Australia
www.massageaustralia.com

Massage Therapist Assn of Alberta
PO Box 24031 RPO Plaza Center
Red Deer, AB T4N 6X6 Canada
403-340-1913; 403-346-2269
www.mtaalberta.com

Massage Therapists Assn of Saskatchewan
PO Box 7841
Saskatoon, SK S7K 4R5 Canada
306-384-7077

Massage Therapists' Assn of British Columbia
34 E 12 Ave 3rd Floor
Vancouver, BC V5T 2G5 Canada
604-873-4467; 604-873-6211

Massage Therapists' Assn of Nova Scotia
PO Box 33103, Quinpool Post Office
Halifax, NS B3L 4T6 Canada
902-429-2190

Massage Therapy Assn of Manitoba
PO Box 63030
Winnepeg, MB R3L 2V8 Canada
204-254 0406

Medical-Aesthetic Education Associates
2049 W Bloomfield Rd., Suite 1
Phoenix, AZ 85029-5543
602-944-6860
www.medical-esthetics.com

Midwives' Alliance of North America
PO Box 175
Newton, KS 67114
888-923-6262; 316-283-4543
www.mana.org

Milton H. Erickson Foundation
3603 N 24th St
Phoenix, AZ 85016 6508
602-956-6196; 602-956-0519
www.erickson-foundation.org

The Nat'l Assn for Holistic Aromatherapy
2000 2nd Ave, Suite 206
Seattle, WA 98121
888-275-6242
www.naha.org

Nat'l Assn of Rubenfeld Synergists
1000 River Rd #8H
Belmar, NJ 07719
800-484-3250; 732-297-1394
www.rubenfeldsynergy.com

Nat'l Athletic Trainers Assn
2952 Stemmons
Dallas, TX 75247-6196
214-637-6282; 214-637-2206
www.nata.org

Nat'l Board for Certified Counselors
3 Terrace Way, Suite D
Greensboro, NC 27403-3660
800-398-6389; 336-547-0607
www.nbcc.org

Nat'l Center for Complementary & Alt Medicine
PO Box 8218
Silver Spring, MD 20907-8215
888-644-6226; 301-495-4957
www.nccam.nih.gov

Nat'l Certification Board for Therapeutic
   Massage & Bodywork
8201 Greensboro Dr, Suite 300
Mc Lean, VA 22102
800-296-0664; 703-610-9015
www.ncbtmb.com

Nat'l Federation of Prof Trainers
PO Box 4579
Lafayette, IN 47903-4579
800-729-6378; 765-447-3648
www.nfpt.com

Nat'l Inst. of Craniosacral Studies
7827 N Armenia Ave
Tampa, FL 33604-3806
813-933-6335; 813-935-0583

Nat'l Accrediting Commission of Cosmetology
   Arts & Sciences
901 N. Stuart St. Ste. 900
Arlington, VA 22203
703-527-7600; 703-527-8811

Nat'l Acup & Oriental Medical Alliance
14637 Starr Rd SE
Olalla, WA 98359
253-851-6896; 253-851-6883
www.acuall.org

Nat'l AIDS Massage Project, Inc.
215 W 24th St
Minneapolis, MN 55404-3202
612-874-9768

Nat'l Assn for Music Therapy
8455 Colecville Rd, Suite 100
Silver Spring, MD 20910
301-589-3300; 301-589-5175
www.musictherpay.org

Nat'l Assn of Myofascial Triggerpoint Therapists
251 Maitland Ave, Suite 312
Altamonte Springs, FL 32701
407-672-2344; 407-331-8825
www.frontiernet.net/~painrel/

Nat'l Assn of Nurse Massage Therapists
PO Box 820
Clarkdale, AZ 86324
800-262-4017; 520-634-5441
http://members.aol.com/nanmt1

Nat'l Assn of Postpartum Care Services
800 Detroit St
Denver, CO 80206
800-453-6852; 303-321-4058
www.napcs.org

Nat'l Assn of Pregnancy Massage Therapy
1007 MoPac Circle, Suite 202
Austin, TX 78746
888-451-4945; 888-323-5925
www.napmt.home.texas.net/

Nat'l Center for Homeopathy
801 N. Fairfax St, Suite 306
Alexandria, VA 22314
877-624-0613; 703-548-7790
www.homeopathic.org

Nat'l Chronic Pain Outreach Assn
7979 Old Georgetown Rd, Suite 100
Bethesda, MD 20814-2429
301-652-4948; 301-907-0745
www.neurosurgery.mgh.harvard.edu/
ncpainoa.htm

Nat'l Coalition of Arts Therapies Assns
8455 Colesville Rd, Suite 1000
Silver Spring, MD 20910
410-751-0103; 410-997-1608
www.ncata.com

Nat'l Guild of Hypnotists
PO Box 308
Merrimack, NH 03054-0308
603-429-9438
www.ngh.net

Nat'l Institutes of Health
Office of Alternative Medicine
PO Box 8218
Silver Spring, MD 20907-8218
888-644-6226; 301-495-4957
www.nih.gov

Nat'l Nurses in Business Assn
56 McArthur
Staten Island, NY 10312
800-331-6534; 718-317-0858
www.greatnurses.com

Nat'l Rehabilitation Assn
633 S Washington St
Alexandria, VA 22314-4109
703-836-0850; 703-836-0848
www.Nationalrehab.org

Nat'l Society of Hypnotherapists
1833 W Charleston Blvd
Las Vegas, NV 89102
702-384-4420
www.trancetime.com/nsh.html

Nat'l Therapeutic Recreation Society
22377 Belmont Ridge Rd
Ashburn, VA 20148
703-858-0784; 703-858-0794
www.nrpa.org/branches/ntrs.htm

The Nat'l Wellness Assn
PO Box 827
Stevens Point, WI 54481-0827
800-244-8922; 715-342-2969
www.wellnessnwi.org/nwa

Naturopathic Medicine in the UK
GCRN Goswell House 2 Goswell Rd
Somerset, BA16 OJG England

New Brunswick Massotherapy Assn
PO Box 21009
Fredericton, NB E3B 7A3 Canada
506-459-5788; 506-459-5656

New Zealand Assn of Ther Massage Practitioners
PO Box 375
Hamilton, Auckland New Zealand

Newfoundland Massage Therapists' Assn
95 Monkstown Road
St. John's, ND A1C 3T7 Canada
709-726-4006; 709-754-0443

North Amer Vodder Assn of Lymphatic Therapy
833 Independence Dr
Longmont, CO 80501
888-462-8258; 303-776-1891
www.navalt.com

Nurse Healers-Professional Associates Int'l
3760 S Highland Dr, Suite 429
Salt Lake City, UT 84106
801-273-3399; 801-273-3352
www.therapeutic-touch.org

Nursing Touch & Massage Therapy Assn
1438 Shortcut, Suite E
Slidell, LA 70458
504-893-8002; 504-892-3493
http://members@aol.com/ntmta

Nutrition Education Assn
3647 Glen Haven
Houston, TX 77225
713-665-2946

Ontario Naturopathic Assn
4174 Dundas St W Ste 304
Toronto, ON M8X 1X3 Canada
416-233 2001; 416-233 2924

Ontario Massage Therapist Assn
365 Bloor St E, Suite 1807
Toronto, ON M4W 3L4 Canada
800-668-2022; 416-968-6818

Ontario Polarity Therapy Assn
135 Aspenwood Dr
Willowdale, ON L3R 9W6 Canada
416-493-3841
polpus@aol.com

The Radiance Technique Int'l Assn
PO Box 40570
St. Petersburg, FL 33743-0570
813-347-3421
www.trt-rpai.org

Reflexology Assn of America
4012 S Rainbow Blvd #K-585
Las Vegas, NV 89103-2059
702-871-9522
www.reflexology-usa.org

Reflexology Assn of Australia
44 Florence Rd
Surrey Hills, VIC 3127 Australia
03-9-899-4760
http://raa.inta.net.au

Reflexology Assn of Canada
Box 110, 541 Turnberry St
Brussels, ON N0G 1H0 Canada
519-887-9991
www.reflexologycanada.com

Reiki Alliance
East 33135 Canyon Road/ PO Box 41
Cataldo, ID 83810-0041
208-682-3535; 208-682-4848
reikialliance@compuserve.com

Rolf Institute of Structural Integration
205 Canyon Blvd
Boulder, CO 80302-4920
800-530-8875; 303-449-5903
www.rolf.org

Rosen Method Professional Assn
PO Box 11144
Berkeley, CA 94712
800-893-2622; 510-644-4166
www.rosenmethod.org

Sacro Occipital Research Society Int'l
PO Box 6067
Leawood, KS 66206
888-245-1011; 913-341-7685
www.sorsi.com

Share Foundation
PO Box 192825
San Francisco, CA 94119
415-882-1530; 415-882-1540
www.igc.org/share

Shiatsu Diffusion Society
320 Danforth Ave E #206
Toronto, ON M4K 1N8 Canada
416-466-8780

Shiatsu Therapists Alliance
238 Davenport Rd #180
Toronto, ON M5R 1J6 Canada
416-410 0174
www.shiatsu-therapists-allaince.on.ca

Shiatsu Therapy Assn of British Columbia
PO Box 37005 / 6495 Victoria Dr
Vancouver, BC V5P 4W7 Canada
604-433-9495
www.shiatsutherapy.bc.ca/home/html

Shiatsu Therapy Assn of Ontario
517 College St, Suite 232
Toronto, ON M6G 4A2 Canada
416-923-7826

Sky Foundation
339 Fitzwater St.
Philadelphia, PA 19147
215-574-9180; 215-574-1210
yogasearch@aol.com

Society of Clinical & Medical Electrologists
132 Great Rd, Suite 200
Stowe, MA 01775
978-461-0313; 978-897-5442
www.scmeweb.org

Society of Clinical Masseurs
PO Box 8060
Camberwell, VIC 3124 Australia
613-9-817-7577
societycm@bigpond.com

Society of Natural Therapists and Researchers
7 Legrande Street, P.O. Box 211
Freshwater, QLD 4870 Australia
www.sunweb.net/kooka/SNTR

Society of Ortho-Bionomy Int'l, Inc.
PO Box 869
Madison, WI 53701
800-743-4890; 608-257-8828

Society of Permanent Cosmetics
655 Enterprise Dr #200
Rohnert Park, CA 94928
888-584-7727; 707-586-2982
www.spcp.org

Somatics Society
1516 Grant Ave #212
Novato, CA 94945-3146
415-892-0617; 415-892-4388
www.somaticsed.com

Sound Healers Assn
PO Box 2240
Boulder, CO 80306-2240
303-443-8181; 303-443-6023
www.members.aol.com/SoundHeals

Spiritual Massage Healing Ministry
6907 Sherman St.
Philadelphia, PA 19119
215-842-0265

Student Canadian Chiropractic Assn
1900 Bayview Ave
Toronto, ON M4G 3E6 Canada
416-482-2340

Tai Chi Assn
4651 Roswell Rd, Suite E402
Atlanta, GA 30342
404-289-5652

Texas Assn of Massage Therapists
801 Handell Ln
Pasadena, TX 77502-4422
800-809-9970; 713-944-4326
www.tamt.org

Therapeutic Touch Network
P.O. Box 85551, 875 Eglington Ave West
Toronto, ON M6C 4A8 Canada
416-658-6284
www.therapeutictouchnetwork.com

Touch for Health Kinesiology Assn
PO Box 392
New Carlisle, OH 45344 0932
800-466-8342; 937-845-3404
www.tfh.org

Touch Research Institute: Tiffany Field
Univ of Miami/School of Medicine/Pediatrics
PO Box 016820
Miami, FL 33101
305-243-6790; 305-243-6488
www.miami.edu/touch-research

Trager Institute
21 Locust Ave
Mill Valley, CA 94941-2806
415-388-2688; 415-388-2710
www.trager.com

U.S. Assn for Body Psychotherapy
7831 Woodmont Ave Ste 294
Bethesda, MD 20814
202-466-1619; 212-629-2039
www.usabp.org

World Chiropractic Alliance
2950 N Dobson Rd #1
Chandler, AZ 85224
800-347-1011; 480-732-9313
www.worldchiropracticalliance.org

World Federation of Chiropractic
3080 Yonge St Ste 5065
Toronto, ON M4N 3N1 Canada
416-484 9978; 416-484 9665
worldfed@sympatico.ca

Worldwide Aquatic Bodywork Assn
PO Box 889
Middletown, CA 95461
707-987-3801; 707-987-9638
www.waba.edu

Yoga Research Society
341 Fitzwater St
Philadelphia, PA 19147
215-592-9642; 215-574-1210
yogasearch@aol.com

The Zero Balancing Assn
PO Box 1727
Capitola, CA 95010
831-476-0665
www.zerobalancing.com

• IRS and SBA Publications •

Both the Small Business Administration (SBA) and the Internal Revenue Service (IRS) offer publications to help you in the management of your business. The publications from the SBA are modestly priced and give a lot of good information, ideas and examples. Contact your local office for a free Business Start-up Kit. The free publications from the IRS assist you in understanding your legal tax requirements and the correct procedures, as well as offer advice and ideas.

Small Business Administration Publications ~~~

409 Third St, SW, Washington, DC 20416;   website http://www.sbaonline.sba.gov
Phone 202-205-6744;   800-827-57228;   Fax 202-205-7064;   TDD 704-344-6640

Emerging Business Series

EB01	$3	Transferring Management / Family Businesses
EB02	$4	Marketing Strategies for Growing Businesses
EB03	$3	Management Issues for Growing Businesses
EB04	$3	Human Resource Management for Growing Businesses
EB05	$3	Audit Checklist for Growing Businesses
EB06	$3	Strategic Planning for Growing Businesses
EB07	$4	Financial Management for Growing Businesses

Financial Management

FM01	$3	ABC's of Borrowing
FM01s	$3	Elementos Basicos Para Pedir Dinero Prestado
FM04	$3	Understanding Cash Flow
FM05	$2	A Venture Capital Primer for Small Business
FM08	$3	Budgeting in a Small Service Firm
FM10	$3	Record Keeping in a Small Business
FM13	$3	Pricing Your Products and Services Profitably
FM14	$3	Financing for Small Business

Management and Planning

MP03	$3	Problems In Managing a Family-Owned Business
MP04	$3	Business Plan for Small Manufacturers
MP05	$3	Business Plan for Small Construction Firms
MP06	$3	Planning & Goal Setting for Small Business
MP09	$3	Business Plan for Retailers
MP11	$4	Business Plan for Small Service Firms
MP12	$3	Checklist for Going Into Business
MP12s	$3	Lista Para Comenzar Su Negocio
MP14	$3	How To Get Started With a Small Business Computer
MP15	$4	Business Plan for Home-Based Business
MP16	$3	How To Buy or Sell a Business
MP21	$3	Developing a Strategic Business Plan
MP22	$2	Inventory Management
MP25	$2	Selecting the Legal Structure for Your Business
MP26	$2	Evaluating Franchise Opportunities
MP28	$3	Small Business Risk Management Guide
MP30	$3	Child Day-Care Services
MP31	$4	Handbook for Small Business
MP32	$3	How to Write a Business Plan

Marketing

MT01	$2	Creative Selling: The Competitive Edge
MT02	$2	Marketing for Small Business: An Overview
MT08	$3	Researching Your Market
MT09	$3	Selling by Mail Order
MT11	$3	Advertising

Personnel Management

PM02	$3	Employees: How to Find and Pay Them

Products/Ideas/Inventions

Videotapes

Department of the Treasury, Internal Revenue Service

Forms Distribution Center, P.O. Box 25866   Richmond, VA 23289

800-829-3676;   website http://www.irs.ustreas.gov/prod/forms_pubs/index.html

Index

B

Balance
2, 30, 32, 34, 36, 37, 45-48, 50, 85, 154, 155, 178-180, 227, 392

Barriers
30-32, 105, 153, 238, 411

Barter
35, 69, 181, 186, 190-194, 221-223, 286, 293

Benefits
12, 21, 22, 24, 33, 52, 53, 58, 91, 94, 99, 99, 101, 105, 255, 257, 264, 265, 269, 272-274, 277, 279, 280, 287, 289-291, 293, 295, 298, 299, 311, 313, 320, 321, 339, 342, 343, 358, 411
See also Insurance

Body Language
218, 238, 310

Bookkeeping
12, 103, 106, 118, 177-187, 190, 212

Booths
286, 303, 304, 349, 358-360

Broadcast Advertising
330, 331

Brochures
92, 118, 172, 252, 269, 277, 278, 281, 286, 289-293, 304, 340, 354, 355, 357, 364, 365, 367

Budget
6, 61, 160, 161, 166, 266, 282, 283, 349, 353, 372, 373, 392

Business Cards
23, 60, 86, 93, 118, 172, 245, 252, 253, 258, 259, 283, 286-289, 304, 315, 317, 339, 354, 355, 358, 362, 367, 389

Business Group
310, 312, 315, 316, 362

Business Name
70, 78, 79, 287, 334, 371

Business Organizations
58, 373, 411, 416

Business Plan
8, 39, 47, 48, 67, 69, 103, 207, 282, 358, 369-375

Buying a Practice
70-73
See also Selling a Practice

C

C Corporations
75-77

Canadian Supplement
212-216

Cancellations
225, 226, 229, 245

Capital Cost Allowance
214

Cash flow
69, 156, 166, 178, 180, 187, 190, 203, 206, 207, 373, 393

Character
11, 59, 62, 86, 138,

CivicSource
56

Classified Ads
320, 328, 329, 358

Clearing
2, 8-10, 22, 26, 32, 42, 44, 46
Exercises
10, 43, 45

Client Files
61, 91, 106, 115, 117, 136, 142, 165, 170, 180, 202, 231-233, 240-242, 367
See also Forms

Client Interviews
196, 218, 219, 233-241, 245, 258, 259, 413, 414

Client Retention
19, 22, 23, 73, 199, 209, 244-252, 298, 364

Clinics
5, 86, 127, 144-146, 163-167

Comment Card
243, 359, 367

Commitment
14, 41, 53, 58, 65, 68, 101, 207, 248, 255, 315-318, 374

Communication
5, 36, 50, 57, 103, 105, 107, 111, 143, 152, 153, 158, 161, 164, 168, 173, 217-228, 230-234, 238, 241, 258, 273, 310, 360, 413, 414

Community Relations
284, 348, 372
See also Social Responsibility

Competition
12, 71, 97, 204, 205, 209, 264-267, 269, 271, 281, 282, 320, 349, 359, 371, 372

Compliance
238

Computers
39, 54, 91, 108, 110-118, 125, 131-133, 178, 182, 200, 214, 229, 250, 287, 295, 301, 318, 319, 332, 333, 356, 359, 373

Conditioning
8, 14, 30

Contracts
70-73, 136-151, 163, 166, 169, 206-209, 232, 353-356, 366

Conventions
142, 143, 286, 303, 304, 349

Cooperative Marketing
92, 265, 349-352, 367

Corporations
74-78, 103, 178, 179, 188-190, 210

Credibility
63, 86, 97, 101, 104, 120, 207, 218, 228, 255, 256, 277, 279, 285, 289, 298, 319, 333, 357, 362-365, 415

Credit Cards
180, 222, 226, 321, 359

Customer Service
49, 52, 164, 199, 239-244, 248, 249, 254, 259

D

Deductions
84, 137, 177, 188, 189, 212, 213

I

Image
30, 37, 42, 57-61, 78-80, 85-87, 144, 146, 152, 157, 159, 160, 163, 167, 229, 257, 265-268, 271, 283, 286-289, 301, 303, 320, 321, 333, 334, 341, 348, 352, 353, 365, 366, 371

Incentives
99, 170, 243, 246, 247, 286, 295, 296, 303, 321, 364

Income
4, 5, 35, 38-40, 93, 97-101, 107, 178-183, 186, 188-190, 193, 195, 196, 199, 209, 212-216, 222, 247, 264, 280, 306, 372-374, 390, 394
See also Finances

Incorporation
75-77

Independent Contractor
136-145, 148-151, 163, 166, 169

Independent Living Resources
415, 417

Insurance Coverage
80, 96, 97, 106, 142, 145, 147, 149

Insurance Reimbursement
119-135, 222, 231, 249, 373
Benefits
121, 122, 126, 128, 130, 132, 133

Integrity
27, 51, 52, 58, 61, 64, 65, 263

Internal Revenue Service (IRS)
35, 74-79, 166, 179, 182, 184, 188, 190, 414, 423, 424

Internet
93, 114, 119, 300, 310, 330, 332, 333

Introductions
312-314, 360

Inventory/Products
71, 90, 105, 152, 157, 160, 179, 182, 184, 200, 206, 249, 372, 373

L

Leases
80, 81, 113, 137

Legal Structure
74-78, 157

Letters
54, 83, 91, 93, 94, 118, 242, 250, 257, 286, 287, 295-302, 339, 344, 360, 361, 365, 367, 374
Letter of Intent
70, 209

Liability
33, 74-78, 96, 106, 137, 139, 140, 142, 144, 145, 147, 149, 150, 180, 188, 410

Licensing
74, 82, 93, 95, 124, 125

Limited Liability Company (LLC)
74, 77, 78

Listening
8, 31, 36, 65, 218-221, 239-241, 265

Location
12, 69, 72, 79-95, 142, 206, 269-271, 282-290, 362, 364, 371

Logistics
73, 162, 167, 171
See also Policies and Procedures

Logo
79, 286, 287, 302, 303, 321, 355, 357, 358, 362, 364, 365, 366

M

Make A Difference Day
55

Management
6, 49, 50, 68, 97, 102-106, 118, 136, 142, 143, 153-155, 157, 163, 164, 171, 242, 248, 371, 373 389, 391, 393, 395, 416, 417, 423, 424
See also Self-Management and Time Management

Marketing
5, 12, 36, 38-40, 46, 49, 50, 56, 65, 72, 73, 92, 93, 118, 142-146, 152, 155, 160-163, 167, 170, 171, 182, 205-209, 212, 239, 244, 263-367, 370-372, 412, 415

Media Interviews
40, 255, 279, 300, 302, 333, 334, 339-350, 362, 363, 367

Medical Codes
128

Mentors
17, 54, 314, 318

Message Systems
110, 11, 230, 231, 357

Mind Mapping
18, 19

Motivation
24, 30, 34, 43, 44, 154, 370

N

Networking
12, 23, 36, 48, 83, 94, 155, 173, 208, 258, 277, 286, 304, 308, 310, 312, 314-317, 319, 358, 360-362, 367, 374

Neuro-Linguistic Programming
219, 220

Newsletters
23, 118, 235, 242, 245, 250, 278, 279, 286, 287, 298-302, 328, 357, 362, 363, 366, 367

Newspaper
38, 40, 61, 68, 79, 93, 208, 255, 278, 279, 284, 286, 298, 300, 320, 334-336, 340-345, 357, 358, 362, 363

No-Shows
245

S

T

V

W

Y

Z

Other Offerings

• About SMA •

Our purpose at Sohnen-Moe Associates, Inc. is to provide you with convenient, affordable access to state-of-the-art information and products for your professional development. Plainly stated, having the technical skills to be an excellent health care practitioner is necessary but not sufficient for business success. It takes very different skills and planning to cultivate a profitable practice. You can gain these skills through studying, taking continuing education courses and working with a successful and experienced coach who knows how to support people in achieving their goals.

Business Coaching

We are pleased to offer a special price on our coaching services to the purchasers of *Business Mastery*. We can assist you in defining your goals and objectives, support you in resolving problems and provide suggestions to implement change for a more efficient, dynamic, successful business. Sometimes people need ongoing support to achieve their goals, particularly when a goal involves a habit to be eliminated or a behavior to be developed. Many people are so intent on "doing it themselves" that they never get it done. Our coaching sessions range from one time to weekly to quarterly and can be done on-site or over the telephone. Our fees are $100 per hour, but you can receive the first hour at only $75 or $35 for the first half hour.

Trainings ～～

Our skill-building seminars and training courses are interactive and experiential. Each seminar is custom designed to achieve the results that you desire. These programs can last from two hours to nine weeks. We offer public seminars to make training available and cost-efficient for individuals. The workshops are also available as an in-house program for your company, organization, school or professional association. *Cherie is approved by the National Certification Board for Therapeutic Massage and Bodywork (NCBTMB) as a Category A continuing education provider.*

Please contact us if you are interested in attending or sponsoring a workshop. Sponsorship is easy! All you need is 10 or more cohorts with goals to reach. Assemble a group of friends or business associates; arrange to co-sponsor a workshop with another business or school; or contact your professional association's education chair. Call us to discuss topics and select dates—we also may be in the process of organizing a workshop in your area. If you are with a company, school or association, please call us directly at 800-786-4774 or 520-743-3936.

• Workshops •

Below is a description of workshops that Cherie Sohnen-Moe commonly presents. Cherie is a dynamic presenter and her workshops are very well-received. Sponsors may mix and match topics from any workshop description to design a seminar that meets their specific goals. Please call us to discuss these workshops in more detail.

Marketing From Your Heart ～～

Discover how to expand your practice by using proven techniques that integrate your values into your business. Effective marketing is the cornerstone to a successful practice. Marketing involves all of the business activities done on a daily basis to attract potential clients to utilize your services and to retain your current clients. Thriving practices combine a good mixture of promotion, advertising, publicity and community relations.

This highly interactive workshop focuses on increasing your success by integrating **YOU** into your marketing. Explore ways to increase your income through client retention, referrals and diversification; learn fun, creative, practical and proven marketing techniques; clarify your differential advantage; identify the people you want as clients; design a concise, engaging introduction; and renew your confidence and enthusiasm.

Even if you are doing well in your practice, you will leave this workshop knowing how to increase the impact of your marketing in your print materials, presentations, networking and advertising. You will also learn how to get free media coverage and expand your visibility through creative marketing techniques and cooperative marketing.

The Business Mastery Workshop ～～

The Business Mastery Workshop is an exciting, interactive workshop where you make a quantitative shift in your relationship to your business. The focus is supporting you in living your life and running your business from your values. You will clarify your vision and learn specific, creative, proven techniques for actualizing your goals.

The Business Mastery Workshop also allows you the opportunity to get feedback on your specific concerns. Topics include business management, increasing client retention, creating effective marketing strategies, networking, diversification, cooperative marketing, self-management, developing a dynamic self-introduction, designing promotional materials, educating your clients, increasing your profits and keeping balance. The Business Mastery Workshop inspires powerful insights and results for seasoned business professionals as well as those just embarking in their field.

Present Yourself Powerfully ∼∼

Public speaking is the key to expanding your business! People become your clients out of their experience of you. Public speaking increases your visibility in the community, educates the public about the benefits of your services, and establishes your credibility.

The Presentation Skills Workshop provides you with the skills to speak powerfully and confidently from informal one-on-one contacts to formal group presentations. This exciting program is fast paced, participative and fun. Discover how to increase your comfort when speaking in public; build your communication strengths; create a presentation outline; expand your practice through educating the public; enhance your delivery through your voice and body language; design a powerful self–introduction; involve and motivate your audience; research, organize and practice your presentations; incorporate demonstrations and audiovisuals; and develop effective workshop marketing techniques.

Therapeutic Communication Skills ∼∼

Effective Communication with Clients, the Public and Other Health Care Providers. Excellent communication skills are integral to a successful practice. As therapists, we need to be able to adapt our style as well as vocabulary when talking with different people such as clients, other health care providers and the general public. The more you enhance your communication abilities, the easier it becomes to build your practice, develop professional affiliations and retain clients.

In this workshop you will learn the keys to effective therapeutic communications and interpersonal interactions. We cover client interactions: how to develop rapport, do great intake interviews (elicit appropriate information, using "buzz" words, understand non-verbal cues), design treatment plans, get feedback during sessions and empower your clients in their well-being. We also explore ways to build professional alliances: developing a team approach to wellness, designing a descriptive promotional package and marketing to physicians and other primary health care providers.

Business Ethics ∼∼

An ethical approach to business promotes an atmosphere of trust. Ethics is really about understanding boundaries. Given the personal nature of this field it's imperative to set clear boundaries and operate from a code of ethics. Most people do not think about ethical dilemmas until they arise.

This workshop gives participants the opportunity to experience real-life ethical dilemmas and discuss various methods of resolution, so participants will be better prepared to solve and hopefully avoid potential problems. Topics covered include: identifying the four steps to resolving an ethical dilemma; distinguishing between laws, morals, values and ethics; and incorporating ethics into policies. Participants will leave with tools to morally and ethically manage their businesses and clientele.

• Professional Development Catalog •

We want you to be successful! So, we've assembled a catalog of products to assist you in the "business" part of your profession. Too often we invest the majority of our time and money enhancing our technical skills and ignore developing our business acumen. The following pages contain a sampling of the items we stock.

Continuing Education Courses Published by SMA ~~~

The Business Mastery Home-Study Course
by **Cherie Sohnen-Moe 12 CEUs $100 #H305 (Only $75 if you have a registered copy of** *Business Mastery³*)
The Business Mastery Home-Study Course is now available! This 12 CEU course helps new practitioners establish thriving practices, and supports seasoned therapists in taking their businesses to the next level. This highly interactive course is filled with information, exercises, examples and resources that provide you with the tools to increase your profits, set goals that get results, effectively market your practice, manage your business, communicate with clients, stay balanced and keep more of the money you earn.
Course Materials: *Business Mastery³* **Assessment:** Test, goal-setting exercise and target market profile exercise

Therapeutic Communications Home-Study Course
by **Cherie Sohnen-Moe 4 CEUs $60 #H404 (Only $40 if you have a registered copy of** *Business Mastery³*)
Excellent communication skills are integral to a successful practice. Therapists need to be able to adapt their style as well as vocabulary when talking with different people such as clients, other health care providers and the general public. The *Therapeutic Communications* home-study course provides you with the tools to improve communications, identify basic learning styles, enhance therapeutic effectiveness, keep appropriate client files, develop treatment plans, set policies, increase client retention, generate referrals and build professional alliances.
Course Materials: Chapter Eight from *Business Mastery³*
Assessment: Test, telephone script exercise and customer service action plan exercise

The Soul of Ethics: Module I—Boundaries and Ethical Decision-Making
by **Cherie Sohnen-Moe and Ben E. Benjamin Ph.D. $39.95 56 pages 8.5 x 11 #E125**
The Soul of Ethics home-study course helps to clarify an often vague, amorphous topic. It is our desire to assist you in developing a solid ethical foundation beyond reproach. This is a highly interactive course filled with information, exercises, models, examples and resources. This course will: guide you in resolving ethical dilemmas; assist you in managing an ethical practice; help create/maintain personal and professional boundaries; clarify the behaviors that constitute boundary violations; and provide insight into your own psychological make-up. Each module is worth three CEUs. This meets the two hour ethics requirement for NCBTMB recertification and the additional CEU can be applied toward ethics hours or general hours under Category A.
Course Materials: 56-page manual
Assessment: Test and ethical dilemma resolution exercise

Other Items Published by SMA ⚏

Business Mastery Supplement

| by Sohnen-Moe Associates, Inc. | | Individual User | $24.95 | #C102 |
| Clinic (up to 5 users) | $59.95 #C102A | School Edition | $129.95 | #C102B |

Work smarter—not harder! Save time and money with this supplement to *Business Mastery*. This text-based computer disk helps you easily update your business plan, save time in creating professional letters and spark creative marketing ideas. It includes a 50⁺ page massage practice business plan and more than 150 letters (including primary care correspondence, cooperative marketing suggestions, resume cover letters, client communications and thank-you notes), announcements, press releases and checklists commonly needed by practitioners in professionally managing their business. Indicate PC or Macintosh on order form.

Don't have a computer? We also offer the software in a Printout form! $29.95   #F102

Present Yourself Powerfully

by Cherie Sohnen-Moe $39.95 77-page manual & 14 handout masters   #F170

Public speaking is one of the best ways to build your business. This presentation kit makes it easy for therapists to give talks, workshops and demonstrations. The kit is designed to take away the hassles of public speaking and to dissipate fear by replacing it with a toolbox of ideas, techniques and reproducible materials. The manual explores topics such as: the keys to giving successful presentations; analyzing the audience's needs and preferences; designing exciting presentations; utilizing audio-visual materials; developing an engaging self-introduction; managing the physical environment; enhancing verbal communication skills; doing fun, effective demonstrations; getting your audience involved; increasing the impact of your non-verbal communications; tips for continuing connections made through your presentations; and how to make money through public speaking.

This kit also includes a variety of checklists to encourage further exploration, connect you with companies that provide products you can sell during your presentations, support the ongoing development of your presentation skills and assist you in remembering all the little things. Additionally, you will find two 20-minute scripted presentations, complete with handout masters.

Available in Autumn 2001 :

The Ethics of Touch by Cherie Sohnen-Moe and Ben E. Benjamin Ph.D.
A comprehensive manual addressing ethical issues involved in boundaries, communication, dual relationships, sexuality, sexual misconduct, abuse and trauma, practice management, and clinical supervision.

Items From Other Publishers ⚏

Finding Your Niche...Marketing Your Professional Service

by B. Brodsky & J. Geis $15.95   272 pages   8.5 x 11   #B139

Finding Your Niche shows you how to market all kinds of services, from accounting to Zen, dance lessons to therapy sessions. Many professionals find it difficult to "sell themselves," to describe what they do in terms that are attractive to prospective clients. This book addresses these needs and covers the entire marketing process: identifying prospective clients; researching your market; getting known; conducting a promotion campaign; writing ad copy; producing flyers and brochures; and how to build sideline careers of writing and lecturing.

Hands Heal: Documentation For Massage Therapy
by Diana Thompson $17.95   80 pages   8.5 x 11   #B160
Hands Heal: Documentation For Massage Therapy, A Guide to SOAP Charting explains and demonstrates all the documentation any bodyworker needs to establish and maintain a system of accurate client/treatment information (as needed by most insurance companies and other health care providers). This step-by-step learning tool is valuable to new practitioners as well as those experienced with filling out insurance reports. Highly recommended regardless of whether you work with insurance reimbursement.

The Inner Manager
by Ron Dalrymple, Ph.D. $8.95   108 pages   5.5 x 8.5   #B108
The Inner Manager: Mastering Business, Home, and Self reveals how you can use your rational, emotional and intuitive resources to successfully manage conflicts, financial worries, problems and many other aspects of your life, helping you gain the respect and success we all need. This book, told in the form of a simple parable, leads you through an 8-step mind development course that is easy and fun to read. It integrates science, psychology and Eastern/ Western philosophies into a powerhouse of pragmatic ideas and techniques designed to help you better manage your life today.

The Insurance Reimbursement Manual For Bodyworkers & Massage Professionals
by Christine Rosche $69.95   280 pages   8.5 x 11   #B135
This concise reference manual contains proven techniques for billing insurance companies nationwide—and getting paid quickly! It helps clarify the often confusing field of insurance reimbursement. It contains information applicable to bodyworkers of all levels of expertise. It describes how to process third-party insurance claims, keep correct charts and records, and establish effective, profitable relationships with other health professionals.

Marketing With Newsletters
by Elaine Floyd $29.95   330 pages   7.25 x 9.25   #B136
Most forms of advertising are inappropriate for health care practitioners, yet a newsletter is viewed by clients as an added service. It's a cost-effective way to stay in touch with clients, while building your image in the community. Increase your practice by producing an informative and promotional publication. Containing 200+ examples, testimonials and cartoons, this easy-to-read book demonstrates how to choose engaging content, write and design an effective newsletter. It's written for practices currently publishing newsletters and those just getting started.

Marketing Without Advertising
by M. Phillips & S. Rasberry $19.00   168 pages   7 x 9   #B106
This book provides you with the philosophical underpinnings for the development of a successful, low-cost marketing plan not based on advertising. Phillips and Rasberry demolish the myth of advertising effectiveness and outline practical steps for marketing your small business. This book is for the business person who is proud of and enjoys providing a quality product or service.

Massage Therapy Career Focus Workbook
by D. Helmer & D. Lemke $19.95   78 pages   8.5 x 11   #B155
Massage therapy is a vast profession with literally thousands of possible career paths. By exploring the possible wellness outcomes provided to the client and how and where those outcomes are provided, this workbook helps the student or practicing professional choose or refine a career path. Real world scenarios illustrate how to employ and communicate this knowledge for professional development and marketing purposes. Also included are exercises to determine which of the 6,000+ practice description combinations will best suit the individual. Ideal for classroom use, guidance counseling and individual study.

Medical Code Manual

by E. Denning & D. Hecht $27.95   74 pages   5.5 x 8.5   #B145

This 3-ring binder handbook was designed specifically for massage therapists. Previously, to use proper medical codes for insurance billing you had to refer to two separate medical code books, at a cost of more than $75 annually. Now the major codes for massage therapy are in this handy reference guide. The book is updated annually. The first update is free and subsequent updates will cost less than $5.

Minding Her Own Business

by Jan Zobel, EA $16.95   208 pages   7 x 10   #B154

Minding Her Own Business: The Self-Employed Woman's Guide to Taxes and Recordkeeping is a down-to-earth, one-stop source of answers to your most pressing questions including: the kinds of records the IRS expects you to keep; what expenses are deductible; which tax forms to use; what are your chances of being audited; and many more.

The Motivated Salon

by Mark D. Foley $19.95   256 pages   6 x 9   #B200

Learn how to apply time-tested practical and psychological strategies to attract and retain clients while prompting them to purchase more of your products and services. This book provides you with hard-hitting sales and marketing methods that are sure to yield more profitable results.

Networking Success

by Ann Boe $14.95   236 pages   5.5 x 8.5   #B115

Networking success: How To Turn Business & Financial Relationships Into Fun and Profit is a "hands on" approach to Boe's dynamic, on-going process of networking principles, skills and techniques. By the time you work through this book, you will know yourself more intimately and be able to approach networking with ease and enthusiasm.

The Partnership Book

by D. Clifford & R. Warner $34.95   240 pages   8.5 x 11   #B105

Many people dream of going into business with a friend. That dream can become a nightmare without a solid partnership contract. This book shows you step-by-step how to prepare an agreement that meets your needs. It covers initial contributions, wages, profit-sharing, buy-out, death or retirement of a partner and disputes. Also includes a PC disk that contains the sample partnership clauses from the book.

Practical Massage Teacher's Guide

by K. Anderson & H. Nicoll $49.95   **Manual, video & handout masters** #FV125

A Complete Planning Kit for Teaching a Beginner's Massage Class in Your Community. Teaching is one of the best ways to educate people about the benefits of massage, reach new clients, and develop an alternate source of income! If you've never taught, the Practical Massage Teacher's Guide can help you get started. This A-Z kit for planning and teaching a massage class in your community uses a seated, clothed routine that's easy to learn and easy to teach in any setting. No special equipment is required. Includes a 47-minute video, detailed teaching instructions, marketing tips, sample ads, class handouts and more!

Small Time Operator

by Bernard Kamaroff, C.P.A. $16.95   216 pages   8.5 x 11   #B110

Small Time Operator: How to Start Your Own Small Business, Keep Your Books, Pay Your Taxes And Stay Out of Trouble! is a step-by-step guide to help you set up the "machinery" of your business. It's written in everyday English so anyone can understand it. *Small Time Operator* is also a workbook that includes bookkeeping instructions and a set of ledgers, especially designed for small businesses. This book has sold over 500,000 copies and is recommended by hundreds of schools, associations and the U.S. Small Business Administration.

Visit our website for up-to-date workshop schedules & descriptions of our full product line: **www.sohnen-moe.com**

Touch, Ink Newsletters

by Craig Quaglia $95.00 per kit   **11 x 17 double-sided, 4 Templates**

Newsletters are a wonderful forum to increase client retention, attract new clients and educate the public. Discover how easy and inexpensive it can be to build and maintain your practice with these newsletters specially designed for massage therapists to give away. These newsletters are tailored to the layperson: they are interesting, informative and beautifully designed. The back of the newsletter has one panel (8.5 x 3.5) that can be left blank or personalized with a note, a description of your services or an announcement about upcoming open houses or specials. Each kit contains 4 newsletter templates, plus a variety of gift certificate templates and 10 brochure templates on massage and: carpal tunnel, overtraining, pregnancy, SCM, arthritis, fibromyalgia, sciatica, stress, ice therapy and what to expect from the therapist. Receive one year's worth of newsletter templates for less than the cost of two massages!

Kit 1 (#F344A): PMS, So What's New?, Exercise Program, What to Look For in a Massage Therapist, Body Mobilization, Workplace Anxiety, Massage—Old Therapy, Massage in the News, Experience of Massage, 10 Ways to Prepare for Massage, Chiropractic and Massage, Gift Certificate Ads.

Kit 2 (#F344B): Exercise and Massage, Move Your Body, Delayed Muscle Soreness, Avoid Heat Stroke, Stress & Aging, Massage in the News, Massage & Cancer Prevention, Choose Health, Waiting to Exhale, Seated Massage, Daily Stretching, Massage Q&A, Carpal Tunnel Syndrome, Use of Ice, Gift Certificate Ads.

Kit 3 (#F344C): Gluteals, Aromaaatherapy, Moist Heat, Massage & Essential Oils, What's the Big Deal About Sports Massage?, Cope with Stress, Repetitive Strain Injury Update, Oh Those Working Quads, Youth in a Barbell, Osteoarthritis and Massage, Seasonal Affective Disorder, Gift Certificate Ads.

Kit 4 (#F344D): Healthy Massage Partnerships, Burnout, Frozen Shoulder, Massage in the News, Summer Precautions, Piriformis Syndrome, No Back Pain, Feet, Complementary Therapies Health Alert, Massage's Role in Surgery, Clean Air, New Millenium Medical Alert, Holiday Gift Certificate Ads.

Kit 5 (#F344E): Headache Relief, Magic of Massage, Exercise Alert, Massage in the News, The Physiological Mystery of Massage, The Pelvis, Massage Therapy: the Circulatory Enhancer, 10 Reasons for Getting a Massage, Scientific Research & Massage, Massage for the Elderly, Massage for Athletes, Massage for Pregnant Moms, Gift Certificate Ads.

The Twig Unbent: Exercises for a Supple Spine

by Stephen Davidson $14.95   **30 pages   6 x 9 Spiral   #B120**

The Twig Unbent offers 20 safe, easy-to-follow, gentle movements and positions to help strengthen and loosen your spine. These are the same stretching exercises that respected Osteopathic Physician, Robert Fulford, developed during 40 years of clinical trial and error to help patients throughout the world! This book is a great product for your practice. You can sell it to your clients or just photocopy the appropriate exercises, use the handy space for personal recommendations, and send them home with your clients. These exercises are so clearly illustrated and described that you'll save hours in repeated demonstration, question and answer time. *Quantity Discounts Available.*

Visit our website for a complete catalog with full-color covers and expanded descriptions!

www.sohnen-moe.com

Order Form

Company: _____
Name: _____
Street: _____
City: _____ State: _____ Zip: _____
Phone: (work) _____ (home) _____
e-mail: _____ website: _____
Type of Business: _____

Qty	Title	Amount
_____	Business Mastery	$ 24.95
_____	Business Mastery Supplement-Individual	
	❏ PC ❏ Mac	$ 24.95
_____	Business Mastery Supplement-Clinic	
	❏ PC ❏ Mac	$ 59.95
_____	Business Mastery Supplement-School	
	❏ PC ❏ Mac	$129.95
_____	Present Yourself Powerfully	$ 39.95
_____	Coaching ❏ ½ Hour ❏ 1 Hour	$ 35/75
_____	_____	_____
_____	_____	_____
_____	_____	_____

Prices Subject to Change Without Notice	
Subtotal:	_____
Sales Tax:	
(5% AZ Residents Only)	_____
Shipping:	_____
Total Due:	_____

Payment Method

❏ Check Enclosed ❏ Visa ❏ MasterCard
Credit card orders complete the following:
Card # _____
Expires: _____
Name on Card: _____
Signature: _____

Your Success Is Our Business!™

Order By Toll-Free Phone

Call 800-786-4774 to place Visa and MasterCard orders, weekdays 9 am to 4 pm M.S.T. (24-hour voice mail).

Order By Fax

Fax your order to us 24 hours a day at 520-743-3656.

Order By Mail

Fill out the order form with the quantities and titles you wish to receive. We ship via UPS in the continental U.S. To ensure prompt delivery please provide your full name and street address. Complete the credit card information or attach a check or money order (payable to Sohnen-Moe Associates, Inc.) and mail to:

Sohnen-Moe Associates, Inc.
3906 W. Ina Road #200 PMB367
Tucson, AZ 85741-2295

Shipping Rates

Continental U.S.: We ship UPS ground; $6 for the first item; and $2 for each additional item.

Hawaii/Alaska: U.S. mail; $6 for the first item; and $2 for each additional item.

Canada: Air mail; $10 for the first item; and $3 for each additional item.

All Others: Call for current rates at 520-743-3936.

Our Guarantee

Your satisfaction is our foremost concern. If any of our products do not meet your needs or expectations, please return them in new condition within 15 days for a refund, credit or exchange.

Business Mastery Registration Card

We want to hear from you. Please let us know if this book meets your needs and offer any suggestions you have for improvement. Fill out and return this card to receive free updates, current catalogs and a 25% discount on subsequent editions of *Business Mastery*.

Company: _____
Name: _____
Street: _____
City: _____ State: _____ Zip: _____
Phone: (work) _____ (home) _____
e-mail: _____ Website: _____
Type of Business: _____ Area of Specialty: _____
How did you hear about this book? _____
Where did you purchase this book? _____
Comments: _____
_____

Return This Card Today & Receive a 10% Discount on Your Next Order!

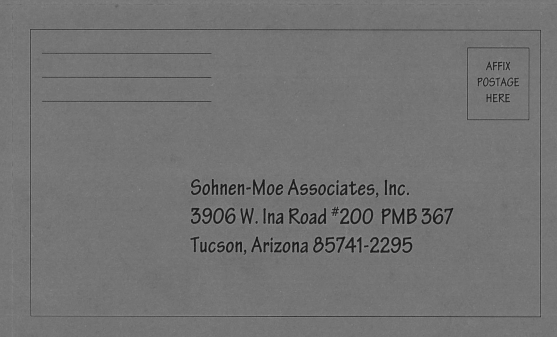

AFFIX
POSTAGE
HERE

Sohnen-Moe Associates, Inc.
3906 W. Ina Road #200 PMB 367
Tucson, Arizona 85741-2295